AF413040

Yearbook of Pediatric Endocrinology 2009

Yearbook of Pediatric Endocrinology 2009

Endorsed by the European Society for Paediatric Endocrinology

Editors

Jean-Claude Carel
Ze'ev Hochberg

Associate Editors

John C. Achermann
Gary Butler
Francesco Chiarelli
Mehul Dattani
Nicolas De Roux
Heiko Krude
Mohamad Maghnie
Ken Ong
Orit Pinhas-Hamiel
Lars Sävendahl
Olle Söder
Martin Wabitsch

KARGER

Sponsored by a grant from Pfizer Endocrine Care

© Copyright 2009 by S. Karger AG, P.O. Box, CH–4009 Basel (Switzerland)
www.karger.com
Printed in Switzerland on acid-free and non-aging paper (ISO 9706) by Reinhardt Druck, Basel
ISBN 978-3-8055-9231-4
ISSN 1662-3391

Heiko Krude

Institute of Experimental Pediatric Endocrinology, Charité
University-Medicine-Berlin, Augustenburgerplatz 1
DE–13353 Berlin, Germany
Tel. +49 30 450 666 039; Fax +49 30 450 566 926; E-Mail heiko.krude@charite.de

Mohamad Maghnie

Department of Pediatrics, IRCCS Giannina Gaslini
University of Genova
Largo G. Gaslini 5, IT–16147 Genova, Italy
Tel. +39 0105 636 574; Fax +39 010 553 8265, E-Mail mohamadmaghnie@ospedale-gaslini.ge.it

Ken Ong

Medical Research Council Epidemiology Unit
Institute of Metabolic Science, Addenbrooke's Hospital, Box 285
Cambridge CB2 0QQ, UK
Tel. +44 1223 769207; Fax +44 1223 330316; E-Mail ken.ong@mrc-epid.cam.ac.uk

Orit Pinhas-Hamiel

Pediatric Endocrine and Diabetes Unit, Safra Children's Hospital
Sheba Medical Center Ramat-Gan, IL–52621 Ramat-Gan, Israel
Tel. +972 3 5305015, Fax +972 3 5305055, E-Mail Orit.Hamiel@sheba.health.gov.il

Lars Sävendahl

Pediatric Endocrinology Unit; Q2:08
Department of Woman and Child Health
Karolinska Institutet and University Hospital, Solna
SE–171 76 Stockholm, Sweden
Tel. +46 8 5177 2369; Fax +46 8 5177 5128; E-Mail lars.savendahl@ki.se

Olle Söder

Pediatric Endocrinology Unit, Q2:08
Department of Woman and Child Health
Karolinska Institutet and University Hospital, Solna
SE–171 76 Stockholm, Sweden
Tel. +46 8 517 75124, Fax +46 8 517 75128, E-Mail olle.soder@kbh.ki.se

Martin Wabitsch

Pediatric Endocrinology, Diabetes and Obesity Unit, Department of Pediatrics and Adolescent Medicine
University of Ulm, Eythstrasse 24
DE–89075 Ulm, Germany
Tel. +49 731 5002 7715; +49 731 50027789; E-Mail martin.wabitsch@uniklinik-ulm.de

Table of Contents

Preface

The *Blue Book*, which is now at its 6th volume, is all about scientific discoveries. Whereas anniversaries may not always justify celebrations, this year is different for three great reasons.

With the rest of the scientific world, we observe 2009 as the *International Year of Astronomy*, 400 years after Galileo made his first telescopic observations. Against a background of dominant Renaissance 'rebirth', which contended that everything worth knowing had already been ascertained by the great Greek and Roman philosophers, Galileo (1564–1642) represents the scientific revolution that sought to make new observations using a scientific approach. He then coined the then avant-garde phrase: '*The grand look of nature* (for him – the universe) *is written in the language of mathematics*'.

The Darwin year 2009 marks 200 years from his birth and 150 years since *On the Origin of Species by Means of Natural Selection* was first published. We can easily understand why Darwin has been so influential – he reported his theory in a book that today we would call popular science. *The Origin of Species* consists of a sustained, strongly argued case with enough stunning examples to convince educated readers without overwhelming them with too much technical detail. As biology and medical research have been drifting toward cellular and molecular biology, those of us who took part in various Darwin events throughout the world were again astonished at nature's splendor and the astuteness of evolution. These events may release a wave of research into organic biology and evolution that may well open new research horizons. This is exemplified in our 2009 selection of the *Yearbook* articles.

It is also 150 years since the philosopher John Stuart Mills (1806–1873) published his *On Liberty*, in which he argued in favor of an open exchange of ideas. By forcing other individuals to reexamine and reaffirm their ideas in the process of scientific publishing and debate, ideas are kept from declining into mere dogmas. This Yearbook applauds Mills' philosophy and makes its best to realize it in the field of pediatric endocrinology.

Finally, 2009 marks the 20th anniversary of the invention of the Web – young but prominent.

Why do we bother to cite these giants of the past in a Yearbook that deals with the most contemporary of all observations? Newton declared that '*we can see farther because we sit on the shoulders of giants*'.

We keenly acknowledge the generous support by Pfizer that makes the Yearbook project possible. The tireless work of our Associate Editors and authors makes this important text for pediatric endocrinologists an indispensible tool in keeping updated with the latest. By reading this collection of the 250 best articles of the year, the reader will recognize the fact that (to paraphrase) *there is no such thing as the best articles, yet this is a book about them*.

Ze'ev Hochberg (Haifa)
Jean-Claude Carel (Paris)

Neuroendocrinology

Lukas Huijbregts, Carine Villanueva and Nicolas de Roux

INSERM U676, Hôpital Robert Debré and Université Paris Diderot, Paris, France

The choice of papers in neuroendocrinology for the Yearbook is a cruel dilemma. The borders of this field are confusing, in particular in clinics. The hypothalamus is the place of central regulation of all endocrine axes as well as metabolic homeostasis. Neuroendocrine dysregulation leading to endocrine disorders is thus rarely detailed without complete analysis of peripheral hormones. Most of these clinical papers are thus reported in other chapters of the Yearbook. This is why we focused our attention on articles which mainly report fundamental research and are therefore considered as being pretty far away from human clinics. Some of these new concepts will probably never be confirmed in human physiology but others represent really new original findings with some rapid application in humans.

New mechanism: maternal feeding determines the risk of obesity in offspring

Maternal high-fat diet and fetal programming: increased proliferation of hypothalamic peptide-producing neurons that increase risk for overeating and obesity

Chang GQ, Gaysinskaya V, Karatayev O, Leibowitz SF
Rockefeller University, New York, N.Y., USA
J Neurosci 2008;28:12107–12119

Background: Recent studies have demonstrated the close association between dietary fat or circulating lipids with stimulation of hypothalamic peptides involved in the control of food intake and body weight. In this study, Chang et al. have tested the hypothesis that a fat-rich diet during pregnancy alters the regulation and synthesis of these peptide systems in utero, leading to postnatal neuronal changes in the offspring that persist after the diet and have long-term consequences.

Methods: Pregnant Sprague-Dawley rats were fed from embryonic day 6 (E6) to birth with a high-fat diet (HFD) or a balanced diet (BD). At birth, offspring were suckled by their own dams and maintained on their respective diets until they were killed at different postnatal ages. A 3rd group, referred to as HFD-BD, was composed of offspring which were removed from their HFD dams and suckled by BD dams that had no prior exposure to the HFD. A 4th BD-HFD group was composed of BD offspring exposed to HFD after birth. The offspring were killed at different postnatal ages (P) by rapid decapitation.

Results: The offspring of dams on a HFD versus BD from E6 to P15 showed an increase in caloric intake, body weight, leptin and insulin, a stronger preference for fat, elevated TG levels and an increased expression of orexigenic peptides, galanin, enkephalin and dynorphin in the paraventicular nucleus and orexin and melanin-concentrating hormone in the perifornical lateral hypothalamus. The increased density of these peptide-expressing neurons was also observed in HFD offspring fostered at birth to BD dams, suggesting events that might be occurring in utero. During gestation, HFD stimulated the proliferation of neuroepithelial and neuronal precursor cells of the embryonic hypothalamic third ventricle. It also stimulated the proliferation and differentiation of neurons and their migration toward hypothalamic areas.

Conclusion: An increase in neurogenesis was observed in offspring from dams fed with HFD. This increase was closely associated with a marked increase in lipids in the blood. It may play a role in producing the long-term behavioral and physiological changes observed in offspring after weaning, including an increase in food intake, preference for fat and higher body weight.

This study reproduces previous studies showing that perinatal HFD increased several hypothalamic parameters involved in the regulation of food intake and fat mass. This difference is only apparent after weaning in offspring exposed prenatally to HFD suggesting that the prenatal period is a critical time in programming expression of these peptides in the hypothalamus. The increase in peptide expression in the hypothalamus was site-specific. The most interesting finding of this paper is the proposed mechanism leading to this increased expression. Rather than an increase in gene expression in specific neurons, they observed an increase in hypothalamic neurons expressing these peptides. This increased neurogenesis related to prenatal diet has never been reported and seems to be site-specific as it did not occur in the arcuate nucleus. It is related to an increase in proliferation rather than an increase in cell survival. Analysis of several markers of cell differentiation indicates that HFD also induces differentiation in post-mitotic neurons. Persistent neurogenesis in the postnatal brain is now well known and mainly occurs in the subventricular zone and dentate gyrus. Similar postnatal neurogenesis is described in the hypothalamus as well. It would be interesting to study whether post-natal neurogenesis is also enhanced by prenatal feeding with HFD and therefore highly determined by prenatal environment.

Finally, this study led us to revise the concept of the transmission of a complex genetic trait such as obesity. The role of environmental factors in obesity is well known. This study suggests that it is necessary to consider maternal feeding during pregnancy as a risk factor of obesity as well. The most dramatic consequence revealed by this study is the irreversible effect of such prenatal maternal feeding on hypothalamic neurogenesis of the offspring.

Concepts revised: the composition of what you eat determines apoptosis of hypothalamic neurons

High-fat diet induces apoptosis of hypothalamic neurons

Moraes JC, Coope A, Morari J, Cintra DE, Roman EA, Pauli JR, Romanatto T, Carvalheira JB, Oliveira AL, Saad MJ, Velloso LA

Department of Internal Medicine, University of Campinas, Campinas, Brazil
PLoS ONE 2009;4:e5045

Background: Recent studies have shown that consumption of dietary fats promotes hypothalamic resistance to leptin and insulin. This resistance is the consequence of diet-induced activation of inflammation in the hypothalamus. Since inflammation can lead to the activation of an apoptotic process, the authors evaluated the effect of high-fat feeding on the induction of apoptosis of hypothalamic cells.

Methods: Adult male rats were submitted to a high-fat diet or control diet for 8 weeks, after which they received intracerebroventricular leptin or insulin to evaluate resistance to those peptides. At the end of the experimental period, the animals were killed by decapitation and hypothalami were extracted for determination of protein expression and immunohistochemistry.

Results: After 8 weeks of HFD, all HFD-fed rats showed functional resistance to insulin and leptin. Gene expression analysis revealed an increase of 57% in 84 apoptosis-related genes in the hypothalamus. Dietary fats induce apoptosis of neurons and a reduction of synaptic inputs in the arcuate nucleus and lateral hypothalamus. This effect is dependent upon diet composition, and not on caloric intake, since pair-feeding is not sufficient to reduce the expression of apoptotic markers. The Toll-like receptor 4 protects cells from further apoptotic signals.

Conclusion: In diet-induced inflammation of the hypothalamus, TLR4 exerts a dual function, on one hand by activating proinflammatory pathways that play a central role in the development of resistance to leptin and insulin, and on the other hand by restraining further damage by controlling the apoptotic activity.

In this paper, Moraes et al. show that high-fat feeding of rats induced an inflammation in the hypothalamus followed by neuronal apoptosis in the arcuate nucleus. The inflammatory process is mediated via activation of the toll-like receptor 4 (TLR4) leading to cytokine secretion such as TNFα in the hypothalamus. This increase in TNFα probably triggers neuronal apoptosis in the arcuate nucleus.

This mechanism is original and must be compared to the induction by HFD of neurogenesis in the hypothalamus. On one hand, there is an increase in neurons and, on the other, HFD induced neuronal apoptosis. Different mechanisms control these two effects which occur in different parts of the hypothalamus. It is interesting to note that such inflammation was not described in the offspring of HFD dams described in the Chang paper (see above) even though triglyceride levels were high at birth. It will be important to investigate the proposed dual role for TLR4 in the hypothalamus, participating in the balance between inflammation and cell survival. Recent studies have shown that insulin and leptin resistance in extra-hypothalamic brain regions may relate to Alzheimer's disease and depression. It will be exciting to evaluate the participation of TLRs and high-fat feeding in these contexts [1].

New hope: NF-κB signaling pathway, a new target in obesity treatment

Hypothalamic IKKβ/NF-κB and ER stress link overnutrition to energy imbalance and obesity

Zhang X, Zhang G, Zhang H, Karin M, Bai H, Cai D
Department of Physiology, University of Wisconsin-Madison, Madison, Wisc., USA

Cell 2008;135:61–73

Background: Chronic metabolic inflammation can be induced by overnutrition, but whether it affects neuronal regulation of energy balance and lead to related diseases is unknown.

Methods and Results: In this study, the authors show that high levels of IKKβ/NF-κB, a major regulator of inflammation, are detected in hypothalamic neurons. Under normal nutritional conditions the IKKβ/NF-κB pathway remains inactive. However, it is strongly activated by overnutrition, due at least partly to an increase in endoplasmic reticulum stress. Chronic activation of hypothalamic NF-κB by a constitutively active IKKβ blunts central insulin/leptin signaling and actions, and site or cell-specific suppression of IKKβ in the whole brain or in the mediobasal hypothalamus only or even more specifically in the hypothalamic agouti-related protein (AgRP) neurons can prevent glucose intolerance and obesity onset. Hypothalamic activation IKKβ/NF-κB leads to an increase in *SOCS3* gene expression, a core inhibitor of insulin and leptin signaling.

Conclusion: These results show that the IKKβ/NF-κB pathway in hypothalamic AgRP neurons is a key mechanism for energy imbalance underlying obesity and that suppressing IKKβ/NF-κB in hypothalamic neurons represents a strategy for counteracting obesity and associated diseases induced by overnutrition.

While chronic inflammation in peripheral metabolic tissues is generally considered a consequence of overnutrition and obesity, this study provides new insights showing that a metabolic inflammatory pathway can be activated in the brain under high-fat diet and participates in insulin and leptin insensitivity, therefore promoting obesity onset and associated diseases. The authors show that this vicious circle can, however, be blocked in mice in which IKKβ/NF-κB signaling is specifically inhibited in hypothalamic orexigenic AgRP neurons (which also express NPY) and therefore prevent them from obesity. Activation of IKKβ by phosphorylation induces phosphorylation of its substrate IκBα, and subsequent proteosomal degradation of IκBα releases NF-κB to translocate into the nucleus where it mediates the transcription of its target genes. These neurons express SOCS3, which is a critical inhibitor for both insulin and leptin in the hypothalamus. This paper shows that IKKβ/NF-κB promotes SOCS3 expression and therefore this upregulation may be the cause of the leptin and insulin resistance in obese mice. This encouraging result could lead to the development of novel anti-inflammatory treatment to prevent overnutrition-induced activation of hypothalamic IKKβ/NF-κB. Because IKKβ/NF-κB normally remains inactive in the CNS, suppressing IKKβ/NF-κB in the hypothalamus is likely a safe approach.

MeCP2, a key contributor to neurological disease, activates and represses transcription

Chahrour M, Jung SY, Shaw C, Zhou X, Wong ST, Qin J, Zoghbi HY
Department of Molecular and Human Genetics, Baylor College of Medicine, Houston, Tex., USA
Science 2008;320:1224–1229

Background: Rett syndrome is a neurodevelopmental disorder caused by the inactivation of the transcriptional repressor methyl-CpG binding protein 2 (MeCP2). Many phenotypes observed in patients with MeCP2 mutations suggest hypothalamic dysfunctions such as sleep abnormalities, abnormal response to stress as measured by increased cortisol levels, episodes of heightened anxiety and growth deceleration. MeCP2 invalidation in mice reproduces many phenotypes seen in patients with Rett syndrome. In this study, the authors sought to examine gene expression patterns in the hypothalamus that either lack or overexpress MeCP2.
Methods: Microarray was performed on the hypothalamic RNA of mice at 6 weeks of age bearing a MeCP2 null allele or overexpressing MeCP2.
Results: In both models, MeCP2 dysfunction induces changes in the expression of thousands of genes but unexpectedly the majority of genes (~85%) appeared to be activated by MeCP2. MeCP2 binding was confirmed on six genes selected by the authors. Furthermore, an association of MeCP2 with the transcriptional activator CREB1 was observed at the promoter of an activated target but not on a repressed gene.
Conclusion: These results suggest that MeCP2 regulates the expression of a wide range of genes in the hypothalamus and it can both function as an activator and a repressor of transcription.

Deletion of Mecp2 in Sim1-expressing neurons reveals a critical role for MeCP2 in feeding behavior, aggression, and the response to stress

Fyffe SL, Neul JL, Samaco RC, Chao HT, Ben-Shachar S, Moretti P, McGill BE, Goulding EH, Sullivan E, Tecott LH, Zoghbi HY
Department of Molecular and Human Genetics, Baylor College of Medicine, Houston, Tex., USA
Neuron 2008;59:947–958

Background: The paper reported above demonstrated that MeCP2 can function as an activator as well as a repressor of gene expression in the hypothalamus. This result was unexpected and opened new horizons to map the neuroanatomic origins of the complex neuropsychiatric behaviors observed in patients with Rett syndrome (RTT). In this second paper, the authors have tried to uncover the endogenous functions of MeCP2 in the hypothalamus.
Methods: MeCP2 was specifically invalidated in Sim1-expressing hypothalamic neurons using Cre-loxP strategy.
Results: Loss of MeCP2 in Sim1-expressing neurons led to increased physiological response to stress similar to what is seen upon MeCP2 dysfunction in the entire brain. Unexpectedly, MeCP2 conditional knockout (CKO) mice were aggressive, hyperphagic and obese. MeCP2 CKO mice express high levels of Npy in the dorsomedial nucleus of the hypothalamus and hypothalamic expression of 2 MC4R downstream targets is decreased.
Conclusion: This study has demonstrated that deletion of MeCP2 in Sim1-expressing neurons results in a subset of phenotypes observed in RTT and related MeCP2 disorders. It also revealed a role for MeCP2 in the MC4R signaling pathway.

Rett Syndrome (RTT) is an autism spectrum disorder caused by loss of function of the methyl-CpG-binding protein 2. The many phenotypes that are seen in patients with RTT stem from MeCP2 dysfunction in neurons throughout the brain. Previous transcriptional profiling studies comparing brain tissue from MeCP2-null and wild-type (WT) mice revealed subtle differences in gene expression. Chahrour et al. thus decided to focus their attention on the hypothalamus since a number of RTT phenotypes (anxiety, growth deceleration, sleep-wake rhythm disturbance and autonomic abnormalities) could be attributed to hypothalamic dysfunction. MeCP2 was originally described as a transcriptional repressor for its capacity to bind methylated DNA. The transcriptional analysis performed by Chahrour et al. clearly revealed that the majority of genes (2,184) differentially expressed between MeCP2 null and WT mice appeared to be activated by MeCP2 at least in the hypothalamus. The transcriptional changes suggest that the duplication phenotype is due to MeCP2 gain of function (hypermorph), rather than loss of function. The hypothesis that MeCP2 represses a repressor from those 2,184 genes is unlikely as there was no such repressor among the MeCP2 repressed genes. The study of Chahrour et al. thus revealed for the first time a dual activity of MeCP2, its interaction with CREB1 protein on promoter of activated genes and its involvement in the hypothalamus physiology. Thus, patients with RTT will have to be treated differently than patients with *MECP2* duplications. The finding that MeCP2 regulates a large number of genes, at least in the hypothalamus, suggests a need for therapeutic strategies that focus on restoring neuronal function rather than restoring the activity of individual gene products affected by MeCP2 dysfunction.

The second paper revealed a critical role for MeCP2 in feeding behavior, aggression and response to stress. Although the increased response to stress is a well-known phenotype of RTT, feeding problems have been reported in RTT patients but they are not included in the classical phenotype of RTT. MeCP2 CKO mice showed higher serum corticosterone after 30 min of restraint when compared to WT mice. This altered corticosterone response to stress might reproduce the increased urinary cortisol excretion in patients with RTT. This point is very interesting as corticotrophin-releasing factor (CRF) is produced by paraventricular neurons and its expression is regulated by cAMP-protein kinase A pathway and therefore possibly by CREB1 protein. Altogether, these results indicate that MeCP2 might be involved in the normal regulation of CRF synthesis in the hypothalamus.

The second unexpected result was the obesity associated with hyperphagia and disruption of MCR4 signaling. Hyperphagia and obesity are characteristics of mice that have disrupted MC4R signaling. Fyffe et al. found a decreased expression of *Bdnf* in the PVN of MeCP2 CKO mice. BDNF was recently associated with food intake and its gene expression decreased in MCR4 invalidated mice. It is thus likely that MeCP2 directly regulates *Bdnf* expression.

A free-interval after birth is a characteristic of RTT. These 2 papers revealed a fundamental role for MeCP2 in some hypothalamic functions which mature after birth. Therefore, these papers highlight the possible role of MeCP2 in the postnatal maturation of the hypothalamus.

New gene and new paradigm: far away does not mean unrelated

Regulation of a remote Shh forebrain enhancer by the Six3 homeoprotein

Jeong Y, Leskow FC, El-Jaick K, Roessler E, Muenke M, Yocum A, Dubourg C, Li X, Geng X, Oliver G, Epstein DJ
Department of Genetics, University of Pennsylvania School of Medicine, Philadelphia, Pa., USA
Nat Genet 2008;40:1348–1353

Background: In humans, SHH haploinsufficiency is responsible for holoprosencephaly (HPE), an anterior midline defect. SHH expression above a critical threshold in the forebrain is very important, but very little is known about the upstream regulators involved.

Methods and Results: In this study, the authors report a rare nucleotide variant located 460 kb upstream of SHH in a HPE patient, and show that this mutation results in the loss of Shh brain enhancer-2 (SBE2) in the hypothalamus of transgenic mouse embryos. The SBE2 sequence was then screened for putative DNA-binding protein using DNA affinity-capture assay, and Six3 and Six6, both members of the homeodomain-containing protein family, were identified as candidate regulators of Shh transcription. Six3 has a reduced binding affinity for the mutant SBE2 sequence compared to the wild-type and Six3 with HPE-causing mutations is unable to bind and activate SBE2.

Conclusion: These data bring evidence of a direct link between Six3 and *Shh* regulation during normal forebrain development and in the pathogenesis of HPE.

The sonic hedgehog Shh encodes a signal that is instrumental in patterning the early embryo. Enhancer sequences play a major role in regional expression of Shh in the mouse central nervous system and previous studies of functional *Shh* regulatory elements have already identified 6 enhancers within a 500-kb interval surrounding the *Shh* gene. Through the identification of single nucleotide variation in the highly conserved SBE2 enhancer leading to an impaired regulation of *SHH* by Six3 in the forebrain causing holoprosencephaly, this article outlines the importance of researching regulatory SNPs modulating gene expression in rare and common diseases and brings a better understanding of the mechanisms underlying Shh regulation by Six3 and therefore the molecular mechanism of HPE due to Six3 mutations. The phenotype of this case included a moderate fusion of the hypothalamus and basal ganglia. The altered expression of SHH observed in this case should thus be investigated in regard of the recent involvement of SHH pathway in hypothalamic patterning [2].

This article is an additional example of the growing new concept that analysis of a candidate region in genetic diseases with Mendelian transmission cannot be restricted to the coding sequence.

New hormone: during the evolution, reproduction of all species is determined by a 'Kiss'

Molecular evolution of multiple forms of kisspeptins and GPR54 receptors in vertebrates

Lee YR, Tsunekawa K, Moon MJ, Um HN, Hwang JI, Osugi T, Otaki N, Sunakawa Y, Kim K, Vaudry H, Kwon HB, Seong JY, Tsutsui K
Laboratory of G Protein-Coupled Receptors, Graduate School of Medicine, Korea University, Seoul, Korea
Endocrinology 2009;150:2837–2846

Background: The KiSS-1/KiSS-1 receptor (GPR54) system plays a fundamental role in the regulation of the central control of reproduction. While KiSS-1/GPR54 pair has mainly been characterized in mammals, little is known about this system in non-mammalian vertebrates and about the molecular evolution history of these proteins. In this study, the authors have cloned Kisspeptin and GPR54 cDNAs from a variety of vertebrate species to analyze molecular evolution.

Methods: The authors based their initial analysis on Blast search information from human, zebra fish and *Xenopus laevis* Kisspeptin-10. For GPR54, they did a blast search using human and bullfrog GPR54.

Results: Blast search revealed two forms of kisspeptin genes in fish, *KiSS-1* and *KiSS-2* while xenopus possesses three forms of kisspeptin genes, *KiSS-1A*, *KiSS-1B* and *KiSS-2*. The non-mammalian KiSS-1 gene was found to be the ortholog of the mammalian *KiSS-1* gene while the *KiSS-2* gene is a novel form encoding a C-terminal amidated dodecapeptide. Two isoforms of the GPR54 gene were found in fish, while xenopus carry three receptor isoforms. Kisspeptins and GPR54 were abundantly expressed in the xenopus brain, notably in the hypothalamus, suggesting that these ligand-receptor pairs play neuroendocrine and neuromodulatory roles. GPR54 isoforms exhibit differential sensitivity towards *KiSS-1-* or *KiSS-2*-derived peptides, indicating differential ligand selectivity.

Conclusion: The authors concluded that two lineages of kisspeptin and GPR54 genes exist in vertebrates.

Lee et al. report in their paper that non-mammalian vertebrate *KiSS* and *GPR54* gene isoforms originate from a common ancestral gene which has been further duplicated. The *KiSS-1*-like gene was designated *KiSS-2* because it encodes a peptide that shares a conserved C-terminal pentapeptide with the peptide encoded by *KiSS-1*. *KiSS-2* peptides are able to activate GPR54. The evolutionary history of *KiSS-1* and *GPR54* is quite long. The authors propose that duplication of an ancestral kisspeptin gene took place early during vertebrate evolution with an additional round of gene/chromosome duplication in the amphibian. The absence of *KiSS-2* in the higher mammalian species such as rodents or primates indicates that *KiSS-2* probably degenerated after divergence of mammalian species.

This paper also reports the characterization of the mature endogenous KiSS-2 peptide in the brain of *X. laevis*. Its structure is composed of 12 residues resulting probably from maturation of the propeptide by a proconvertase at an arginine residue located 2 amino acids upstream of the mature peptide N-terminal end. The exact structure of the KiSS-1 peptide in the brain remains unknown, and it is quite difficult to speculate about this structure as there is no consensus sequence that may lead to cleavage by a proconvertase immediately upstream of the N-terminal end of primate and rodent Kp-10.

All Kisspeptin and GPR54 isoforms are expressed in the hypothalamus suggesting a neuroendocrine function for all of them. The Kisspeptin form involved in the regulation of the gonadotropic axis remains unknown in fish. This very complex regulation of the Kisspeptin system in fish must be compared to the GnRH system. Three GnRH isoforms have been described in several vertebrate species as well as 2 or 3 GnRH receptor isoforms. Although two types of GnRH receptors were characterized in primates, GnRHR2 is a pseudogene in humans. Its physiological role, if any, is not known. The hypothesis that each kisspeptin/GPR54 pair is specific to one type of GnRH neuron needs to be explored.

Discovery of potent kisspeptin antagonists delineate physiological mechanisms of gonadotropin regulation

Roseweir AK, Kauffman AS, Smith JT, Guerriero KA, Morgan K, Pielecka-Fortuna J, Pineda R, Gottsch ML, Tena-Sempere M, Moenter SM, Terasawa E, Clarke IJ, Steiner RA, Millar RP
Medical Research Council Human Reproductive Sciences Unit, Queen's Medical Research Institute, Edinburgh, UK
J Neurosci 2009;29:3920–3929

Background: Kisspeptin activation of GPR54 was recently described as the most powerful GnRH secretagogue. Natural loss of function mutations of GPR54 as well as genetic invalidation in mice of Kisspeptin and GPR54 have revealed that this Kisspeptin/GPR54 activity is necessary for the reactivation of the gonadotropic axis at puberty as well as for normal reproduction in adult. However, the effects of Kisspeptin functional inactivation has never been reported in adult animals bearing no genetic defects.

Method: The authors developed kisspeptin antagonists by in vitro and in vivo studies to determine the direct role of kisspeptin neurons in the central regulation of the gonadotropic axis in absence of any genetic defects. Various models were used: female rhesus monkey, female ewes and adult male rodents (rat or mice).

Results: One kisspeptin antagonist, Peptide 234, was defined by its capacity to totally block kp-10-induced IP intracellular accumulation. The IC_{50} of the peptide 234 is 7 nM. It blocked Kp-10 stimulation of GnRH neuron firing as well as Kp-10 stimulation of GnRH pulsatile secretion in pubertal female rhesus monkey. It inhibited kp-10-induced LH release in male rats and mice and the LH increase after castration in sheep, rats and mice. However, basal LH was kept within the normal range.

Conclusion: The experiments with Kisspeptin antagonists provide an interesting contribution to the explanation of the neuroendocrine role of Kisspeptin in the regulation of the hypothalamic-pituitary-gonadal axis, namely their fundamental role in pubertal onset and their role as targets for the negative feedback actions of steroids. These antagonists could be a novel approach in therapeutic treatments of reproduction disorders.

This is the first published report of a direct study of kisspeptin function using kisspeptin antagonists. The results confirm the essential role of kisspeptin in the central regulation of the gonadotropic axis and puberty onset, and give some supplemental data. Surprisingly, the kisspeptin antagonist did not inhibit basal LH, suggesting that other factors regulate basal GnRH and LH secretion in all studied species. These results are discordant with the very low LH and FSH basal levels observed in some patients with loss of function mutation of GPR54. These results might highlight differences between species in the regulation of basal levels of LH and FSH, or indicate that GPR54 has an effect on LH and FSH release independent of Kisspeptin. The more severe gonadotropic deficiency in $GPR54^{-/-}$ mice when compared to $KiSS-1^{-/-}$ mice supports the hypothesis of a Kp-10-independent activation of GPR54. This study suggests that the Kp-10 antagonist could be a novel therapeutic approach in reproductive disorders associated with abnormal LH pulse frequency or amplitude such as infertility, polycystic ovarian syndrome, endometriosis, uterine fibroids, excessive menstrual bleeding, delayed and precocious puberty, and breast, prostatic, and ovarian cancers. Potent and specific kisspeptin antagonists offer potential novel treatments for these conditions.

Kisspeptin-54 at high doses acutely induces testicular degeneration in adult male rats via central mechanisms

Thompson EL, Amber V, Stamp GW, Patterson M, Curtis AE, Cooke JH, Appleby GF, Dhillo WS, Ghatei MA, Bloom SR, Murphy KG
Department of Investigative Medicine, Hammersmith Hospital, Imperial College London, London, UK

Br J Pharmacol 2009;156:609–625

Background: KiSS-1/GPR54 inactivation results in gonadotropic deficiency and this system is a key regulator of pubertal maturation and reproduction. Acute central or peripheral administration of kisspeptin to rodents or primates stimulates the gonadotropic axis. Secondary effects of this injection have not been studied with regard to testicular damage. The authors evaluated the consequences of high doses of Kisspeptin-54 (Kp-54) sustained injection in the rat.

Methods: Histology analyses and hormonal dosage after Kp-54 administration in adult male Wistar rats were made. Different conditions were tested: subcutaneous administration from 6 h up to 3 days; single subcutaneous administration of 0.5 to 50 nmol Kp-54, and before or after pre-administration of a GnRH-receptor antagonist (cetrorelix). The results were compared to the testicular histology in rats after intracerebroventricular injections of 5 nmol Kp-54 to determine whether the cause of testicular degeneration is of central origin or not.

Results: Continuous subcutaneous administration of Kp-54 caused testicular degeneration after only 12 h, when gonadotropins were still markedly high, suggesting that the degeneration is independent of the desensitization of the HPG axis to Kp-54. Furthermore, a single subcutaneous injection of Kp-54 caused dose-dependent testicular degeneration. Thus, continuous Kp-54 administration is not required to cause testicular degeneration. Pretreatment with cetrorelix blocked kisspeptin-induced testicular degeneration, and a single intracerebroventricular injection of Kp-54 caused testicular degeneration, suggesting it is GnRH-mediated.

Conclusion: The mechanisms of Kp-54-induced testicular degeneration are acute and centrally regulated. A dose dependent GnRH-mediated effect of kisspeptin on the testes can cause damages with loss of Sertoli and germ cells. If kisspeptins represent a potential therapeutic tool for reproductive and pubertal disorders, this study alerts us regarding the choice of the doses used.

Kp-54 induced testicular degeneration in adult male rats. The authors show that it is not the continuous administration of kisspeptin that is responsible for the testicular damage, as had previously been published. An acute single high dose of Kp-54 (50 nmol) is sufficient to alter testis histology whereas a low dose of 0.5 nmol kisspeptin has no effect. This effect on the testes was apparent before the desensitization of the gonadotropic axis which came later after kisspeptin administration.

Kisspeptin was initially described as the most powerful secretagogue of GnRH. As shown in the paper of Roseweir et al. (see above), a kisspeptin antagonist blocks GnRH release as well as LH increase in gonadectomized animals. The main effect of kisspeptin is thus the regulation of GnRH release. The results reported by Thompson et al. were unexpected. The authors interpret their results as an acute hyper-stimulation of the HPG axis. However, acute stimulation of the gonadotropic axis by GnRH agonists is frequently used in medicine and such a very rapid effect on the testes is uncommon. The understanding of this side effect of kisspeptin injection on testes needs probably prior understanding of the kisspeptin effect on the pituitary. Testicular degeneration could also be due to an association of central and peripheral mechanisms.

New mechanism: interaction between negative and positive regulators of GnRH release

Gamma-aminobutyric acid B receptor mediated inhibition of gonadotropin-releasing hormone neurons is suppressed by kisspeptin-G protein-coupled receptor 54 signaling

Zhang C, Bosch MA, Ronnekleiv OK, Kelly MJ
Department of Physiology and Pharmacology, Oregon Health and Science University, Portland, Oreg., USA
Endocrinology 2009;150:2388–2394

Background: GnRH neurons express both γ-aminobutyric acid (GABA) class of receptors, $GABA_A$ which is a ligand-gated chloride channel, and $GABA_B$, which is a metabotropic $G\alpha_{i,o}$–coupled receptor known to activate postsynaptic K^+ channels or inhibit presynaptic Ca^{2+} channels. Recent studies have shown that Cl currents are activated by GABA in GnRH neurons and that these effects are blocked by the $GABA_A$ receptor antagonist bicuculline. However, the potential role of $GABA_B$ receptor signaling in GnRH neurons remains unknown.

Methods and Results: The authors used whole cell electrophysiological recordings from mouse eGFP-expressing GnRH neurons to show that GnRH neurons were hyperpolarized in a concentration-dependent manner by baclophen, a $GABA_B$ receptor antagonist, through the activation of an inwardly rectifying K^+ current. The presence of 17β-estradiol did not have any impact on this activation. However, addition of a selective $GABA_B$ receptor antagonist, CGP52432, abrogated this effect. In a similar manner, the $GABA_A$ receptor antagonist picrotoxin also hyperpolarized GnRH neurons. The authors next assessed whether G-protein-coupled receptor 54 (GPR54) agonist Kisspeptin-10 (Kp10) could alter $GABA_B$-mediated response and showed that, indeed, baclophen in the presence of submaximal concentrations of Kp10 no longer hyperpolarized GnRH neurons.

Conclusion: Kp10 can desensitize the $GABA_B$-mediated response, suggesting that the $GABA_B$ receptor may lower GnRH release pulses during 17β-estradiol negative feedback and that this effect is inhibited by kisspeptin during positive feedback.

The authors show that a majority of GnRH neurons express mRNA of both subunits R1 and R2 of the $GABA_B$ receptor and that baclophen, a selective agonist of the $GABA_B$ receptor, induces a strong hyperpolarization of GnRH neurons. Therefore, GABA may provide a strong inhibitory effect on GnRH neurons to support 17β-estradiol-mediated negative feedback. Another important result in this study comes from the observation that kisspeptin counters the $GABA_B$-mediated response through the activation of GPR54, thus providing a better understanding of how GnRH neurons could become excited during the preovulatory phase and how kisspeptins can modulate GnRH pulses.

New genes: a novel unexpected neuropeptide in the central regulation of the gonadotropic axis

TAC3 and TACR3 mutations in familial hypogonadotropic hypogonadism reveal a key role for neurokinin B in the central control of reproduction

Topaloglu AK, Reimann F, Guclu M, Yalin AS, Kotan LD, Porter KM, Serin A, Mungan NO, Cook JR, Ozbek MN, Imamoglu S, Akalin NS, Yuksel B, O'Rahilly S, Semple RK
Cukurova University, Faculty of Medicine, Department of Pediatric Endocrinology and Metabolism, Balcali, Adana, Turkey
ktopaloglu@cu.edu.tr
Nat Genet 2009;41:354–358

Background: The reactivation of the GnRH pulse at pubertal onset is a fundamental event. This reactivation drives the increase in gonadotropin secretion and then, gonadal steroid secretion and gametogenesis. Several genes are now associated with isolated gonadotropic deficiency, but a few familial cases still remain unlinked to those genes. In this paper, Topaloglu et al. have performed genome mapping in informative families with isolated gonadotropic deficiency.

Methods: Nine consanguineous Turkish families with normosmic hypogonadotropic hypogonadism (nIHH) were subjected to genome-wide SNP analysis after ruling out sequencing mutations in the known hypogonadotropic hypogonadism genes.

Results: A candidate region was found on chromosome 4. Among candidate genes, homozygous loss of function mutations in TACR3 (neurokinin receptor) were identified in 3 families and in TAC3 (neurokinin) in 1 other pedigree. None of the TAC3R mutations were found in 100 ethnically matched controls nor in the 6 other analyzed families or in 50 individuals with nIHH from various ethnic groups. The tachykinin neurokinin B (TAC3) is expressed in kisspeptin neurons, namely in the arcuate nucleus, and its receptor (TACR3) is found in rodent GnRH-expressing neurons localized within the median eminence of the hypothalamus.

Conclusion: nIHH may be due to inactivating mutations of TAC3 or TAC3R. These findings suggest that the TAC3/TACR3 system is a key positive regulator of the central neuroendocrine control of the reproductive axis.

Hypogonadotropic hypogonadism may or may not be associated with anosmia (respectively nIHH or Kallmann syndrome). Human genetics enabled the discovery of some essential genes implicated in the central control of the gonadotropic axis (Kal1, FGFR1, PROK2/PROKR2, GnRHR, KiSS-1/GPR54, etc.). The description of the TAC3/TACR3 inactivation mutation discovered a new gene in the cascade and a new cause of normosmic hypogonadotropic hypogonadism.

The TAC3 mutations were associated with a phenotype of mild learning disability in both affected subjects in this report, but patients with TACR3 mutations were normal. The mechanisms of the gonadotropic axis regulation by neurokinin B remains to be established. This role in rodents has never been suspected because TACR3 invalidated mice are fertile. A probable action at the level of hypothalamic GnRH release is suspected as neurokinin B is expressed in *KiSS-1* neuron axons located in apposition with GnRH neurons expressing both GPR54 and TACR3.

Finally this report opens the way for new pharmacological approaches in the control of reproduction and other hormonally related diseases such as breast and prostate cancer.

Concept revised: involvement of additional genes in the postnatal maturation of the hypothalamus

Developmental profiles of neuroendocrine gene expression in the preoptic area of male rats

Walker DM, Juenger TE, Gore AC
Institute for Neuroscience, University of Texas at Austin, Austin, Tex., USA

Endocrinology 2009;150:2308-2316

Background: Reproductive function is controlled by GnRH neurons and their steroid-sensitive regulatory inputs. The proper maturation of this system is critical to sexual development at puberty and maintenance of adult reproductive function. Regulation of GnRH release is the main central mechanism regulating reproduction. However, molecular mechanisms underlying this regulation are poorly understood as it is a dynamic process, with sex dimorphism and highly regulated by gonadal hormones. In this study, Walker et al. designed a protocol to analyze differential expression in preoptic area (POA) of 5 genes that form a critical part of the neural circuit controlling reproduction, and they also performed a low-density array.

Methods: A developmental profile of the 5 genes, GnRH, estrogen receptor (ER)α, ERβ, androgen receptor (AR) and progesterone receptor (PR), from postnatal day P1 through P60 in the POA was performed in male Sprague-Dawley rats. Serum hormones were measured. A TaqMan low-density array (TLDA) was performed on 48 genes belonging to the estrogen-signaling pathway.

Results: Of the 5 targeted genes, only AR and PR changed robustly (7- and 3- to 4-fold increases, respectively) between P1 and P60. All of the gonadal serum hormones changed markedly: testosterone decreased from P1 to P30 and then increased to P60; progesterone peaked at P30, and estradiol decreased from P1 to P30 and then stayed low until P60. Using the TLDA, the authors identified several genes that dramatically changed in the POA, particularly G protein-coupled receptor 30, IGF-I, vitamin D receptor, estrogen-related receptor-α, and thyroid receptor-α.

Conclusion: These data demonstrate postnatal variations in genes expressed in the POA, particularly AR and PR. Moreover, the relationships between hormones and their corresponding receptors undergo dynamic changes across postnatal development in the hypothalamus of male rats.

Several groups have tried to characterize transcriptomic changes in the hypothalamus between birth and puberty. The analysis reported in this paper is novel because previous studies tested a single gene or used microarray on the whole hypothalamus to perform the initial screening. In this study, Walker et al. have restricted their analysis to POA and used the TLDA screening technique. TLDA is a PCR method which is very sensitive and specific. They found a small but significant increase in GnRH mRNA through classical quantitative PCR analysis but a small decrease using the TLDA technique. These contradictory results reinforce the concept that translational and posttranslational regulation of GnRH is responsible for the pubertal increase in pulsatile GnRH release at puberty. The large increase in AR suggests that prenatal POA regulation by androgens is not dependant on AR. This result is in line with the concept that masculinization of the POA involves the action of estradiol in early postnatal development. The characterization of PR mRNA increasing in POA is new. This increase is associated with an increase in progesterone levels. The role of progesterone in the postnatal maturation of the hypothalamus needs to be explored. TLDA analysis also revealed a decrease in GPR30 and IGF-1 gene expression. GPR30 encodes a cell membrane estrogen receptor. Its function remains obscure, it probably is involved in negative and positive feedback of estradiol on GnRH neurons. The decrease in IGF-1 was unexpected. This growth factor is better known as an activator of the gonadotropic axis than an inhibitor. However, this decrease may be related to the estradiol decrease observed in this study. The large variation in vitamin D receptor expression with a peak at P45 is new and suggests a role in mechanisms immediately preceding the pubertal initiation. The confirmation of such a scenario in humans is difficult but again analysis of the specific phenotype might be very informative.

New concept: maternal care determines the age of the sexual maturity

Maternal programming of sexual behavior and hypothalamic-pituitary-gonadal function in the female rat

Cameron N, Del Corpo A, Diorio J, McAllister K, Sharma S, Meaney MJ
Sackler Program for Epigenetics and Psychobiology, McGill University, Montreal, Que., Canada
PLoS ONE 2008;3:e2210

Background: In many species, maternal effects lead to phenotypic variations in reproductive functions and it is well established that in humans, parental care has a strong influence on the age of puberty, sexual activity during adolescence, and the age at first pregnancy. However, the biological mechanisms involved remain largely unknown, especially during female reproductive development.

Methods and Results: The authors hypothesized that hypothalamic-pituitary-ovarian axis function might be altered by parental care. To assess this hypothesis, they focused on the female offspring of rat mothers with high versus low pup licking and grooming (LG) over the first week postpartum. Compared to those from high LG mothers, adults from low LG mothers showed several differences in sexual comportment, including an increase in the lordosis rating reflecting a higher sexual receptivity, increased LH and progesterone levels at proestrus, an increase in positive feedback of estradiol on LH and GnRH expression in the medial preoptic area, and finally higher levels of estrogen receptor α (ERα) expression in the anteroventral periventricular nucleus. Cross-fostering studies, consisting of removing pups from their biological mother and placing them under the care of mother with the same or different LG phenotype brings clear evidence of a postnatal effect of maternal care but did not rule out an influence of prenatal environment. This is indeed supported by the fact that testosterone levels on embryonic day 20 were higher in fetuses from high LG mothers compared to those from low LG mothers.

Conclusion: This study shows that maternal care in rats has an impact on the hypothalamic-pituitary-ovarian axis development leading to differences in sexual behavior of the female offspring, and that it could result from variations in ERα expression in the anteroventral periventricular nucleus of the hypothalamus.

The age at sexual maturation is highly variable. It is determined by genetic factors as well as environmental factors. The paper of Cameron et al. highlights the consequences of maternal care in the maturation of the function of reproduction. The advanced age of offspring of LG mothers suggests that in adverse conditions, the optimal strategy for the survival of the species is to maximize reproduction by an earlier age at sexual maturity and the number of offspring. As described in the paper of Chang et al. showing the effect on offspring of maternal feeding during pregnancy (see above), the effect of low maternal care on offspring may be interpreted as a genetic trait. In fact, the response to adverse conditions will be similar across generations and therefore transmitted from mothers to daughters. It is well known that adopted children from developed countries are more prone to advanced puberty. The low maternal care provided to these children under an adverse environment may be one explanation.

References
1. Pasinetti GM, Eberstein JA: Metabolic syndrome and the role of dietary lifestyles in Alzheimer's disease. J Neurochem 2008;106:1503–1514.
2. Szabo NE, Zhao T, Cankaya M, Theil T, Zhou X, Alvarez-Bolado G: Role of neuroepithelial sonic hedgehog in hypothalamic patterning. J Neurosci 2009;29:6989–7002.

Pituitary

Mohamad Maghnie[a], Andrea Secco[a] and Sandro Loche[b]

[a]Department of Pediatrics, Istituto di Ricovero e Cura a Carattere Scientifico, Giannina Gaslini, University of Genova; [b]Ospedale Regionale per le Microcitemie, Cagliari; Italy

Important for clinical practice
Midline defects and pituitary: awaiting for more genes

Congenital hypopituitarism: clinical, molecular and neuroradiological correlates

Mehta A, Hindmarsh PC, Mehta H, Turton JP, Russell-Eggitt I, Taylor D, Chong WK, Dattani MT
Developmental Endocrinology Research Group, Institute of Child Health and Great Ormond Street Hospital for Children, University College London, London, UK
Clin Endocrinol (Oxf) 2009; Epub ahead of print

Background: Many studies have recently described mutations in genes encoding transcription factors involved in hypothalamic pituitary (HP) development which result in various degrees of pituitary function impairment (ranging from isolated GH deficiency IGHD, to combined pituitary hormone deficiency, CPHD) and structural HP abnormalities detected by brain MRI. However, none of these previous studies compared subjects affected by hypopituitarism with or without optic nerve hypoplasia (ONH). The aim of the present study was to investigate a large number (n = 170) of children with congenital hypopituitarism and/or septo-optic dysplasia (SOD) for their clinical, MRI and genetic findings.
Methods: This is a retrospective analysis of clinical, hormonal, MRI and genetic data relative to 170 children with congenital hypopituitarism, or with ONH, who are at risk of pituitary endocrine defects, in order to determine predictors of hypopituitarism
Results: ONH showed a significant relationship with the absence of septum pellucidum (OR 31.5, p<0.001), anomalies of corpus callosum (OR 10.5, p < 0.001) and pituitary stalk (OR 2.3, p = 0.009). Markers for a high risk of hypopituitarism were ectopic posterior pituitary (OR 27.2, p < 0.001), anterior pituitary hypoplasia (OR 3.1, p = 0.006) and pituitary stalk abnormalities (χ^2 20.11, p < 0.001), while CPHD was observed to be more frequently associated with abnormal corpus callosum (OR 6.1, p = 0.008) and pituitary stalk (OR 2.8, p = 0.006). Gender prevalence of hypopituitarism was 3.3:1 for males with normal optic nerve and 1.2:1 for males with ONH. Vasopressin, TSH and ACTH deficiencies showed a higher prevalence in subjects with ONH compared to idiopathic hypopituitarism. Pituitary transcription factor mutations were found in only 5 of 170 subjects, confirming them as a rare condition in patients with sporadic hypopituitarism.
Conclusion: Based on the reported data, ONH is often associated with other neuroradiologic abnormalities and represents a risk factor for the development of pituitary hormone defects, the severity of which is correlated with specific MRI alterations. The high correlation between midline anomalies and pituitary defects is likely compatible with a common genetic origin of both of these disorders, an origin that in most of cases remains largely undefined.

This is a comprehensive study on midline defects, optic nerve involvement and pituitary defects that is worth reading. It shows that gene identifiable mutations are rare in sporadic hypopituitarism in a large cohort from a single center. The study confirms previous reports suggesting that neuroradiological findings of septum pellucidum agenesis in association with optic nerve hypoplasia with or without abnormalities of the corpus callosum and structural hypothalamic-pituitary abnormalities are risk factors for severe pituitary dysfunction. Early identification of such CNS malformations can predict the outcome in terms of the number of pituitary hormone deficiencies and will allow clinicians a better surveillance of evolving pituitary hormone defects including ACTH deficiency.

Endocrine manifestations of the rapid-onset obesity with hypoventilation, hypothalamic, autonomic dysregulation, and neural tumor syndrome in childhood

Bougnères P, Pantalone L, Linglart A, Rothenbühler A, Le Stunff C
Department of Pediatric Endocrinology, Hôpital Saint Vincent de Paul, Paris, France bougneres@paris5.inserm.fr
J Clin Endocrinol Metab 2008;93:3971–3980

Background: ROHHADNET is a new syndrome characterized by early- and rapid-onset obesity with hypoventilation, hypothalamic dysregulation, and neural tumor. It is associated with hypothalamic-pituitary dysfunction, which can be similar to syndromes observed in forms of genetic obesity. The syndrome can cause cardiorespiratory arrest. Early recognition of the syndrome is crucial for the prevention of fatal events. This study reports the clinical and laboratory characteristics of 6 patients with ROHHADNET and discusses differential diagnoses with other endocrine diseases such as pseudo-Cushing syndrome, hypopituitarism, glucocorticoid insufficiency, and adrenal tumors.

Methods: Thorough endocrine investigations were carried out on 6 patients who presented with early-onset obesity associated with growth deceleration as seen in 5 of them. These patients were ultimately diagnosed as having ROHHADNET. Five patients with Cushing disease and a group of obese children served as controls.

Results: All of the patients were apparently normal in their first 2–4 years of life. The initial manifestation of obesity began between 1.5 and 4.3 years, and at the same time growth velocity started to decelerate. Clinical examination was normal in all patients. Investigation of the pituitary adrenal axis revealed a Cushing-like profile in 1 patient, glucocorticoid deficiency with normal ACTH in 2 others and normal findings in the remaining 3. Four patients showed GH deficiency with low IGF-I, 4 had hypogonadotropic hypogonadism, 6 showed hyperprolactinemia, and 5 had various degrees of pituitary/thyroid dysfunction. Pituitary MRI was normal in all but 1 patient who had a Rathke's cleft cyst. CT scan of the adrenals revealed adrenal tumors in 5 patients. Ganglioneuromas were diagnosed 4.5–16 years after the onset of obesity. Hypernatremia was observed in all patients. Three patients manifested cardiorespiratory arrest, and 2 of them died at age 8.5 and 12 years. One patient had symptomatic obstructive sleep apnea. All 6 patients had alveolar hypoventilation. Symptoms of autonomic dysregulation included hyper- or hypothermia, papillary dysfunction, and gastrointestinal dysmotility.

Conclusion: This study shows that the ROHHADNET syndrome can be associated with various hypothalamic pituitary dysfunctions. ROHHADNET syndrome should be considered in all cases of isolated rapid and early-onset obesity, and when ROHHADNET syndrome is suspected, all children with early-onset obesity should be tested for alveolar hypoventilation.

This study focuses on the clinical presentation, laboratory investigation and follow-up of a rarely made diagnosis of a syndrome of early-onset and severe obesity. The syndrome, named ROHHADNET, is associated with hypoventilation, hypothalamic autonomic dysregulation and neural tumor. The syndrome can be distinguished from all other known genetic syndromes with early-onset obesity. ROHHADNET mimics congenital leptin deficiency with undetectable leptin concentrations. Given the possibility of fatal cardiorespiratory arrest in a syndrome with pleiotropic features, it is important to recognize any and all possible symptoms that may indicate such a diagnosis or other types of hypothalamic obesity. It is conceivable that a substantial subgroup of patients with 'simple obesity' might have hypothalamic obesity.

Prenatal MR imaging of the normal pituitary stalk

Righini A, Parazzini C, Doneda C, Arrigoni F, Triulzi F
Radiology and Neuroradiology Department, Children's Hospital V. Buzzi, ICP, Milan, Italy
AJNR Am J Neuroradiol 2009;30:1014–1016

Background: Although occasional cases of pituitary stalk (PS) detection by fetal MRI have been reported, well-established data about prenatal MR imaging of the hypothalamic-pituitary area are still lacking. These data would allow an early diagnosis of congenital pituitary disorders. The aim of the present study is the systematic identification and description of PS in healthy fetuses of different gestational ages (GAs) by means of single-shot fast-spin echo T2-weighted images.
Methods: The authors investigated 73 fetuses with GAs between 19 and 37 weeks, normal prenatal MRI and clinical follow-up after birth. Three-plane 4-mm MRI sections with 1.25 × 1.25 mm in-plane resolution were analyzed in consensus by 2 pediatric neuroradiologists to search for PS, defined as a linear isointense structure connecting the hypothalamic region with the floor of the sella turcica. When it was detectable on sagittal images, the angle between the intersection of the PS and the sellar plane (SP) was measured (PS-SP angle).
Results: The PS was identified at GA between 19 and 25 weeks in at least 1 coronal or sagittal section in 30 of 42 cases (sensitivity 71.4%), while a 100% sensitivity (PS identification in all 31 cases) was observed in the successive gestational ages. The PS-SP angle showed a significant decrease with GA, reaching values below 90° in all fetuses with GA ≥25 weeks.
Conclusion: The authors conclude that MRI, at the current available resolution for clinical prenatal evaluations, is an accurate method for the detection of PS after a GA of 25 weeks. A missing PS after this age could represent an early marker of congenital structural pituitary abnormalities.

Prenatal imaging has benefited from rapid technological progress in the last 10 years. Ultrasound remains the standard screening method for fetal malformations, but it can be hindered by the bony structure of the skull. In particular, it can be difficult to distinguish between white and grey matter, and MRI represents a complementary method to ultrasound for detecting brain malformations. In particular, MRI is needed to detect associated malformations and to obtain a precise diagnosis when ultrasound examination shows ventricular dilation.

Prenatal diagnosis of absent septum pellucidum has been made as early as 22 weeks of gestation and sonographic demonstration of isolated absence of the septum pellucidum with fusion of the frontal horns of the lateral ventricles is a clue for the diagnosis of septo-optic dysplasia [1]. This study reinforces the need for thorough knowledge of normal and abnormal neuroanatomy and shows that fetal MRI can identify the pituitary stalk and that such identification might have an impact on the evaluation of congenital CNS malformations related to pituitary endocrinopathies.

Although a clinical course and development still cannot be predicted based on MRI findings alone, the identification of pituitary stalk agenesis in fetuses with associated brain malformations could be helpful both for the early management of neonatal hypopituitarism and for counseling parents.

Treatment of pituitary-dependent Cushing's disease with the multireceptor ligand somatostatin analog pasireotide (SOM230): a multicenter, phase II trial

Boscaro M, Ludlam WH, Atkinson B, Glusman JE, Petersenn S, Reincke M, Snyder P, Tabarin A, Biller BM, Findling J, Melmed S, Darby CH, Hu K, Wang Y, Freda PU, Grossman AB, Frohman LA, Bertherat J
Division of Endocrinology, Polytechnic University of Marche, Ancona, Italy
J Clin Endocrinol Metab 2009;94:115–122

Background: Cushing's disease is caused by a corticotropin-secreting pituitary adenoma. Surgical resection of the adenoma via the transphenoidal route is, so far, the only available effective treatment. Therapeutic trials with different compounds, including somatostatin (SS) analogs have been disappointing. Human corticotroph adenomas express multiple SS receptors (SSR) with a predominance of SSR5. This study reports the results of a phase-II, open-label, multicenter trial in patients with persistent or recurrent Cushing's disease treated with pasireotide, a novel SS analog with high affinity for SSR5.
Methods: Thirty-nine patients with either de novo Cushing's disease or with persistent or recurrent disease participated in the trial. The patients self-administered pasireotide subcutaneously at a dose of 600 µg twice daily for 15 days. The primary efficacy outcome was normalization of mean urinary free cortisol (UFC) after 15 days of treatment. Secondary endpoints were normalization of serum ACTH and cortisol levels.
Results: 22/29 patients (76%) in the primary efficacy analysis showed a reduction in UFC levels after 15 days of treatment. Among them, 5 showed normalization of UFC. These changes were paralleled by a reduction of both serum ACTH and cortisol concentrations.
Conclusion: Treatment with pasireotide produced a reduction of UFC and ACTH in about two thirds of patients with Cushing's disease. This compound opens a new field of investigation for the medical treatment of corticotropin-secreting adenomas.

Cushing's disease is a rare condition in children. It is associated with most of the features of the adult disease and, in addition, it causes growth arrest in virtually all patients. Transphenoidal surgery is a difficult therapeutic procedure, even more so in children. Therefore, a medical approach to treatment of Cushing's disease in the pediatric age would be most desirable. Pasireotide is a novel multireceptor ligand somatostatin analog with high binding affinity for four of the five known somatostatin receptors (1–3 and 5) and has a 40-fold higher affinity for SSR5 than octreotide. Corticotroph adenomas express multiple SS receptors with high abundance of SSR5. Studies in vitro and in experimental animals have shown that pasireotide effectively inhibited ACTH secretion. The results of this study in adult subjects treated with the somatostatin analog pasireotide are promising.

OTX2 mutation in a patient with anophthalmia, short stature, and partial growth hormone deficiency: functional studies using the IRBP, HESX1, and POU1F1 promoters

Dateki S, Fukami M, Sato N, Muroya K, Adachi M, Ogata T
Department of Endocrinology and Metabolism, National Research Institute for Child Health and Development, Setagaya, Tokyo, Japan
J Clin Endocrinol Metab 2008;93:3697–3702

Background: While the role of the transcription factor gene OTX2 for eye development is well known, its relevance in pituitary function regulation is not completely understood. The objective of the present study was to assess the involvement of OTX2 in pituitary function development by means of functional studies.

Methods: A Japanese girl affected by bilateral anophthalmia and short stature (−3.3 SDS), was diagnosed with isolated GH deficiency (GH peaks of 3.1 and 9.7 µg/l after insulin and arginine administration, respectively, with IGF-I 37 µg/l) at the age of 3 years and 9 months. No significant structural pituitary abnormalities were found on brain MRI. DNA samples from the patient and her parents were analyzed for mutation of OTX2, HESX1, and POU1F1.

Results: A novel OTX2 heterozygous frameshift mutation (c.402insC) was detected, which conserved the homeodomain but lost the transactivation domain. In fact, functional analysis revealed that both the wild-type and the mutant Otx2 proteins showed analogous binding capability to their nuclear target sequence within the interstitial retinoid-binding protein (IRBP), HESX1 and POU1F1 promoters. The wild-type Otx2 protein markedly transactivated the promoters of IRBP (approximately 27-fold), HESX1 (approximately 4.5-fold), and POU1F1 (approximately 19-fold), while the mutant Otx2 protein barely retained transactivation activities, without dominant-negative effects.

Conclusion: This study confirms a significant role for OTX2 in pituitary function regulation, demonstrating that a heterozygous OTX2 loss-of-function mutation can cause GH deficiency and short stature with a mechanism related to decreased HESX1 and POU1F1 transactivation.

A novel dominant negative mutation of OTX2 associated with combined pituitary hormone deficiency

Diaczok D, Romero C, Zunich J, Marshall I, Radovick S
Division of Pediatric Endocrinology, Johns Hopkins University School of Medicine, Baltimore, Md., USA
J Clin Endocrinol Metab 2008;93:4351–4359

Background: Mutations in different transcription factors involved in pituitary cell lineage differentiation and regulation of gene expression were described in patients affected by combined pituitary hormone deficiency (CPHD). Mutation of OTX2, a bicoid class homeodomain protein active in forebrain development and transactivation of HESX1 promoter, has not yet been definitively associated with CPHD. The aim of this study was to identify novel mutations of pituitary specific transcription factors in CPHD patients.

Methods: Genomic DNA obtained from 19 patients with hypopituitarism and 50 control subjects was sequenced for HESX1, LHX3, LHX4, OTX2, PITX2, POU1F1, PROP1, and SIX6. Thirty-one additional CPHD patients were studied for mutations in exon 3 of the OTX2 gene. Novel mutations were structurally and functionally characterized.

Results: Two unrelated children, presenting with neonatal hypoglycemia, CPHD and ectopic posterior pituitary with anterior pituitary hypoplasia at MRI, were found to be heterozygous for a novel OTX2 mutation (N233S). Mutant protein did not lose its ability to bind to the bicoid-binding sites, but showed a significant decrease in HESX1 transactivation, suggesting a dominant negative effect of mutant Otx2 on the binding and action of the OTX2 wild-type copy at the HESX1 promoter.

Conclusion: A new heterozygous OTX2 mutation could have a dominant negative inhibitor effect on HESX1 gene expression, leading to both impairment of the correct spatiotemporal sequence required for pituitary cell lineage differentiation and, consequently, to absence or underdevelopment of the anterior pituitary gland with reduced hormonal expression.

OTX2 loss of function mutation causes anophthalmia and combined pituitary hormone deficiency with a small anterior and ectopic posterior pituitary

Tajima T, Ohtake A, Hoshino M, Amemiya S, Sasaki N, Ishizu K, Fujieda K
Department of Pediatrics, Hokkaido University School of Medicine, Sapporo, Japan
tajeari@hokudai.med.ac.jp
J Clin Endocrinol Metab 2009;94:314–319

Background: The OTX2 (orthodenticle homeobox 2) transcription factor is required for normal ocular and forebrain development. Heterozygous mutations of OTX2 were previously described in patients with severe ocular malformations.

Table 1. Summary of the main characteristics of three novel OTX2 mutations associated with hypopituitarism (molecular consequences, inheritance, clinical, biochemical and neuroradiologic phenotypes)

	Dateki et al. [J Clin Endocrinol Metab 2008;93:3697–3702]	Diaczok et al. [J Clin Endocrinol Metab 2008;93:4351–4359]	Tajima et al. [J Clin Endocrinol Metab 2009;94:314–319]
Mutation	c.402insC	A698G (N233S)	c.576-577insCT (S136fsX178)
Type of mutation	Frameshift	Substitution	Frameshift Premature stop codon (codon 178)
Functional consequences	Loss of the transactivation domain Conservation of the homeodomain	Reduced transactivation activity Multiple bicoid binding site promoter	Severely reduced or absent transactivation of POU1F1 and HESX1, respectively Normal nuclear localization
Inheritance	De novo heterozygous mutation No dominant negative effects	De novo heterozygous mutation	De novo heterozygous mutation No dominant negative effects
Subjects	One Japanese female patient	Two unrelated children (case 1 male, case 2 female)	One Japanese male patient
Familial cases	None	None	None
Eye phenotype	Bilateral anophthalmia Optic nerve hypoplasia	Normal	Bilateral anophthalmia Optic nerve hypoplasia
Clinical phenotype	Cleft palate Short stature	Neonatal hypoglycemia hyperbilirubinemia, and poor feeding (case 1) Neonatal respiratory distress, hypoglycemia and seizures (case 2)	Neonatal hypoglycemia, hyperbilirubinemia and failure to thrive Short stature Severe developmental delay
Hormone defects	GH	GH TSH LH, FSH ACTH	GH TSH LH, FSH ACTH
MRI phenotype	Normal	APH EPP Absent or severely hypoplastic PS	APH EPP Absent PS Chiari malformation

APH = Anterior pituitary hypoplasia; EPP = ectopic posterior pituitary; PS = pituitary stalk.

Methods: This study offers a functional characterization of an OTX2 mutation associated with structural hypothalamic-pituitary abnormalities, combined pituitary hormone deficiency (CPHD) and anophthalmia. This mutation was found in a Japanese patient with short stature, anophthalmia, severe developmental delay and CPHD (GH, TSH, ACTH and gonadotropin deficiency). Brain MRI showed ectopic posterior pituitary, anterior pituitary hypoplasia, pituitary stalk agenesis and Chiari malformation.

Results: The patient carried a heterozygous two-base insertion [S136fsX178(c.576–577insCT)] in exon 3 of OTX2 (leading to a premature stop codone introduction), not detected in the patient's parents or in 50 Japanese healthy controls. This mutation determined a loss of function of Otx2 protein, which correctly localized to the nucleus but did not activate transcription of HESX1 and POU1F1 genes. A dominant negative effect was not involved in the pathogenesis of pituitary damage, because co-transfection of cultured cells with vectors containing both mutant and wild-type Otx2 lead to a normal HESX1 and POU1F1 expression.

Conclusion: OTX2 mutation is responsible in this patient for CPHD and structural pituitary abnormalities. Further studies of more patients with OTX2 defects could likely shed new light on the pathophysiology of ocular and pituitary diseases related to OTX2 mutations.

These three studies describe four children with heterozygote mutations of OTX2 associated with isolated or multiple pituitary hormone deficiencies (MPHD), as well as brain abnormalities. The studies focus on the role of OTX2, not only in eye development, but also in pituitary organogenesis and function (table 1).

The Otx-family of homeobox genes are vertebrate orthologs to the *Drosophila orthodenticle* homeobox gene and include the *Otx1* and *Otx2* genes. After gastrulation, *Otx2* is expressed in the prosencephalon, mesencephalon and cerebellum of the developing central nervous system. In addition, OTX2 mRNA has been found in the retinal pigment epithelium of human fetal retina, and to a lesser extent in the neural retina. Studies on heterozygous *Otx2*-deficient mice (*Otx2+/–*) report various phenotypes including eyes lacking a lens, cornea, and iris, as well as anophthalmia or microphthalmia [2]. Indeed, mice homozygous for a null allele of Otx2 are embryonic lethal due to severe brain abnormalities [2].

At this point, OTX2 represents an additional gene to be added to the long list of genes (LHX3, LHX4, HESX1, Prop1 and POU1F1, SOX2 and SOX3) that have previously been characterized and whose loss of function causes MPHD, either associated or not with extra-endocrine abnormalities. It is worth pointing out that in the presence of eye abnormalities and pituitary dysfunction, a differential diagnosis between OTX2 and SOX2 mutations and deletion of chromosome 14 del (14) (q22.1q23.1) should be ruled out [3, 4]. Whether OTX2 mutation might be associated with isolated GH deficiency, as reported in one of the studies' 4 patients, remains to be determined during follow-up for evolving pituitary hormone deficiencies.

Overhydration is harmful

Osmotic and nonosmotic regulation of arginine vasopressin during prolonged endurance exercise

Hew-Butler T, Jordaan E, Stuempfle KJ, Speedy DB, Siegel AJ, Noakes TD, Soldin SJ, Verbalis JG
Department of Human Biology, University of Cape Town, Cape Town, South Africa
tamara.hew@chw.edu

J Clin Endocrinol Metab 2008;93:2072–2078

Background: Exercise-associated hyponatremia (EAH) is a relatively frequent condition caused by excessive fluid intake in relation to the kidneys' ability to eliminate excess fluid. The mechanisms involved in the regulation of maximal renal excretory ability during exercise are still not completely known. This study evaluated first the spontaneous secretion of pituitary, natriuretic and adrenal steroid hormones, and cytokines immediately before and after running an ultramarathon. In addition, the authors studied the mechanisms of osmotic and nonosmotic stimulation of arginine vasopressin (AVP) secretion in order to better understand hormonal control of fluid homeostasis during prolonged endurance exercise.

Methods: This was an observational study performed on 82 runners participating in a 56-km ultramarathon. They subjects underwent plasma sodium (Na^+), plasma volume (estimated by a plasmatic protein based method) and plasma AVP [(AVP)p] measurements before and after the race, without any limitations on fluid intake.

Results: Mean marathon duration was 356 ± 4 min. During this time no significant variations were seen in plasma Na^+ (139.3 ± 0.3 mmol/l before and 138.1 ± 0.4 mmol/l after the race), though there was a significant reduction in plasma volume ($-8.5 \pm 0.1\%$, $p < 0.01$) and significant increases (all $p < 0.0001$) in (AVP)p (3.9-fold), oxytocin (1.9-fold), brain natriuretic peptide (4.5-fold), and IL-6 (12.5-fold). Brain natriuretic peptide, oxytocin, and corticosterone variations accounted for 47% of the variance registered in (AVP)p and 13% of the variance in plasma Na^+ in pathway analyses.

Conclusion: An important increase in (AVP)p during ultramarathon was found despite unchanged plasma Na^+, suggesting a non-osmotic limitation of AVP suppression (i.e. osmotic independent AVP stimulation) during exercise, in which some hormones or cytokines may play a significant role. This mechanism may explain the frequent onset of EAH in athletes ingesting fluids in excess in relation to fluid output during prolonged endurance exercise.

Exercise-associated hyponatremia (EAH) has recently emerged as the most common life-threatening complication of endurance exercise. Although the primary cause of EAH is a relative overconsumption of fluids beyond the ability of the kidneys to excrete excess fluid, the mechanisms that limit maximum renal excretory ability during exercise remain unknown. Detailed balance studies performed during recovery from an ultramarathon race show that runners with EAH excreted a large volume of dilute urine in contrast to finishers with normonatremia who excreted a small volume of highly concentrated urine; both groups had equivalent sodium losses as reflected by positive sodium balances during recovery. The change in serum sodium concentration after endurance exercise was inversely proportional to the change in body weight, and the athletes with EAH tended to gain weight during exercise. In fact, most runners with EAH are overhydrated as a result of excessive and perhaps ill-advised water ingestion over an extended race during which water excretion is limited by osmotically stimulated AVP secretion [5]. In the past, several athletes died from mismanagement of EAH until the use of a 3% hypertonic saline was established as the standard treatment [6]. This study explains the mechanism by which osmotic and nonosmotic regulation of arginine vasopressin during prolonged endurance exercise are associated with alterations in water homeostasis leading to EAH. Understanding the pathophysiology of water imbalance during exercise is of great importance for differentiating between dehydrated and overhydrated athletes and for managing those with symptomatic EAH so as to avoid unnecessary deaths.

The role of neurotransmitters in somatotroph proliferation

Neuronal M3 muscarinic acetylcholine receptors are essential for somatotroph proliferation and normal somatic growth

Gautam D, Jeon J, Starost MF, Han SJ, Hamdan FF, Cui Y, Parlow AF, Gavrilova O, Szalayova I, Mezey E, Wess J
Molecular Signaling Section, Laboratory of Bioorganic Chemistry, National Institute of Diabetes and Digestive and Kidney Diseases, National Institutes of Health, Bethesda, Md., USA
Proc Natl Acad Sci USA 2009;106:6398–6403

Background: The molecular pathways involved in the proliferation and maintenance of pituitary cell lineages are not yet well understood. Pharmacological studies suggest that muscarinic cholinergic pathways play an important role in the control of GH secretion in both animals and humans. However, due to the presence of 5 distinct muscarinic receptor subtypes and their spreading distribution in the CNS, it has been difficult to elucidate their specific contribution by means of classic pharmacological tools. To better understand the role of the cholinergic system in the control of somatotroph function and GH secretion, the authors generated a set of mutant mice lacking the muscarinic type 3 receptor (Br-M3-KO).
Methods: Br-M3-KO mice were generated using Cre/loxP technology. These mice lack M3 receptors only in the brain as shown by combined radiological and binding/immunoprecipitation studies.
Results: Br-M3-KO mice did not display any significant changes in body composition or in glucose metabolism. They are dwarfs and show reduced serum GH and IGF-I levels, normal thyroid hormone and sex steroid concentrations and increased corticosterone and ACTH levels. They show pronounced hypoplasia of the anterior pituitary with normal brain weight. The pituitary content of GH and prolactin was markedly reduced with normal LH, FSH and TSH content. Stimulation with GHRH caused a markedly reduced GH response compared to control animals. M3 receptor expression was found in GHRH neurons, and hypothalamic GHRH and somatostatin levels were significantly reduced in Br-M3-KO mice. Treatment with a GHRH analog was effective in preventing the various hormonal and morphological characteristics of Br-M3-KO mice.
Conclusion: Mice lacking M3 muscarinic receptors have dramatic anterior pituitary hypoplasia associated with reduced pituitary GH and prolactin content. As a consequence, serum GH and IGF-I were markedly reduced leading to greatly reduced postnatal growth. These results revealed that M3 receptors play an important role in somatotroph proliferation and function and represent a potential pharmacologic target.

GH secretion is under the dual control of hypothalamic GHRH and somatostatin release. The release of these two hypothalamic hormones is, in turn, regulated by a complex network of neurotransmitters and neuropeptides. GHRH is also a trophic hormone for the somatotrophs. Animals and humans lacking GHRH or its receptors show GH deficiency associated with marked pituitary hypoplasia and reduced pituitary GH content. The cholinergic system plays an important role in the control of GH secretion in humans. Several pharmacological studies have documented that central muscarinic cholinergic pathways play a role in stimulating GH release in humans. However, due to the presence of 5 diverse muscarinic receptors subtypes and to their overlapping distribution throughout the CNS, it was previously impossible to establish their exact role and relative contribution by means of classical pharmacological tools. This study elegantly shows that mice selectively lacking muscarinic receptor type 3 in the brain show profound anterior pituitary hypoplasia associated with reduced pituitary GH and prolactin content and reduced serum GH and IGF-I concentration. As a result, these animals show reduced longitudinal growth in postnatal life. Treatment with a GHRH analog is capable of preventing such alterations. These results are important in elucidating the role of the muscarinic receptor pathways in the control of GH secretion, and open a new window for a potential pharmacologic target.

New paradigms
New weapons for gene hunting

Identification of candidate genes for human pituitary development by EST analysis

Ma Y, Qi X, Du J, Song S, Feng D, Qi J, Zhu Z, Zhang X, Xiao H, Han Z, Hao X
Center for Clinical Laboratory Medicine of PLA, Xijing Hospital, Fourth Military Medical University, Xi'an, PR China
cmbmayy@fmmu.edu.cn

BMC Genomics 2009;10:109

Background: During embryonic development, the 6 specific pituitary cell types originate and differentiate under the control of various mechanisms. It is suggested that a large number of signal molecules and transcription factors essential for pituitary development are still unknown, and that there are important differences in gene expression profiles between mice and humans. This study reports differentially expressed genes from expressed sequence tag (EST) in fetal and adult pituitaries.

Methods: Total RNA was extracted from 2 human male fetal pituitaries. A cDNA library was constructed from a 16-week-old male fetal pituitary. All the ESTs were grouped into clusters of sequences thought to encode for one gene. The gene and ESTs were localized on chromosomes by searching the UniGene database.

Results: The transcription maps derived from the EST analysis revealed that developmentally relevant genes (Sox4, ST13 and ZNF185) were dominant in the cDNA library of the fetal pituitary, while hormones and hormone-associated genes (GH1, GH2, POMC, LH, CHGA, and CHGB) were dominant in the adult pituitary. Forty novel ESTs were identified.

Conclusions: The results of this study suggest a distinct pattern of gene expression between fetal and adult pituitaries. The transcriptome approach was proven to be an effective way of identifying novel genes involved in pituitary development.

Pituitary development, differentiation, and function are under the regulation of a complex network of transcription factors and, ultimately, depend on the secretion and function of hypothalamic releasing and inhibiting hormones. A number of transcription factors are expressed at different times in embryogenesis and affect the development of multiple cell lineages. It is likely that a large number of factors essential for pituitary development and cell differentiation and function have yet to be completely understood. In this study, a transcriptome approach using EST analysis revealed differences in gene expression between fetal and adult pituitaries but, most importantly, pituitary tissue was shown to express cytokines and their receptors, transcription factors, and those involved in the cell cycle, DNA replication and signal transduction, as well as 40 novel ESTs. These ESTs most probably reflect the expression of some yet unknown genes and microRNAs, particularly in fetal pituitary cells, which are involved in pituitary development and function.

p21(Cip1) restrains pituitary tumor growth

Chesnokova V, Zonis S, Kovacs K, Ben-Shlomo A, Wawrowsky K, Bannykh S, Melmed S
Department of Medicine, Cedars-Sinai Medical Center, Los Angeles, Calif., USA

Proc Natl Acad Sci USA 2008;105:17498–17503

Background: Pituitary tumorigenesis can be caused by disruption of the mechanisms controlling normal cell cycle. A number of genetic factors have been implicated in the formation of pituitary adenomas in humans and animals. Pituitary tumor-transforming gene (Pttg) is a mammalian securin that facilitates sister-chromatid separation during metaphase, and its overexpression causes cell transformation and promotes tumor formation. P21$^{Cip/Kip}$ is a transcriptional target of p53 and acts to constrain cell cycle, and may mediate either suppression or promotion or cell proliferation.

Methods: Triple mutant Rb$^{+/-}$Pttg$^{-/-}$p21$^{-/-}$ mice were generated. Seventy-nine human pituitary adenomas of various phenotypes were analyzed for PTTG and p21 expression.

Results: p21 deletion restores pituitary tumor development in Rb$^{+/-}$Pttg$^{-/-}$ mice and enhances pituitary cell proliferation. It also increases growth and transformation of Rb$^{+/-}$Pttg$^{-/-}$ mouse embryonic fibroblasts. P21 is induced in GH3 cells overexpressing PTTG and in human pituitary tumors. GH-secreting pituitary adenomas also expressed markers of senescence.

Conclusions: This study shows that a proto-oncogene switches between oncogenic and tumor-suppressive modes depending on the genetic context. PTTG is abundantly expressed in human pituitary tumors, and behaves as either a tumor suppressor or oncogene depending on p21 status which controls cell cycle stability. Either deletion or overexpression of Pttg promotes pituitary cell aneuploidy and senescence. High levels of PTTG cause defective cell cycle progression and chromosomal instability, and promote pituitary tumor formation. Activation of pituitary DNA damage pathways triggers p21, which may restrain further growth and carcinogenesis.

Cell cycle control of pituitary development and disease

Quereda V, Malumbres M
Cell Division and Cancer Group, Centro Nacional de Investigaciones Oncologicas, Madrid, Spain

J Mol Endocrinol 2009;42:75–86

This is a comprehensive review on the mechanisms controlling pituitary development. One of the key issues in tumorigenesis is loss of control of cell cycle. This article clearly describes how pituitary cells develop and differentiate as controlled by a number of factors, and how disruption of some of these pathways results in genomic instability leading to disease or tumor formation.

Understanding how cell cycle regulation controls pituitary cell homeostasis may help us to find new therapeutic strategies against pituitary diseases.

Regulation of the cell cycle is controlled by a number of factors, some of which are tissue- and cell-specific. These studies show that factors which play an important role in the control of cell cycle are involved in pituitary disease and tumorigenesis. Although pituitary adenomas are rare in children, it is believed that they are somehow more aggressive than in adult subjects. Prolactinomas, corticotropinomas or somatotroph adenomas may have serious adverse consequences on growth, puberty, bone formation, and cardiovascular and reproductive function. The diagnosis is often delayed. Understanding how these factors control pituitary development and how cell cycle regulation controls pituitary biology may help us to find new diagnostic and therapeutic tools.

Pituitary autoimmunity: 30 years later

Caturegli P, Lupi I, Landek-Salgado M, Kimura H, Rose NR
Department of Pathology, Johns Hopkins University School of Medicine, Baltimore, Md., USA
pcat@jhmi.edu
Autoimmun Rev 2008;7:631–637

This is a review addressing the complex issues related to pituitary autoimmunity, a heterogeneous condition ranging from histologically confirmed lymphocytic hypophysitis to the incidental detection of pituitary autoantibodies in otherwise healthy subjects. The most frequent clinical presentation of this increasingly recognized condition is a sellar mass at pituitary MRI, which requires differential diagnosis from other nonfunctioning pituitary masses, primary among them pituitary adenoma. Noteworthy is the temporal association between hypophysitis and pregnancy or immunotherapies blocking CTLA-4. Many efforts have been made to identify pituitary autoantigens that could shed light on the pathophysiology of autoimmune hypophysitis, as well as be used for its diagnosis; it emerges from this review that even with these efforts, many challenges still remain. The authors of the review describe both the steps forward taken so far for comprising this condition and the several questions that remain unanswered as yet.

Novel autoantigens in autoimmune hypophysitis

Lupi I, Broman KW, Tzou SC, Gutenberg A, Martino E, Caturegli P
Department of Pathology, Johns Hopkins University, School of Medicine, Baltimore, Md., USA
Clin Endocrinol (Oxf) 2008;69:269–278

Background: Pituitary autoantibodies are associated with autoimmune hypophysitis and various other conditions. They have no extensive clinical application, principally because of a current lack of accurate laboratory methods for their detection. Such methods need to be based on the specific pituitary autoantigens against which autoimmune response is raised. Subsequently, the identification of pituitary autoantigens will lead to the construction of antigen-specific immunoassays.

Methods: The aim of the present study was to search for new pituitary autoantigens using sera as probes in proteomic assays. A comparison was also made between the immunoblotting and immunofluorescence methods to determine which was the most accurate for diagnosis of autoimmune hypophysitis. The authors analyzed 28 sera from subjects with autoimmune hypophysitis (14 histologically confirmed and 14 clinically suspected) and matched them with 98 control sera, obtained from 14 patients with pituitary adenomas, 15 with Graves' disease, 33 with Hashimoto's thyroiditis, and 36 healthy subjects. All sera were incubated with human pituitary cytosolic proteins separated by one-dimensional (1D) gel electrophoresis in order to identify the molecular weight regions which were more frequently recognized by hypophysitis sera. The corresponding proteins were then sequenced by means of immunoblotting and mass spectrometry. Furthermore, an immunofluorescence test was performed to evaluate the binding between sera and *Macaca mulatta* pituitary sections.

Results: Hypophysitis sera recognized a band in the 25- to 27-kDa region more frequently than healthy subjects (p = 0.004) or pituitary adenoma patients (p = 0.044). The band contains two proteins: chromosome 14 open reading frame 166 (C14orf166) and chorionic somatomammotrophin. Immunoblotting positivity for the 25-to 27-kDa region showed better sensitivity (64 vs. 57%) and specificity (86 vs. 76%) than immunofluorescence for identifying subjects with histologically confirmed hypophysitis; its performance, however, was not sufficiently accurate to justify the introduction of immunoblotting into routine clinical practice.

Conclusion: Two candidate pituitary autoantigens were identified in this study, but the demonstration of their possible pathogenetic role in autoimmune hypophysitis and the development of an accurate laboratory assay for their detection both require further investigation.

T regulatory cells distinguish two types of primary hypophysitis

Mirocha S, Elagin RB, Salamat S, Jaume JC
Department of Medicine, School of Medicine and Veterans Affairs Medical Center, University of Wisconsin-Madison, Madison, Wisc., USA
Clin Exp Immunol 2009;155:403–411

Background: Primary hypophysitis is a frequently recognized condition, though further insights into its pathophysiology are needed to reach the goal of administering etiology-based treatment. The present study aimed to conduct further research into the pathogenesis of primary hypophysitis.
Methods: The authors used immunohistochemistry to characterize the immune cells detected at histological examination in pituitary biopsies performed for suspected 'lymphocytic' hypophysitis. In particular, they analyzed 2 cases at the clinical, cellular and molecular levels, showing that at least 2 main types of lymphocytic hypophysitis exist. The first case was a 29-year-old female subject presenting with diabetes insipidus, headache, menstrual irregularities, galactorrhea and an enlargement of the anterior pituitary and pituitary stalk at MRI. The second was a 52-year-old man with headache, combined pituitary hormone deficiencies (including suspected diabetes insipidus for polyuria and polydipsia) and a pituitary mass dislocating the optic chiasm. These subjects underwent transsphenoidal pituitary resection and histological examination revealed lymphocytic hypophysitis in both cases.
Results: The first entity is compatible with the classical description of autoimmune lymphocytic hypophysitis associated with an imbalance between T-helper and T-regulatory cell response in favor of T-helper (particularly the so-called 'Th 17 cells', expressing IL-17). On the other hand, the second picture is more complex, with a predominant role of T-regulatory cells that could act in the control of an immune response directed against non-self antigens, suggesting an homeostatic immune process of either infectious or infiltrative etiology.
Conclusion: These data focus attention on two different pathogenetic mechanisms of primary hypophysitis. In light of a possible medical treatment for this condition, the authors showed that in a particular case, active autoimmune process could benefit from immunosuppressive treatment, whereas in the immune homeostatic process, immunosuppression is not indicated. Naturally, to identify the type of autoimmune process involved in a single case and to establish a pathogenetic-driven treatment, pituitary biopsy is needed. Thus, these preliminary data may in the future induce all of us to revise our diagnostic and therapeutic algorithms for suspected hypophysitis.

These 3 papers address comprehensively the role of autoimmunity in determining anterior and posterior pituitary dysfunction in a condition encompassing comparable, albeit less common, pediatric and adult entities. Indeed, the hypothalamic-pituitary stalk and posterior pituitary-anterior pituitary unit have been reported as targets of autoimmune processes, i.e. lymphocytic hypophysitis, lymphocytic infundibulo-hypophysitis or lymphocytic infundibulo-neurohypophysitis, affecting both anterior and posterior pituitary function. Despite histological evidence of tissue lymphocyte infiltration, the role of humoral autoimmunity in lymphocytic hypophysitis has been debated since the first description in the early 1980s of vasopressin cell autoantibodies by Scherbaum and Bottazzo [7]. Moreover, the precise pathogenetic role of these autoantibodies has never been demonstrated, regardless of the high number of clinical studies that report a high prevalence of both anterior pituitary autoantibodies and antibodies against vasopressin cells. One pitfall may be ascribed to the methodology of detecting and measuring these autoantibodies, and the other one to the fact that specific autoantigens have not yet been recognized.

In the study by Caturegli's group, the identification of two candidate autoantigens which might play a direct role in autoimmune hypophysitis on the one hand, and the recent experimental induction of lymphocytic hypophysitis in mice on the other hand [8], open the door to the development of accurate assays for the detection of autoantibodies. In addition, drug induction of autoimmune hypophysitis by cytotoxic T-lymphocyte-associated antigen-4 blockage using the human anti-CTLA4 monoclonal antibody CP-675,206 for the treatment of melanoma [9] is a confirmation of the direct role of T-cell immunity. Finally, the identification by Mirocha et al. of two different potential pathogenetic mechanisms, i.e. one potentially directed against self-antigens and the other against non-self antigens (post-infection), both of which induce primary hypophysitis, adds another piece to the puzzle of these intriguing conditions. Thus, patients with an autoimmune-driven hypophysitis would benefit from steroids or other immunosuppression treatment, whereas immunosuppression may exacerbate conditions that are not autoimmune. Pituitary biopsy, although invasive, is currently the only option we have to determine the exact pathogenesis and may be warranted in some cases in order to provide correct treatment.

Not only for steroidogenesis

Central nervous system-specific knockout of steroidogenic factor 1

Kim KW, Zhao L, Parker KL
Departments of Internal Medicine and Pharmacology, UT Southwestern Medical Center, Dallas, Tex., USA

Mol Cell Endocrinol 2009;300:132–136

Background: Steroidogenic factor-1 (SF-1) is a member of the nuclear hormone receptor family of transcriptional regulators and is an essential regulator of the enzymes involved in the steroidogenic pathway. SF-1 is also important in the establishment and function of endocrine axes. Analysis of global SF-1 KO mice confirmed its role in endocrine development in the ventromedial hypothalamus (VMH), adrenals, and gonads. The VMH regulates sexual behavior, energy homeostasis, thermogenesis, and cardiovascular function, and is the only region of SF-1 expression in the mouse brain. This review discusses the functional role of SF-1 in the brain.
Methods: To understand the specific role of SF-1 in the brain, CNS-specific SF-1 KO mice were generated using Cre-loxP technology.
Results: SF-1 KO mice have increased anxiety-like behavior, and a number of novel SF-1-responsive genes related to anxiety-like behavior were identified, including corticotrophin-releasing hormone receptor 2 (crhr2). This finding indicates that crhr2 may be a direct target of SF-1 in the VMH. Cannabinoid receptor 1 (CB1R) was also found to be a SF-1-responsive gene in the VMH, indicating that SF-1 is implicated in energy homeostasis at the level of the VMH.
Conclusions: This paper has defined specific roles of SF-1 in the function of the VMH in anxiety-like behavior and in energy homeostasis, independent of any effects on steroid hormones.

Genetic modification of experimental animals has been helpful for elucidating diverse aspects of physiology. Generation of animal models that selectively lack the expression of one or more genes, either globally or in selected areas, is extending our understanding of endocrine physiology. Steroidogenic factor-1 (SF-1; officially named NR5A1) was originally identified and characterized as an essential regulator of the enzymes that make steroid hormones in steroidogenic cell lines. Subsequently, several groups have reported that SF-1 is a key regulator in the establishment and function of endocrine organ axis. It is now assigned with a new CNS function. This review reports the results of studies in mice selectively lacking SF-1 in the VMH, showing that this regulator of transcription participates in the control of anxiety-like behavior and energy homeostasis, independent of any effects on steroid hormones.

More on the fetal origin hypothesis

Early postnatal nutrition determines somatotropic function in mice

Kappeler L, De Magalhaes Filho C, Leneuve P, Xu J, Brunel N, Chatziantoniou C, Le Bouc Y, Holzenberger M
Institut National de la Santé et de la Recherche Médicale, Centre de Recherche Saint Antoine, Paris, France
laurent.kappeler@inserm.fr

Endocrinology 2009;150:314–323

Background: Abundant evidence suggests that early life events have consequences for later disease. A number of diseases seem to have a developmental origin in both humans and animals. Epidemiological studies in humans have shown a correlation between perinatal food deprivation and obesity, type II diabetes, hypertension, alterations in pituitary-adrenal-axis function, and cardiovascular disease. Likewise, prenatal and postnatal events in experimental animals can determine adult diseases. A general notion is that the growth-retarded fetus will adapt to the intrauterine environment by modifying endocrine and metabolic pathways, and these modifications may persist postnatally. This study investigated the effects of early postnatal underfeeding or overfeeding on the growth and GHRH/GH/IGF-I axis function in mice.

Methods: Under- or overfeeding was induced in mice by cross-fostering. Endocrine regulation of growth and the development of specific adult diseases were investigated.

Results: The first effects of food restriction or overfeeding were growth retardation and deceleration, respectively. Differences in body weight and length persisted into adulthood despite normal feeding after weaning. Blood glucose was lower in the underfed than in the overfed animals, and serum insulin and leptin were markedly low in food-restricted mice and very high in those that were overfed. Glucose and leptin concentrations normalized with free access to food, while insulin concentrations did not readily normalize. Both overfeeding and underfeeding led to reduced glucose tolerance and hypertension later in life, suggesting long-term modifications in energy metabolism and cardiovascular impairment. The effects of food restriction and overfeeding on growth were paralleled by changes in pituitary GH content, circulating IGF-I and ALS, and hypothalamic GHRH gene expression. These alterations were consistent with the observed phenotypes, and persisted throughout adulthood.

Conclusion: This study shows that early postnatal food restriction or overfeeding induces permanent alterations in growth and the GHRH/GH/IGF-I axis. In addition, metabolic and cardiovascular alterations were also observed, consistent with the hypothesis that early perinatal nutritional events may be linked to adult disease.

This is an elegant study which lends further support to the 'fetal origin of adult health and disease hypothesis'. A number of epidemiological studies in humans have linked fetal malnutrition to postnatal growth and adult disease. This study shows that in mice adverse effects on growth may be mediated by modifications in GHRH/GHII/GF-I axis function, and that these modifications persist up to adulthood. In addition, features of the metabolic syndrome were reproduced in this experimental model of under- or overfeeding. Most children with IUGR catch up, and show no subsequent growth disorder, but it may initiate a process that eventually leads to an increased incidence of the metabolic syndrome. These findings may have clear implications for children with intrauterine growth retardation.

References
1. Malinger G, Lev D, Kidron D, Heredia F, Hershkovitz R, Lerman-Sagie T: Differential diagnosis in fetuses with absent septum pellucidum. Ultrasound Obstet Gynecol 2005;25:42-49.
2. Larsen KB, Lutterodt M, Rath MF, Moller M: Expression of the homeobox genes PAX6, OTX2, and OTX1 in the early human fetal retina. Int J Dev Neurosci 2009;27:485–492.
3. Kelberman D, Rizzoti K, Avilion A, Bitner-Glindzicz M, Cianfarani S, Collins J, et al: Mutations within Sox2/SOX2 are associated with abnormalities in the hypothalamo-pituitary-gonadal axis in mice and humans. J Clin Invest 2006;116:2442–2455.
4. Lemyre E, Lemieux N, Decarie JC, Lambert M: Del(14)(q22.1q23.2) in a patient with anophthalmia and pituitary hypoplasia. Am J Med Genet 1998;77:162–165.
5. Verbalis JG, Goldsmith SR, Greenberg A, Schrier RW, Sterns RH. Hyponatremia treatment guidelines 2007: expert panel recommendations. Am J Med 2007;120(suppl 1):S1–S21.
6. Moritz ML, Ayus JC: Exercise-associated hyponatremia: why are athletes still dying? Clin J Sport Med 2008;18:379–381.
7. Scherbaum WA, Bottazzo GF: Autoantibodies to vasopressin cells in idiopathic diabetes insipidus: evidence for an autoimmune variant. Lancet 1983;i:897–901.
8. Tzou SC, Lupi I, Landek M, Gutenberg A, Tzou YM, Kimura H, et al: Autoimmune hypophysitis of SJL mice: clinical insights from a new animal model. Endocrinology 2008;149:3461–3469.
9. Blansfield JA, Beck KE, Tran K, Yang JC, Hughes MS, Kammula US, et al: Cytotoxic T-lymphocyte-associated antigen-4 blockage can induce autoimmune hypophysitis in patients with metastatic melanoma and renal cancer. J Immunother 2005;28:593–598.

Thyroid

Heiko Krude

Institute of Experimental Pediatric Endocrinology, Charité University Medicine Berlin, Berlin, Germany

In this year's overview of thyroid research the beauty of science was revealed in one paper from the far North of Europe, from Iceland. In the darkness of hypothesis-free genome-wide association studies, where nowadays over 300,000 common genetic variants can be tested for an association with a given phenotype, the colleagues from Iceland found two luminous variants which increase the risk of thyroid differentiated cancer (papillary and follicular PTC and FTC, respectively). These two variants are located close to two transcription factor genes which are known for their role in thyroid growth, proliferation and differentiation, i.e. FOXE1 (formerly TTF2) and NKX2.1 (formerly TTF1). Although the search for the underlying molecular impact of these variants on gene function, either gain or loss, needs to be determined now, it is an illuminating moment when a hypothesis-free experiment, which is based on the genotyping of more than 300,000 SNPs in 15,000 individuals, leads to such a conceptionally consistent result.

Besides this wonderful paper there were more than 3,000 publications related to thyroid research in the past 12 months, 18 are summarized in this chapter. Since this chapter will be the last one in the series of my contribution to the *Yearbook*, I will take the opportunity to apologize not only to the authors of the 2,982 papers not mentioned this year but also to the more than 15,000 publications of the last 5 years for not having referred to their work in these thyroid chapters – it was a very subjective choice!

Concept of the year: thyroid cancer meets thyroid development

Common variants on 9q22.33 and 14q13.3 predispose to thyroid cancer in European populations

Gudmundsson J, Sulem P, Gudbjartsson DF, Jonasson JG, Sigurdsson A, Bergthorsson JT, He H, Blondal T, Geller F, Jakobsdottir M, Magnusdottir DN, Matthiasdottir S, Stacey SN, Skarphedinsson OB, Helgadottir H, Li W, Nagy R, Aguillo E, Faure E, Prats E, Saez B, Martinez M, Eyjolfsson GI, Bjornsdottir US, Holm H, Kristjansson K, Frigge ML, Kristvinsson H, Gulcher JR, Jonsson T, Rafnar T, Hjartarsson H, Mayordomo JI, de la Chapelle A, Hrafnkelsson J, Thorsteinsdottir U, Kong A, Stefansson K
deCODE Genetics, Reykjavik, Iceland
julius.gudmundsson@decode.is
Nat Genet 2009;41:460–464

Background: Thyroid carcinoma is the most common endocrine malignancy. It has been estimated that the risk of thyroid cancer has a greater genetic component than the risk of any other cancer.
Methods: In order to search for sequence variants conferring risk of thyroid cancer, a genome-wide association study in 192 and 37,196 Icelandic cases and controls, respectively, was conducted followed by a replication study in individuals of European descent.
Results: The data show that two common variants, located on 9q22.33 and 14q13.3, are associated with the disease. Overall, the strongest association signals were observed for rs965513 on 9q22.33 (OR = 1.75; p = 1.7×10^{-27}) and rs944289 on 14q13.3 (OR = 1.37; p = 2.0×10^{-9}). The genes nearest to the 9q22.33 locus are FOXE1 (TTF2) and NKX2-1 (TTF1), which are among the genes located at the 14q13.3 locus. Both variants contribute to an increased risk of both papillary and follicular thyroid cancer. Approximately 3.7% of individuals are homozygous for both variants, and their estimated risk of thyroid cancer is 5.7-fold greater than that of noncarriers. In a study on a large sample set from the general population, both risk alleles are associated with low concentrations of thyroid-stimulating hormone (TSH), and the 9q22.33 allele is associated with low concentration of thyroxine (T_4) and high concentration of triiodothyronine (T_3).

Conclusion: Sequence variants in two genes that are known for their critical role in thyroid development are associated with an increased risk for thyroid carcinoma.

The genetic contribution to the pathogenesis of medullary thyroid cancer (MTC), frequently as part of MEN syndrome, was among the first clinically relevant genetic findings in endocrinology. Nowadays, prophylactic thyreoidectomy after the molecular diagnosis of activating RET gene mutations helps to prevent cancer-related death in thousands of patients worldwide. The differentiated thyroid cancer types like papillary (PTC) and follicular (FTC) thyroid cancer are less likely to be associated with a genetic predisposition as MTC but still have a high familial risk in first-degree relatives. How this risk is inherited has not been determined so far. This paper of the year in the thyroid chapter used the power of the Iceland genotyping project to unravel the common genetic variants that are associated with an increased risk for PTC and FTC. Compared to the common susceptibility variants recently discovered for complex diseases, thyroid cancer may not be as complex. Out of 304,083 single nucleotide polymorphisms (SNP), only 2 (!) were found to be associated with an increased risk. The incidence of thyroid cancer, i.e. 4.6 and 12.1 in 100,000 males and females, respectively, is 5.7-fold greater in individuals with double homozygosity for the two predisposing SNP variants AA and TT. This result does not reach a clinical relevance as the finding of an activating mutation in the RET gene which renders the carrier at risk to develop MTC is 100%. The double homozygous SNP variant carriers will most probably *not* develop PTC or FTC: only 47 of 100,000 will have cancer and therefore the data have no clinical relevance in terms of prophylactic thyreoidectomy!

However, the beauty of the study is the nature of the genes in which the identified variants are located: both genes, FOXE1 (also named initially TTF2) and NKX2.1 (initially named TTF1) are well known for their role in thyroid development and as candidate genes for syndromic thyroid dysgenesis. From the extremely large number of possible genes related to cell growth and cell cycle regulation which could potentially be linked to cancer susceptibility, only these two genes, which are established key transcription factors for thyroid cell growth and differentiation [1], were located closely to the risk SNPs. These data might tell us that the transcriptional regulation of embryogenesis of the thyroid gland is closely related to the transformation process of differentiated thyroid follicular cells into less differentiated cancer cells. The question is how the two variants in FOXE1 and NKX2.1 increase the thyroid cancer risk. In principle, SNPs outside the coding region of genes can either increase or decrease the function of the gene by modification of transcription and translation. Both transcription factor genes are involved in thyroid growth and differentiation. Therefore, loss or gain of function could contribute to tumorigenesis. If loss of function caused the increased cancer risk, patients with CH and loss of function in FOXE1 and NKX2.1 would harbor a so far unrecognized thyroid cancer risk.

The following study, which was published before the Iceland thyroid cancer SNP data, already gives some answers to these critical questions.

A germline mutation (A339V) in thyroid transcription factor-1 (TTF-1/ NKX2.1) in patients with multinodular goiter and papillary thyroid carcinoma

Ngan ES, Lang BH, Liu T, Shum CK, So MT, Lau DK, Leon TY, Cherny SS, Tsai SY, Lo CY, Khoo US, Tam PK, Garcia-Barceló MM
Department of Surgery, University of Hong Kong, Pokfulam, Faculty of Medicine, Hong Kong, SAR, China
engan@hku.hk
J Natl Cancer Inst 2009;101:162–175

Background: To determine the molecular basis of the risk of papillary thyroid carcinoma (PTC) among patients with multinodular goiter (MNG), the authors hypothesized that mutations in the gene that encode NKX2.1 (TTF-1) are a genetic determinant of MNG/PTC predisposition.
Methods: 20 unrelated PTC patients with a history of MNG (MNG/PTC), 284 PTC patients without a history of MNG (PTC), and 349 healthy control subjects were screened for germline mutation(s) in TTF-1/NKX2.1 by sequencing of amplified DNA from blood. The effects of the mutation on the growth and differentiation of thyroid cells were demonstrated by ectopic expression of wild-type (WT) and mutant proteins in PCCL3 normal rat thyroid cells, followed by tests of cell proliferation, activation of cell growth pathways, and transcription of TTF-1 target genes.

Results: A missense mutation (1016C>T) was identified in TTF-1/NKX2.1 that led to a mutant TTF-1 protein (A339V) in 4 of the 20 MNG/PTC patients (20%). These patients developed substantially more advanced tumors than MNG/PTC or PTC patients without the mutation (p = 0.022, Fisher exact test). Notably, this germline mutation was dominantly inherited in two families, with some members bearing the mutation affected with MNG, associated with either PTC or colon cancer. The mutation encoding the A339V substitution was not found among the 349 healthy control subjects nor among the 284 PTC patients who had no history of MNG. Overexpression of A339V TTF-1 in PCCL3 cells, as compared with overexpression of WT TTF-1, was associated with increased cell proliferation including thyrotropin-independent growth (average A339V proliferation rate = 134.27%, WT rate = 104.43%, difference = 34.3%, 95% CI = 12.0–47.7%, p = 0.010), enhanced STAT3 activation, and impaired transcription of the thyroid-specific genes Tg, TSH-R, and Pax-8.

Conclusion: This is the first germline mutation identified in MNG/PTC patients. It could contribute to predisposition for MNG and/or PTC and to the pathogenesis of PTC. Joined with the Iceland data, one might expect that the SNPs in the NKX2.1 gene that increase the risk for thyroid cancer more likely lead to an increased expression of the gene.

Before knowing the results from Iceland, the colleagues from Hong Kong followed a candidate concept for the genetics of PTC and speculated that those PTC that develop in goiter glands would more likely be linked to a genetic germline predisposition in a gene of thyroid growth regulation like NKX2.1. They identified a likely gain of function germline mutation in a rather high number of patients with PTC and goiter. According to these data, it seems likely that activation of the NKX2.1 gene leads to increased proliferation and dedifferentiation, and might cause thyroid cancer. These will pave the way for further experiments that will focus on the functional relevance of the NKX2.1 gene-associated SNPs in the Iceland study. For pediatric patients with loss of function mutations in NKX2.1, who are affected by thyroid dysfunction and movement defects, these data represent a relief; it is unlikely that their loss of NKX2.1 function renders them susceptible for thyroid cancer.

In the following sections the two themes of the paper of the year, thyroid cancer and thyroid development, will be dwelled upon and interesting papers focusing on thyroid childhood cancer and thyroid development will be discussed.

Clinical concepts in childhood thyroid cancer

Ultrasound screening for thyroid carcinoma in childhood cancer survivors: a case series

Brignardello E, Corrias A, Isolato G, Palestini N, Cordero di Montezemolo L, Fagioli F, Boccuzzi G
Transition Unit for Childhood Cancer Survivors, San Giovanni Battista Hospital, Turin, Italy
ebrignardello@molinette.piemonte.it
J Clin Endocrinol Metab 2008;93:4840–4843

Background: Childhood cancers are at risk for developing late-onset complications of cancer therapy, including thyroid carcinoma in childhood cancer survivors. How to screen for thyroid cancer in these patients is a matter of debate.

Methods: A total of 129 subjects who had received radiotherapy to the head, neck, or upper thorax for a pediatric cancer were studied in the setting of a long-term follow-up unit. Thyroid ultrasound usually began 5 years after radiotherapy and was repeated every third year, if negative. Median follow-up time since childhood cancer diagnosis was 15.8 years (range 6.1–34.8). Solid thyroid nodules were found in 35 patients. Fine-needle aspiration was performed in 19 patients, of which 14 had nodules >1 cm. The main outcome measure was the finding of not palpable thyroid cancers.

Results: Cytological examination of specimens diagnosed papillary carcinoma in 5 patients who underwent surgery. The cytological diagnosis of papillary thyroid carcinoma was confirmed in all cases by histological examination. Notably, only 2 of these patients had palpable nodules; the other 3 were <1 cm and were detected only by ultrasound. However, histological examination showed nodal metastases in 2 of these.

Conclusion: Although ultrasound screening for thyroid cancer in the general population is not cost-effective and could lead to unnecessary surgery, due to false positives, they believe that in childhood cancer survivors who received radiotherapy involving the head, neck, or upper thorax, it would be worthwhile.

With the increasing use of thyroid ultrasound as a screening tool for thyroid nodules, a new cohort of 'potential' patients is being diagnosed without a clear concept of how to treat and how to follow these children with 'thyroid incidentalomas'. Population-based nodule screening by palpation or by ultrasound revealed a prevalence of 0.6% single nodules in children and adolescents [2]. Even though this is by far less than in the adult population [3], we do not want to biopsy 6 in 1,000 children. Because few studies with preselected patients claimed a high rate of malignancy in childhood thyroid nodules, the diagnosis of a nodule is causing for the most part severe concern and fear in the patients and their families. However, the reported malignancy rate of up to 20% of childhood thyroid nodules is not affirmed by population-based calculations of reported thyroid cancer cases in childhood and a far lower rate can be expected. Moreover, with the advancement of ultrasound techniques, more and more smaller nodules are being detected and their malignancy potential is not clear. The available data does not justify the screening of all children for thyroid nodules but some groups of patients with an increased risk of thyroid malignancy should be followed more carefully. This paper presents data about a group of children with primary malignancies and head and neck irradiation as part of their treatment. Even in this thyroid cancer-prone group of patients, only a small number of cases with thyroid cancer was identified by the ultrasound screening program (5 of 129). These results are different from a recent large thyroid FNA study which showed that about 30% of patients having thyroid nodules with a cytological diagnosis of follicular neoplasm had histologically confirmed malignancy [4]. Moreover, the identified secondary thyroid cancers did not develop distant metastases, and belong therefore to the group of PTC with a very good prognosis given that therapy with radioiodine is performed. The histologically diagnosed thyroid cancers were adequately prediagnosed by fine-needle aspiration. In the particular group of patients with primary cancer and irradiation an ultrasound screening for secondary thyroid cancer seems to be useful to identify PTCs that have a good prognosis before they develop distant metastasis.

Three of the 5 diagnosed thyroid cancers were <1 cm and therefore fulfilled the criteria of 'microcarcinoma'. These very small tumors are difficult to diagnose by FNA and their clinical course is very difficult to predict. The following nice review was published with a summary of available data for microcarcinoma, and it turns out that the estimated risk for a less favorable course with higher recurrence risk is related mainly to a younger age <45 years (but childhood was not covered), a lymph node infiltration and a clinical sign of palpability. However, we need to keep in mind that about half of the ultrasound-detected nodules >1.5 cm were not palpated by 21st century endocrinologists [5]. Since the data are generated mainly for adults, microcarcinomas in children will further lead to uncertainty, but in general microcarcinomas have a more benign course.

Thyroid papillary microcarcinoma: a descriptive and meta-analysis study

Roti E, degli Uberti EC, Bondanelli M, Braverman LE
Institute of Endocrinology, University of Milan, Milan, Italy
elio.roti@unimi.it
Eur J Endocrinol 2008;159:659–673

Background: Microcarcinomas of the thyroid are frequent and prediction of the course of further growth and malignancy of the tumors are of utmost clinical importance.

Methods/Results: The authors review anatomical, clinical characteristics and prevalence of thyroid microcarcinoma. Diagnostic procedures and risk factors of aggressiveness at diagnosis and during follow-up are also covered. The possible clinical, pathologic and therapeutic risk factors are analyzed by meta-analysis study. Treatment procedures by different authors and guidelines suggested by societies are reported.

Conclusion: Papillary thyroid microcarcinoma has in general a benign course and sophisticated diagnostics and aggressive treatment appear unnecessary.

For normal thyroid development, precursor cells require an intrinsic regulatory cascade, of which we know three transcription factors, e.g. FOXE1, NKX2.1 and PAX8, which are affected by loss of function mutations in patients with thyroid dysgenesis. However, the developing thyroid precursor cells need to be embedded in a growth and differentiation-promoting environment, which is defined by a variety of different growth factors. In the last year, three papers, which are summarized below, described pathways which are involved in these external signals. These signals are required for the thyroid precursor to find its way to the lateral neck position and to grow appropriately. Members of these growth factor cascades are already known from areas of other organ developments and are involved in complex genetic diseases like the CATCH 22 syndrome, a disease that rarely involves thyroid dysgenesis like hemithyroid. The major candidate gene within the Catch22-deleted region in Tbx1 and Tbx1 knockout mouse resembles the asymmetric hypoplastic thyroid phenotype of some Catch22 patients. Altogether, we have learned a lot about the complexity of mesodermal signaling cascades that are involved in thyroid development, but diseases of such factors are rare and result in much more complex syndromes than thyroid dysgenesis itself. We still need to learn more about the critical steps of thyroid development to find the key for the pathogenesis of congenital hypothyroidism. The findings are summarized in figure 1.

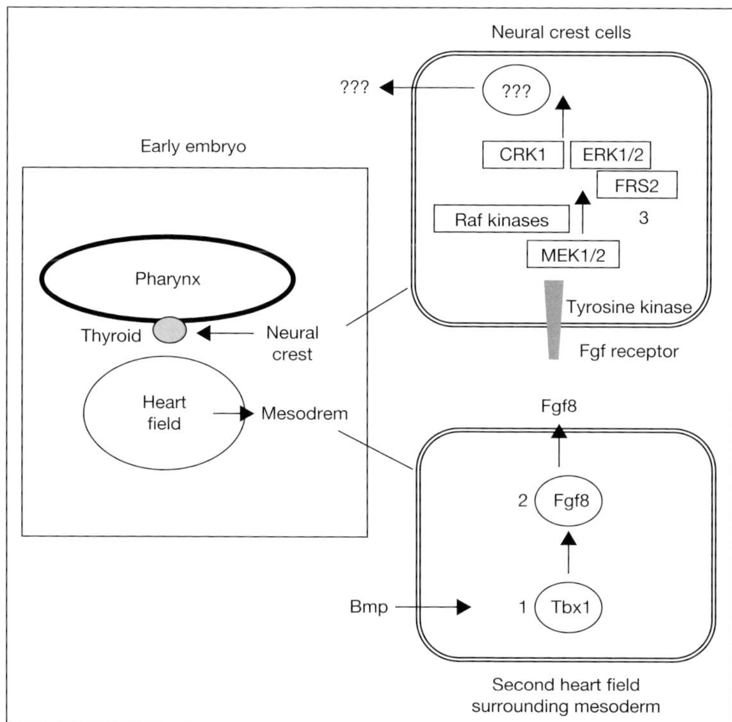

Fig. 1. Summary of signal pathways that are involved in thyroid growth and proper localization during early steps of embryogenesis. In addition to transcription factors that are expressed within the thyroid primordium itself, several regulatory factors were described in the last years, which are involved in the 'external' growth promotion and localization of the primordium. The first of these factors was Tbx1 – located within the deleted region of Catch22 patients. Tbx1 knockout mice have a misplaced single-lobed thyroid gland, as it was reported for few patients with Catch22 deletions. The three papers summarized have now described the Tbx1 signal cascade in more detail. Lania et al. demonstrated that within the Tbx1-positive mesodermal cells, Fgf8 is one downstream effector because Tbx1 cell-specific Fgf8 knockout revealed the same asymmetric and hypoplastic thyroid phenotype as Tbx1 knockout itself. Most likely, but not conclusively proven, one target of the Fgf8 signal are neural crest cells in the surrounding of Tbx1-positive cells because in these cells several components of the Fgf-receptor signal cascade are involved in thyroid shaping as well (as shown by Kameda et al. for FRS2α and by Newbern et al. for Erk1/2). How these signals are transferred to the thyroid primordium and how the mesodermal cascade is initiated remains unclear.

Early thyroid development requires a Tbx1-Fgf8 pathway

Lania G, Zhang Z, Huynh T, Caprio C, Moon AM, Vitelli F, Baldini A
Telethon Institute of Genetics and Medicine, and University Federico II, Naples, Italy
Dev Biol 2009;328:109–117

Background: The thyroid develops within the pharyngeal apparatus from endodermally-derived cells. The many derivatives of the pharyngeal apparatus develop at similar times and sometimes from common cell types, explaining why many syndromic disorders express multiple birth defects affecting different structures that share a common pharyngeal origin. Thus, different derivatives may share common genetic networks during their development. Tbx1, the major gene associated with DiGeorge syndrome, is a key player in the global development of the pharyngeal apparatus, being required for virtually all its derivatives, including the thyroid.

Methods/Results: The authors show by studying a variety of different knockout mouse lines that Tbx1 regulates the size of the early thyroid primordium through its expression in the adjacent mesoderm. Because Tbx1 regulates the expression of Fgf8 in the mesoderm, they postulated that Fgf8 mediates critical Tbx1-dependent interactions between mesodermal cells and endodermal thyrocyte progenitors. Conditional ablation of Fgf8 in Tbx1-expressing cells caused an early thyroid phenotype similar to that of Tbx1 mutant mice. In addition, expression of an Fgf8 cDNA in the Tbx1 domain rescued the early size defect of the thyroid primordium in Tbx1 mutants.

Conclusion: The authors have established that a Tbx1→Fgf8 pathway in the pharyngeal mesoderm is a key size regulator of mammalian thyroid.

Mouse and human phenotypes indicate a critical conserved role for ERK2 signaling in neural crest development

Newbern J, Zhong J, Wickramasinghe RS, Li X, Wu Y, Samuels I, Cherosky N, Karlo JC, O'Loughlin B, Wikenheiser J, Gargesha M, Doughman YQ, Charron J, Ginty DD, Watanabe M, Saitta SC, Snider WD, Landreth GE
Neuroscience Center, University of North Carolina, Chapel Hill, N.C., USA
Proc Natl Acad Sci USA 2008;105:17115–17120

Background: Disrupted ERK1/2 (MAPK3/MAPK1) MAPK signaling has been associated with several developmental syndromes in humans; however, mutations in ERK1 or ERK2 have not been described.

Results: The authors demonstrate haplo-insufficient ERK2 expression in patients with a novel approximately 1 Mb microdeletion in distal 22q11.2, a region that includes ERK2. These patients exhibit conotruncal and craniofacial anomalies that arise from perturbation of neural crest development and exhibit defects comparable to the DiGeorge syndrome spectrum. Remarkably, these defects are replicated in mice by conditional inactivation of ERK2 in the developing neural crest. Inactivation of upstream elements of the ERK cascade (B-Raf and C-Raf, MEK1 and MEK2) or a downstream effector, the transcription factor serum response factor resulted in analogous developmental defects including thyroid malpositioning.

Conclusion: The findings demonstrate that mammalian neural crest development is critically dependent on a RAF/MEK/ERK/serum response factor signaling pathway and suggest that neural crest autonomous ERK2 signaling is important for normal thyroid development.

FRS2α is required for the separation, migration, and survival of pharyngeal-endoderm derived organs including thyroid, ultimobranchial body, parathyroid, and thymus

Kameda Y, Ito M, Nishimaki T, Gotoh N
Department of Anatomy, Kitasato University School of Medicine, Sagamihara, Kanagawa, Japan
kameda@med.kitasato-u.ac.jp
Dev Dyn 2009;238:503–513

Background: The docking protein FRS2α plays an important role in fibroblast growth factor (FGF)-induced intracellular signal transduction by linking FGF receptors (FGFRs) to a variety of intracellular signaling pathways. Given the potential role of Fgf10 and Fgf8 in normal thyroid development, FRS2α might also be involved in normal thyroid organogenesis.

Results: In FRS2α(2F/2F) mutant mice at embryonic day (E)18.5, in which the Shp2-binding sites of FRS2α were disrupted, the thyroid glands were aplastic or hypoplastic. C cells were absent or present in low numbers and rarely formed a compact mass of cells. Parathyroid glands were mostly connected to thymus tissues. At E10.5, the formations of pharyngeal pouches and thyroid primordium were normally initiated in the mutant mice. At E11.5–E12.5, the thyroid primordium of wild-type embryos was located close to the aortic sac, and the epithelial buds of pharyngeal-derived organs, including the parathyroid gland, thymus and ultimobranchial body, were separated from the epithelium and began to migrate to their final destinations. In the FRS2α(2F/2F) mutants, however, the thyroid primordium became hypoplastic and the pharyngeal-derived organ primordia remained affiliated with the pharyngeal epithelium. At these stages, organ-specific differentiation markers (i.e., Nkx2-1/TTF1 for the thyroid lobe and ultimobranchial body; Pax8 for the thyroid lobe; parathormone (PTH), chromogranin A, P75(NTR), and S100 protein for the parathyroid gland, and p63 for the thymus) were normally expressed in the mutant issues.

Conclusion: The separation, migration, and survival of the pharyngeal organs including the thyroid were impaired in the FRS2α(2F/2F) mutants.

Thyrotropin-independent induction of thyroid endoderm from embryonic stem cells by activin A

Ma R, Latif R, Davies TF
Thyroid Research Unit, Mount Sinai School of Medicine, James J. Peters Veterans Affairs Medical Center, New York, N.Y., USA
risheng.ma@mssm.edu
Endocrinology 2009;150:1970–1975

Background: Studies with embryonic stem cells can further unravel relevant factors for early embryogenesis. To model the differentiation of thyroid epithelial cells, the authors examined embryoid bodies derived from undifferentiated murine embryonic stem cells treated with activin A to induce endoderm differentiation, the germ layer from which thyroid cells occur.

Methods: Resulting endodermal cells were then further exposed to TSH and/or IGF-I for up to 21 days.

Results: Oct-4 and REX1 expression, required to sustain stem cell self-renewal and pluripotency, were appropriately downregulated, whereas GATA-4, and α-fetoprotein, both endodermal-specific markers, increased as the embryonic stem cells were exposed to activin A. By day 5 culture, TSH receptor (TSHR) and sodium iodide symporter (NIS) gene and protein expression were markedly induced. Cells isolated by the fluorescence-activated cell sorter simultaneously expressed not only TSHR and NIS proteins but also PAX8 mRNA, an expression pattern unique to thyroid cells and expected in committed thyroid progenitor cells. Such expression continued until day 21 with no influence seen by the addition of TSH or IGF-I.

Conclusion: The sequence of gene expression changes observed in these experiments demonstrated the emergence of definitive thyroid endoderm. The activin A induction of thyroid-specific markers, NIS and TSHR, occurred in the absence of TSH stimulation, and, therefore, the emergence of thyroid endoderm in vitro parallels the emergence of thyroid cells in TSHR knockout mice. Activin A is clearly a major regulator of thyroid endoderm.

This last paper in the series of relevant factors in thyroid development is unique in that a reverse approach is taken. The authors are pioneers in establishing the experimental settings to generate thyroid cells from embryonic stem cells. Applying this strategy, growth factors can be tested in vitro for their contribution to thyroid differentiation and commitment. Employing this experimental setting, the authors demonstrate that activin A, a growth factor known to play a pivotal role in the organogenesis of other endodermal areas, seems to have the potential for thyroid determination. The overall concept of early organ determination within a developmental field like the anterior endoderm is based on the assumption that a gradient of growth factors defines a particular concentration that will direct the uncommitted cell to start an organ-specific program. For the thyroid gland, one of the early growth factors could be activin A.

Since the introduction of newborn screening for congenital hypothyroidism the key question remains if an early postnatal treatment with thyroid hormone can enable a completely normal cognitive outcome and if the fetal hypothyroidism itself does cause a noncompensable defect of mental development. The early reports of final cognitive outcome in young adult patients diagnosed in screening programs have shown a remarkably normal outcome but still with a gap of 8 IQ points less compared to appropriate control groups [6, 7]. However, in these cohorts, treatment started later, within the second week of life and consisted of doses <10 µg/kg. Now the first cohort that was treated very early and with a high initial dose is reported from Switzerland.

Children with congenital hypothyroidism: long-term intellectual outcome after early high-dose treatment

Dimitropoulos A, Molinari L, Etter K, Torresani T, Lang-Muritano M, Jenni OG, Largo RH, Latal B
Child Development Center, University Children's Hospital Zurich, Zurich, Switzerland
Pediatr Res 2009;65:242–248

Background: Outcome studies in patients with congenital hypothyroidism (CH) diagnosed in newborn screening programs revealed a significant 6- to 10-point difference in IQ. The question remains if a very early and high-dose treatment can close this gap in cognitive development.
Methods: 63 prospectively followed children with CH were assessed at age of 14 years with the Wechsler Intelligence Scale for Children-Revised and compared with 175 healthy controls. Median age at onset of treatment was 9 days (range 5–18) and median starting dose of levothyroxine (L-T_4) was 14.7 µg/kg/day (range 9.9–23.6).
Results: Full-scale intelligence quotient (IQ) was significantly lower than in controls after adjustment for socioeconomic status (SES) and gender (101.7 vs. 111.4; p < 0.0001). Children with athyreosis had a lower performance IQ than those with dysgenesis (adjusted difference 7.6 IQ scores, p < 0.05). Lower initial thyroxine (T_4) levels correlated with poorer IQ (r = 0.27, p = 0.04). Lower SES was associated with poorer IQ, in particular in children with CH (interaction, p = 0.03). Treatment during childhood was not related to IQ at age 14 years.
Conclusion: Adolescents with CH manifest IQ deficits when compared with their peers despite early high-dose treatment and optimal substitution therapy throughout childhood.

Thus, the gap still exists! Obviously these data are a drawback for the hope of completely normal IQ in patients with congenital hypothyroidism. But, some important questions still need to be answered. As it was shown that congenital hypothyroidism can be part of more complex endocrine developmental diseases like pseudohypoparathyroidism and the more recently described gene mutations that are important for thyroid as well as brain development (FOXE1 and NKX2.1, see above), a more detailed analysis of the cases which did not reach satisfactory outcome, and which might have decreased the overall IQ level of the patient cohort, are mandatory. Based on these findings of associated brain defects, an alternative explanation for the IQ gap in patients with congenital hypothyroidism is that subgroups of patients are affected by associated and not directly causally related genetic brain defects, and that these deficits persist independently of the thyroid hormone treatment efforts. A more thorough search for such defects and an exclusion of these cases from the outcome cohorts might end up with IQ levels showing no gap.

Early and high-dose treatments are only part of the strategy, which this study addresses. Quite as important is the maintenance throughout childhood of normal TSH.

The principal message to parents with a newborn with congenital hypothyroidism is that for most children cognitive development will be within the normal range, provided that therapy is given using a full dose and TSH is monitored often enough.

Although the gap still exists, the question whether a higher dose is beneficial compared to a lower dose is not further answered by this new publication. The evidence for the use of a higher dose is still low, and the only existing prospective randomized study, comparing 37 and 50 µg/day is in favor of a higher dose [8]. Nevertheless, the next report from the Cochrane Collaboration this year shows our limits of evidence and makes it obvious that the evidence for the higher dose is not strong enough to be officially recommended.

High versus low dose of initial thyroid hormone replacement for congenital hypothyroidism

Ng SM, Anand D, Weindling AM

School of Reproductive and Developmental Medicine, University of Liverpool, Liverpool Women's Hospital, Liverpool, UK

ngszemay@yahoo.com
Cochrane Database Syst Rev 2009;CD006972

Background: The authors aimed to determine the evidence for effects of high versus low dose of initial thyroid hormone replacement for congenital hypothyroidism.

Methods: Randomized controlled trials were identified by searching The Cochrane Library, MEDLINE and EMBASE and reference lists of published papers. Randomized controlled clinical trials investigating the effects of high versus low dose of initial thyroid hormone replacement for congenital hypothyroidism were included. Both authors independently selected trials, assessed risk of bias and extracted data.

Results: The initial search identified 1,014 records, which identified 13 publications for further examination. After screening the full text of the 13 selected papers, only one study evaluating 47 babies finally met the inclusion criteria. Using the same cohort at two different time periods, the study investigated the effects of high versus low dose thyroid hormone replacement in relation to (1) time taken to achieve euthyroid status and (2) neurodevelopmental outcome. The study reported that a high dose is more effective in rising serum thyroxine and free thyroxine concentrations to the target range and earlier normalization of thyroid-stimulating hormone compared to a lower dose. Similarly, full-scale intelligence quotient (IQ) was noted to be significantly higher in children who received the high dose compared to the lower dose. However, the verbal IQ and performance IQ were similar in both groups. Growth and adverse effects were not reported in the included trial.

Conclusion: There is currently only one randomized controlled trial evaluating the effects of high versus low dose of initial thyroid hormone replacement for CHT. There is inadequate evidence to suggest that a high dose is more beneficial compared to a low dose initial thyroid hormone replacement in the treatment of CHT.

What should we do? First, we need more studies which compare the outcome in relation to the initial treatment dose and large enough to define subgroups with different forms of the disease including the exemption of genetic syndromic defects. Due to the low incidence of the disease, such studies can only be conducted in a multicentered, international effort. So far, almost all outcome studies of congenital hypothyroidism come from single centers and patient groups are too small to allow significant conclusions. Until then, we should continue with the actual recommendations since the available studies are in favor of a better outcome with the higher dosage and no relevant side effects of the higher dose have been reported. It will take many years and births of thousands of children with congenital hypothyroidism until we will have enough data for evidence-based decisions. It would be unethical to treat until then with a lower dose.

Concepts revised: course and causes of 'subclinical' thyroid dysfunction

Neonatal thyroid function in Seveso 25 years after maternal exposure to dioxin

Baccarelli A, Giacomini SM, Corbetta C, Landi MT, Bonzini M, Consonni D, Grillo P, Patterson DG, Pesatori AC, Bertazzi PA

Department of Environmental Health, Harvard School of Public Health, Boston, Mass., USA

abaccare@hsph.harvard.edu
PLoS Med 2008;5:e161

Background: Neonatal hypothyroidism has been associated in animal models with maternal exposure to several environmental like 2,3,7,8-tetrachlorodibenzo-*p*-dioxin (TCDD), a persistent and widespread toxic environmental contaminant.

Methods/Results: Between 1994 and 2005, in individuals exposed to TCDD after the 1976 Seveso accident, we conducted: (i) a residence-based population study on 1,014 children born to the 1,772 women of reproductive age in the most contaminated zones (A, very high contamination; B, high contamination), and 1,772 age-matched women from the surrounding noncontaminated area (reference); (ii) a biomarker study on 51 mother-child pairs for whom recent maternal plasma dioxin measurements were available. Neonatal blood thyroid-stimulating hormone (b-TSH) was measured on all children. We performed crude and multivariate analyses adjusting for gender, birth weight, birth order, maternal age, hospital, and type of delivery. Mean neonatal b-TSH was 0.98 µU/ml (95% CI 0.90–1.08) in the reference area (n = 533), 1.35 µU/ml (95% CI 1.22–1.49) in zone B (n = 425), and 1.66 µU/ml (95% CI 1.19–2.31) in zone A (n = 56) (p < 0.001). The proportion of children with b-TSH >5 µU/ml was 2.8% in the reference area, 4.9% in zone B, and 16.1% in zone A (p < 0.001). Neonatal b-TSH was correlated with current maternal plasma TCDD (n = 51, β = 0.47, p < 0.001) and plasma toxic equivalents of coplanar dioxin-like compounds (n = 51, β = 0.45, p = 0.005).

Conclusion: The data indicate that environmental contaminants such as dioxins have a long-lasting capability to modify neonatal thyroid function after the initial exposure.

Almost all available epidemiological studies failed to demonstrate a significant impact of environmental factors on the incidence of congenital hypothyroidism. The only example of a strong environmental influence was found in extreme maternal and fetal iodine deficiency that led to cretinism; but this is of no concern in countries with iodine supplementation and newborn-screening programs. However, in contrast to manifest hypothyroidism, slight elevations of TSH have been monitored in areas with milder iodine deficiency. In the paper by Baccarelli et al., a new cause of neonatal TSH change – however in the normal range! – was described in a population of neonates from mothers with dioxin exhibition in the Seveso nuclear accident 30 years ago. Due to the extremely long half-life of digoxin, the authors could still measure relevant levels of the toxin in the maternal blood and it seems that the fetal thyroid axis is mildly influenced by the toxin; the neonatal TSH correlated with the level of maternal toxin load. While it remains to be determined how digoxin affects thyroid function, the good news is that even in highly exposed women, children are *not* born with congenital hypothyroidism and so far there is no evidence to argue that a mildly elevated TSH within the normal range may cause harm to the developing child.

This discussion of cognitive outcome and mild neonatal differences in thyroid function has seen a significant improvement by the following study of a large cohort of children tested for cognitive function in relation to neonatal T_4 values.

Neonatal thyroxine, maternal thyroid function, and child cognition

Oken E, Braverman LE, Platek D, Mitchell ML, Lee SL, Pearce EN
Department of Ambulatory Care and Prevention, Harvard Medical School, Boston, Mass., USA
emily_oken@hphc.org
J Clin Endocrinol Metab 2009;94:497–503

Background: Thyroid hormone is essential for normal brain development. Limited data are available regarding whether thyroid function in neonates influences later cognitive development.

Methods: The authors studied cognitive test scores at ages 6 months and 3 years in participants in Project Viva, a cohort study in Massachusetts with a total of 500 children born 1999–2003 at 34 weeks or more.

Results: Mean newborn T_4 at a mean age of 1.94 days was 17.6 (SD 4.0) µg/dl, and levels were higher in girls [1.07 µg/dl; 95% CI 0.38, 1.76] and infants born after longer gestation (0.42 µg/dl; 95% CI 0.17, 0.67 per week). Newborn T_4 levels were not associated with maternal T_4, TSH, or thyroid peroxidase antibody levels. On multivariable linear regression analysis, adjusting for maternal and child characteristics, higher newborn T_4 was unexpectedly associated with poorer scores on the visual recognition memory test among infants at age 6 months (–0.5; 95% CI –0.9, –0.2), but not with scores at age 3 years on either the Peabody Picture Vocabulary Test (0.2; 95% CI –0.1, 0.5) or the Wide Range Assessment of Visual Motor Abilities (0.1; 95% CI –0.2, 0.3). Maternal thyroid function test results were not associated with child cognitive test scores.

Conclusions: Newborn T_4 concentrations within a normal physiological reference range are not associated with maternal thyroid function and do not predict cognitive outcome in a population living in an iodine-sufficient area.

The very important and clear message of this study is that irrespective of the TSH level – unfortunately we do not even know the TSH levels of the investigated children – the cognitive development of neonates is *not* related to the concentration of neonatal T$_4$ as long as it is within the normal range. It seems to make no difference if a child was born with a high normal or low normal T$_4$ and this correlates to a wide range from 6.4 to 35.7 µg/dl. Moreover, the neonatal T$_4$ value and cognitive development of the newborns did not correlate with maternal thyroid function in the first trimester. Obviously these data do not completely exclude those children with mild thyroid dysfunction in terms of isolated TSH elevation and normal T$_4$ ('hyperthyreotropinemia') who will all have a normal cognitive outcome. But concerns about children with mild TSH elevation, as long as T$_4$ is normal, need to be downgraded. Moreover, the trend to lower TSH cut-off levels in neonatal screening programs [9] needs to be reconsidered in regard to the normal outcome of these 500 studied newborns.

Beside the very sensitive question of hyperthyreotropinemia in newborns, elevated TSH in older children is a very frequent cause to seek a pediatric endocrinologist, and data are needed to have good ground for clinical decisions what to do with these children of mostly incidental findings of elevated TSH. Two studies were published in the last 12 months that contribute significantly to this important clinical question.

Prospective evaluation of the natural course of idiopathic subclinical hypothyroidism in childhood and adolescence

Wasniewska M, Salerno M, Cassio A, Corrias A, Aversa T, Zirilli G, Capalbo D, Bal M, Mussa A, De Luca F
Department of Pediatrics, University of Messina, Messina, Italy
wasniewska@yahoo.it
Eur J Endocrinol 2009;160:417–421

Background: The authors aimed to prospectively evaluate the course of subclinical hypothyroidism (SH) in children and adolescents with no underlying diseases and no risk factors, which might interfere with the progression of SH.
Methods: Clinical status, thyroid function, and autoimmunity were prospectively evaluated at entry and after 6, 12, and 24 months in 92 young patients (mean age 8.1 ± 3.0 years) with idiopathic SH.
Results: During the study, mean TSH levels showed a trend toward a progressive decrease while FT$_4$ levels remained unchanged. Overall, 38 patients normalized their TSH (group A): 16 patients between 6 and 12 months, and 22 patients between 12 and 24 months. Among the remaining 54 patients, the majority maintained TSH within the baseline values (group B), whereas 11 exhibited a further increase in TSH >10 mU/l (group C). Baseline TSH and FT$_4$ levels were similar in the patients who normalized TSH, compared with those with persistent hyperthyrotropinemia. Even in the patients of group C, both TSH and FT$_4$ at entry were not different with respect to those of groups A and B. No patients showed any symptoms of hypothyroidism during follow-up and no changes in both height and body mass index were observed throughout the observation period.
Conclusion: The natural course of TSH values in a pediatric population with idiopathic subclinical hypothyroidism is characterized by a progressive decrease over time; the majority of patients (88%) normalized or maintained unchanged their TSH, and TSH changes were not associated with either FT$_4$ values or clinical status or auxological parameters.

Natural history of thyroid function tests over 5 years in a large pediatric cohort

Lazar L, Frumkin RB, Battat E, Lebenthal Y, Phillip M, Meyerovitch J
The Jesse Z. and Sara Lea Shafer Institute for Endocrinology and Diabetes, National Center for Childhood Diabetes, Schneider Children's Medical Center of Israel, Petah Tikva, Israel
J Clin Endocrinol Metab 2009;94:1678–1682

Background: Because clinical manifestations of thyroid disorders are variable and subtle in children and adolescents, thyroid function tests are often repeated in patients with nonspecific symptoms. The objective of the study was to determine the natural history of initial abnormal TSH and define populations at greater risk for developing a subsequent thyroid dysfunction.
Methods: A total of 121,052 of 1.043 million outpatients aged 0.5–16 years insured by the Clalit Health Medical Organization had a TSH determination in 2002 and follow-up to 2007. Extracted from the

Clalit Health Medical Organization database were their demographic data, referral diagnoses, and laboratory results (TSH, free T$_4$, thyroid antibodies). Excluded were patients with overt hypothyroidism or hyperthyroidism on initial testing.

Results: Results of 96.5% of initial serum TSH concentrations were normal (0.35–5.5 mIU/l), 0.2% were low (<0.35 mIU/l), 2.9% elevated (>5.5 to ≤10 mIU/l), and 0.4% highly elevated (>10 mIU/l). The frequency of TSH testing increased with age and female gender. During follow-up, repeated (two to more than four) TSH tests were performed in 45.7% of the patients. In the second TSH determination, normal TSH was documented in 40, 73.6, and 78.9% of those whose initial serum TSH was highly elevated, elevated, and low, respectively, and in 97% of those with normal initial TSH. Predictive factors for a sustained highly elevated TSH were initially TSH >7.5 mIU/liter (p = 0.014) and female gender (p = 0.047).

Conclusion: In the pediatric population, initial normal or slightly elevated TSH levels are likely to remain normal or spontaneously normalize without treatment. Patients with initial levels >7.5 mIU/l, particularly girls, are at a greater risk for sustained abnormal TSH levels.

Both studies give evidence that an elevated TSH in the range of 5–10 and higher while T$_4$ is normal seems not to be a cause for concern in children. Based on a prospective follow-up study of 92 patients – including measurement of antibodies and thyroid ultrasound – from Italy as well as a huge study from Israel based on 121,052 (!) children, the authors all together demonstrated that almost all children did not develop overt thyroid disease within the study period of 0.5–16 years and that 50–70% of elevated TSH normalized just by 'observation'. Those children who maintained with an elevated TSH mostly did not further increase and only 2% developed autoimmune thyroiditis in the Italian study and 0.4% developed manifest hypothyroidism in the study from Israel.

As a conclusion, we have again to accept that Nature is not exact. TSH levels vary and the arithmetic border of normal, which defines a TSH >2 standard deviations as 'unnormal', does *not* define a disease for itself. We should be conservative in our management of elevated TSH while T$_4$ is normal.

Extreme longevity is associated with increased serum thyrotropin

Atzmon G, Barzilai N, Hollowell JG, Surks MI, Gabriely I
Department of Medicine, Division of Endocrinology, Albert Einstein College of Medicine, Bronx, New York, N.Y., USA
J Clin Endocrinol Metab 2009;94:1251–1254

Background: The distribution of serum TSH shifts progressively to higher concentrations with age. The aim of the study was to determine whether the population shift in TSH distribution to higher concentrations with aging extends to people of exceptional longevity, namely centenarians, and to assess the relationship between concentrations of TSH and free T$_4$ (FT$_4$).

Methods: The authors analyzed TSH, FT$_4$, and TSH frequency distribution curves in thyroid disease-free Ashkenazi Jews with exceptional longevity (centenarians; median age 98 years), in younger Ashkenazi controls (median age 72 years), and in a population of thyroid disease-free individuals (median age 68 years) from the US National Health and Nutrition Examination Survey 1998–2002 (NHANES controls).

Results: Serum TSH was significantly higher in centenarians [1.97 (0.42–7.15) mIU/l] than in Ashkenazi controls [1.55 (0.46–4.55) mIU/l] and NHANES controls [1.61 (0.39–6.29) mIU/l] (median 2.5 and 97.5 centiles) (p < 0.001). The TSH frequency distribution curve of centenarians was relatively similar in shape to controls but shifted significantly to higher TSH, including TSH concentration at peak frequency. The TSH distribution curve of the NHANES control group was superimposable to and not significantly different from the Ashkenazi controls. FT$_4$ was similar in centenarians and Ashkenazi controls, and there was a significant inverse correlation between FT$_4$ and TSH in both groups.

Conclusions: The TSH population shifts to higher concentrations with age appear to be a continuum that extends even to people with exceptional longevity. The inverse correlation between TSH and FT$_4$ in these populations suggests that changes in negative feedback may contribute to exceptional longevity.

Although pediatric endocrinologists are not frequently confronted with patients older than 100 years of age, it might be interesting for our community to know that higher TSH levels do not seem to be a cause for concern when thinking of a long life expectancy. The lucky individuals who reach such exceptionally old age seem to have higher TSH levels. However we do not know if higher TSH values are essential for reaching such an old age, but at least they do not seem to detain a long life expectancy.

New hope: to predict the outcome of Graves' disease in children

Predictors of autoimmune hyperthyroidism relapse in children after discontinuation of antithyroid drug treatment

Kaguelidou F, Alberti C, Castanet M, Guitteny MA, Czernichow P, Léger J, French Childhood Graves' Disease Study Group
Institut National de la Santé et de la Recherche Médicale U690, Hôpital Robert Debré, Paris, France
J Clin Endocrinol Metab 2008;93:3817–3826

Background: There is debate about how Graves' disease (GD) should be treated in children. The aim of this study was to identify predictors of relapse after antithyroid drug (ATD) treatment in children with GD.
Methods: The authors conducted a prospective, multicenter cohort study of children (n = 154) with GD treated with carbimazole for an intended duration of 24 ± 3 months. After the end of treatment, patients were followed up for at least 2 years. The primary outcome was hyperthyroidism relapse. Cox's regression analysis was used and a prognostic score was constructed.
Results: The overall estimated relapse rate for hyperthyroidism was 59% (95% CI 52–67%) at 1 year and 68% (95% CI 60–76%) at 2 years after the end of treatment. Multivariate survival analysis showed that the risk of relapse was higher for patients of non-Caucasian origin [hazard ratio (HR) = 2.54, p < 0.001], with high serum thyroid-stimulating hormone receptor antibodies (HR = 1.21 by 10 U, p = 0.03) and free T_4 (HR = 1.18 by 10 pmol/l, p = 0.001) levels at diagnosis. Conversely, relapse risk decreased with increasing age at onset (HR = 0.74 per 5 years, p = 0.03) and duration of first course of ATD (HR = 0.57 per 12 months, p = 0.005). A prognostic score was constructed, allowing the identification of three different risk groups, with 2-year relapse rates of 46, 77, and 98%.
Conclusion: A longer initial duration of euthyroid state with ATD seems to be the only variable related to the risk of hyperthyroidism relapse in children that can be manipulated. Ethnic origin, age, and severity of the disease at diagnosis may guide long-term disease management decisions.

Since the initial and provocative publication by Barbara Lippe in 1987 which claimed a close correlation of initial duration of antithyroid drug treatment and long-term outcome of Grave's disease, no final proof for that hypothesis was contributed to the field. Although not closing the gap of evidence, the French release of follow-up data from 154 children with Grave's disease – which represents the largest pediatric cohort published ever – is very good ground to prolong medication before deciding for definite treatment by surgery or radioiodine. The retrospective data show that medical treatment for over 24 months can reduce the 'relapse prediction score' from 98 to 44%. This needs to be confirmed in a prospective intervention study comparing 24 versus 24+ months of treatment. However, this study has been due since Lippe's data in 1987 – let's do it now!

Whoever will do this study and whoever treats children with antithyroid drugs, it should be methimazole and not propylthiouracil. This statement is based on the 'papers' that appeared as a report of a meeting rather than a meta-analysis study in the *JCEM* and in the *NEJM*. The authors reported data that were collected from different US institutions showing that liver failure as a severe adverse event of antithyroid drug treatment only occurred when PTU was given. Although the number of liver failures was very low with an incidence of 1 in 2,000–4,000 treated cases, all cases were under PTU and it seems that this side effect can be circumvented by prescribing methimazole. Regardless of the fact that no official study has been conducted, the two releases have such a clinical impact that they are cited here in the Yearbook.

Putting propylthiouracil in perspective

Cooper DS, Rivkees SA
Division of Endocrinology and Metabolism, Johns Hopkins University, Baltimore, Md., USA
J Clin Endocrinol Metab 2009;94:1881–1882

Ending propylthiouracil-induced liver failure in children

Rivkees SA, Mattison DR
N Engl J Med 2009;360:1574–1575

References

1. De Felice M, Di Lauro R: Thyroid development and its disorders: genetics and molecular mechanisms. Endocr Rev 2004;25:722–746.
2. Rallison ML, Dobyns BM, Keating FR Jr, et al: Thyroid nodularity in children JAMA 1975;233:1069–1072.
3. Reiners C, Wegscheider K, Schicha H, et al: Prevalence of thyroid disorders in the working population of Germany: ultrasonography screening in 96,278 unselected employees. Thyroid 2004;14:926–932.
4. Yang J, Schnadig V, Logrono R, Wasserman PG: Fine-needle aspiration of thyroid nodules: a study of 4,703 patients with histologic and clinical correlations. Cancer 2007;111:306–315
5. Eden K, Mahon S, Helfand M: Screening high-risk populations for thyroid cancer. Med Pediatr Oncol 2001;36:583–591
6. Overbeck B, Sundet K, Kase B, Heyerdahl S: Congenital hypothyroidism: Influence of disease severity and L-thyroxine treatment on intellectual, motor and school-associated outcomes in young adults. Pediatrics 2003;112:923–930.
7. Rovet JF: Children with congenital hypothyroidism and their siblings: Do they really differ? Pediatrics 2005;115:e52–e57.
8. Selva KA, Harper A, Downs A, Blasco PA, Lafranchi SH: Neurodevelopmental outcomes in congenital hypothyroidism: comparison of initial T_4 dose and time to reach target T_4 and TSH. J Pediatr 2005;147:775–780.
9. Corbetta C, Weber G, Cortinovis F, Calebiro D, Passoni A, Vigone MC, Beck-Peccoz P, Chiumello G, Persani L: A 7-year experience with low blood TSH cutoff levels for neonatal screening reveals an unsuspected frequency of congenital hypothyroidism. Clin Endocrinol (Oxf) 2009, Epub ahead of print.

Growth and Growth Factors

Evelien F Gevers[a,b] and Mehul T Dattani[a]

[a]Developmental Endocrine Research Group, Clinical and Molecular Genetics Unit, Institute for Child Health, London, UK
[b]Division of Molecular Neuroendocrinology, National Institute for Medical Research, London, UK

When we were asked to select papers for this year's chapter on *Growth and Growth Factors*, it felt as if we had only just finished last year's selection, and that it would be a challenge to find papers that were of comparable quality to the previous 2 years. It was only when we prioritized the eligible papers that we realized that once again there was far too much new high-quality material in the field of growth and growth factors to include in the chapter. Examples include a paper on the IGF-independent involvement of IGFBP4 in cardiac development and work on the choice of signalling pathways by specific activation of the growth hormone receptor.

We have clearly entered the era of genome-wide associations, with two further papers on associations and height, in this chapter and in the chapter on *Population genetics, pharmacogenomics*, that follow up the work which we discussed last year [1–5]. Another recurring theme this year is imprinting and disorders thereof – imprinting has made the translational jump into clinical pediatric endocrinology, with major advances in our understanding of complex and heterogeneous conditions such as Beckwith-Wiedemann syndrome, Silver-Russell syndrome and Prader-Willi syndrome.

New genome-wide associations

Meta-analysis of genome-wide scans for human adult stature identifies novel loci and associations with measures of skeletal frame size

Soranzo N, Rivadeneira F, Chinappen-Horsley U, Malkina I, Richards JB, Hammond N, Stolk L, Nica A, Inouye M, Hofman A, Stephens J, Wheeler E, Arp P, Gwilliam R, Jhamai PM, Potter S, Chaney A, Ghori MJ, Ravindrarajah R, Ermakov S, Estrada K, Pols HA, Williams FM, McArdle WL, van Meurs JB, Loos RJ, Dermitzakis ET, Ahmadi KR, Hart DJ, Ouwehand WH, Wareham NJ, Barroso I, Sandhu MS, Strachan DP, Livshits G, Spector TD, Uitterlinden AG, Deloukas P
Human Genetics Department, Wellcome Trust Sanger Institute, Hinxton, Cambridge, UK
panos@sanger.ac.uk
PLoS Genet 2009;5:e1000445

Background: Recent genome-wide association (GWA) scans have identified several independent loci affecting human stature. This study analyzes their contribution through the different skeletal components of height.

Methods and Results: GWA scans in 2 large cohorts were performed. Seventeen genomic regions associated with height were identified. Two other regions were entirely novel (in CATSPER4 and in TMED10) and two had previously been described with weak statistical support (in NPR3 and JAZF1). One locus (at GNA12) identifies the first height eQTL. The contribution of height loci to the upper- (trunk) and lower-body (hip axis and femur) skeletal components of height were assessed and evidence was obtained for several loci associated with trunk length (most significant for GPR126 and LCORL), hip axis length (LCORL and UQCC), and femur length (PRKG2 and HIST1H1D). Finally, conditional analyses were used to explore a possible differential contribution of the height loci to these different skeletal size measurements.

Conclusions: This study has validated four novel loci controlling adult stature, and has successfully assessed the contribution of genetic loci to specific skeletal components of height.

In this large study, the authors searched for correlation of height-related SNPs, found in previous GWA studies [2–5], with spine length, femur length and hip axis length (femoral greater trochanter to inner pelvic rim distance which correlates with total frame size), which is of interest since the regulation of growth varies for these skeletal components. Interestingly, apart from *SOCS2*, no genes from the GHRH-GH-IGF1 axis show major associations with height, possibly reflecting the contribution of non-endocrine processes to growth. Two novel loci associated with total height were found in CATSPER4 (a cation channel, 0.45 cm/allele) and TMED10 (involved in cellular protein trafficking, 0.34 cm/allele). The strongest association signals were at HGMA2 and UQCC which confirms previous GWA data. HGMA2 is of interest not only because it is involved in proliferation but overexpression results in pituitary adenomas, and UQCC is involved in the FGF pathway, well known for its involvement in bone development. The first quantitative trait locus described is in GNA12, a gene involved in modulating signaling pathways of G-protein-coupled receptors. NPR3 encoding for natriuretic peptide receptor, which plays a key role in bone development and growth [6] and the mutation of which results in acromesomelic dysplasia type Maroteaux, was unexpectedly mostly associated with trunk height. Other genes associated specifically with trunk length, leg length or hip axis length are involved in multiple processes like G-protein-coupled receptor signaling, proliferation and chondrogenesis.

This and other GWA studies give a wealth of data and are paramount in unraveling the physiology and genetics of growth, and may help to find gene abnormalities in children with short stature. They also emphasize that frequent recording of height and other auxological parameters in short children may pay off! One thing to remember though is that these studies do not prove a relation between the SNP and the gene that it lies in or is in close proximity, especially when a SNP is in between two genes, since DNA elements can regulate genes at a long distance.

New mutations – with imprinting issues

Prader-Willi phenotype caused by paternal deficiency for the HBII-85 C/D box small nucleolar RNA cluster

Sahoo T, del Gaudio D, German JR, Shinawi M, Peters SU, Person RE, Garnica A, Cheung SW, Beaudet AL
Molecular and Human Genetics, Baylor College of Medicine, Houston, Tex., USA
abeaudet@bcm.edu
Nat Genet 2008;40:719–721

Background: Prader-Willi syndrome (PWS) is characterized by the presence of neonatal hypotonia, feeding difficulties, failure to thrive in infancy, hyperphagia and severe obesity in childhood, hypogonadism, developmental delay, small hands and feet and a tendency to pick skin. It maps to chromosome 15q11–q13 and is caused by deficiency of one or more paternally expressed imprinted transcripts within this region, including SNURF-SNRPN and multiple small nucleolar RNAs (snoRNAs). This may be due to large interstitial deletions, imprinting defects or maternal uniparental disomy 15. Balanced chromosomal translocations that preserve expression of SNURF-SNRPN and centromeric genes but separate the snoRNA HBII-85 cluster from its promoter also cause PWS.

Methods: A de novo paternally inherited microdeletion within 15q11–q13 was identified in a boy with several features of PWS by array-based comparative genomic hybridization (array-CGH) using a BAC array, followed by FISH analysis. DNA methylation analysis of the PWS-imprinting center and a karyotype revealed no abnormalities. Subsequently a combination of high-resolution oligonucleotide-based array CGH and quantitative real-time PCR was used to define the deletion more precisely.

Results: A deleted segment of just under 175 kB was identified and contained the entire HBII-85 snoRNA cluster as well as approximately half the HBII-52 cluster and one of the two copies of HBII-438.

Conclusion: Since previous studies showed that a paternally inherited microdeletion of the entire HBII-52 cluster was not associated with PWS, the authors suggested that deficiency of HBII-85 snoRNAs causes the key characteristics of the PWS phenotype, although some atypical features in the proband suggest that other genes in the region may make more subtle phenotypic contributions.

Prader-Willi syndrome is associated with significant morbidity and mortality and is extremely difficult to manage. It is an imprinted disorder with the loss of paternally expressed genes at 15q11–13. It is considered a contiguous gene syndrome resulting from deletion of the paternal copies of the imprinted SNRPN and necdin genes, and possibly other genes within the chromosome region. This paper has implicated the non-coding HBII-85 small nucleolar RNAs (snoRNAs) in the etiology of the syndrome. This observation is all the more important as PWS is the first human disorder to be associated with loss of expression of noncoding snoRNAs. However, the commentary by Peters [7] suggests a degree of caution in that the data are based on a single patient with a microdeletion, with some atypical features including relatively tall stature and a head circumference above the normal range. The HBII-85 cluster is made up of C/D box snoRNAs that are predominantly expressed in the brain. The role of most C/D box sno-RNAs is to base pair with their target sequences in ribosomal RNA (rRNA) or small nuclear RNA (snRNA) and to methylate the ribose 2' -hydroxyl group of specific nucleotides. To date the targets of the HBII-85 remain unidentified; it would now be highly important to identify these so that work could begin on developing potential therapies for this debilitating condition.

Germline mutation in NLRP2 (NALP2) in a familial imprinting disorder (Beckwith-Wiedemann Syndrome)

Meyer E, Lim D, Pasha S, Tee LJ, Rahman F, Yates JR, Woods CG, Reik W, Maher ER
Department of Medical and Molecular Genetics, Institute of Biomedical Research, University of Birmingham, Birmingham, UK
e.r.maher@bham.ac.uk
PLoS Genet 2009;5:e1000423

Background: Beckwith-Wiedemann syndrome (BWS) is a fetal overgrowth syndrome characterized by prenatal and postnatal overgrowth, macroglossia and anterior abdominal wall defects and other variable features such as organomegaly, hemihypertrophy, neonatal hypoglycemia and embryonal tumors. It is a human imprinting disorder resulting from the deregulation of a number of genes, including IGF2 and CDKN1C, a candidate tumor suppressor that negatively regulates the cell cycle, in the imprinted gene cluster on chromosome 11p15.5. Most cases are sporadic and result from epimutations at either of the two 11p15.5 imprinting centers (IC1 and IC2). 5–10% of sporadic BWS cases have hypermethylation of the *H19* DMR at IC1 resulting in biallelic expression of *IGF2*. IC2 is a DMR located in intron 10 of the *KCNQ1* gene and is known as KvDMR1; loss of methylation at this locus is observed in up to 50% of sporadic BWS and is associated with biallelic expression of *KCNQ1OT1* and silencing of maternal *CDKN1C* expression. Most BWS patients with IC2 methylation defects appear to have an epimutation of unknown cause. However, rare familial cases may be associated with germline 11p15.5 deletions causing abnormal imprinting in cis. The authors report a consanguineous family with 2 children affected with BWS and an IC2 epimutation; affected siblings had inherited different parental 11p15.5 alleles excluding an in cis mechanism.
Methods: Methylation status of IC1 and IC2 was determined. Linkage studies were performed with a genome-wide linkage scan using the Affymetrix 250k SNP microarray.
Results: Molecular analysis revealed loss of maternal allele KvDMR1 (IC2) methylation in both affected children, but not in an unaffected sibling. Using a positional-candidate gene approach, they found that the mother was homozygous for a frameshift mutation in exon 6 of *NLRP2*. Analysis of methylation levels at the TND (6q24), *SNRPN* (15q13) and *PEG1* (7q32) differentially methylated regions (DMRs) revealed that both affected siblings had normal methylation levels at the TND and *SNRPN* DMRs, but child 2 demonstrated partial loss of methylation at the *PEG1* DMR.
Conclusions: While germline mutations in *NLRP7* have previously been associated with familial hydatidiform mole, this is the first description of *NLRP2* mutation in human disease and the first report of a trans mechanism for disordered imprinting in BWS. These observations are consistent with the hypothesis that *NLRP2* plays a previously unrecognized role in establishing or maintaining genomic imprinting in humans, in keeping with previous data suggesting that mutations in *NLRP7* can cause imprinting disorders in which epimutations at imprinted loci result from a *trans* effect.

This is potentially a highly important study that sheds a novel insight on the etiology of BWS, a disorder of imprinting. The familial case with an IC2 epimutation, with a homozygous mutation in the maternal *NLRP2* gene, reveals a role for this gene in the regulation of genomic imprinting in humans. Of note, homozygous inactivating mutations in the related gene *NLRP7*, which incidentally does not have a rodent homolog, are associated with abnormal imprinting and recurrent hydatidiform moles [8]. *NLRP2* and *NLRP7* encode members of the NLRP (nucleotide-binding oligomerization domain, leucine-rich repeat and pyrin domain) family of CATERPILLER proteins, of which 14 members have been identified and are encoded by two gene clusters on 11p15 and 19q13.4 (including *NLRP2* and *NLRP7*). Some NLRP proteins are components of the inflammasome that is implicated in sensing of, and inflammatory reaction to, extracellular pathogens and intracellular noxious compounds. It is important to note that the 2 family members who were homozygous for a *NLRP2* truncating mutation in this study did not show any evidence of an immune or autoinflammatory disorder. However, most NLRP family proteins are widely expressed, including the immune system, in human oocytes, and in embryos at an early stage of development. In particular, *NLRP2* and *NLRP7* expression progressively decreases from oocytes to day-3 embryos, and then increases sharply on day 5, suggesting a similar role for the 2 genes in early development/imprinting establishment. Interestingly, the methylation defects in FHM are specific for imprinted loci, and DNA methylation at non-imprinted genes and genes subject to X-inactivation is unaffected. It would appear that NLRP2 mutations have a less severe effect on imprinting than *NLRP7* inactivation. Further study of these genes will shed further light on their role in human development and imprinting.

Severe intrauterine growth retardation and atypical diabetes associated with a translocation breakpoint disrupting regulation of the insulin-like growth factor 2 gene

Murphy R, Baptista J, Holly J, Umpleby AM, Ellard S, Harries LW, Crolla J, Cundy T, Hattersley AT
Institute of Clinical and Biomedical Sciences, Peninsula Medical School, Exeter, UK
andrew.hattersley@pms.ac.uk
J Clin Endocrinol Metab 2008;93:4373–4380

Background: IGF2 is an imprinted gene (predominantly transcribed from the paternally inherited allele), which plays an important role in fetal growth in mice, although no mutations have to date been identified in humans with IUGR. *IGF2* gene expression is regulated by a complex system of enhancers and promoters that determine tissue-specific and development-specific transcription.

Methods: A woman of short adult stature (height –3 SDS), born with severe intrauterine growth retardation (birth weight –5.4 SDS), atypical diabetes secondary to insulin resistance, a body mass index of 21.1at the age of 23 years and lactation failure, was found to harbor a balanced chromosomal translocation t(1;11) (p36.22; p15.5). Both chromosomal break points were identified using fluorescent in situ hybridization. Sequence, methylation, and expression of the *IGF2* gene were examined.

Results: The 11p15.5 break point mapped 184 kb telomeric of the *IGF2* gene on the paternally derived chromosome 15p. High-density array CGH confirmed the balanced nature of the translocation. *IGF2* gene sequence and methylation were normal, but expression of the gene was reduced in her mesoderm-derived lymphoblast cells. Hyperinsulinemic, euglycemic clamp studies were performed with glucose tracers, and revealed marked hepatic and total insulin resistance. MRI of the thorax, pelvis and abdomen were performed and revealed an excess of subcutaneous fat.

Conclusion: A breakpoint was identified 184 kb upstream of the paternally derived *IGF2* gene, in a gene-poor region that contains nonskeletal muscle mesodermal-specific enhancers of *IGF2*, with other mesoderm-specific enhancers located between +188 and +273 kB. In the mouse, enhancers of *IGF2* gene expression are located up to 260 kB telomeric to the gene, and this suggests that the breakpoint separates the gene from some telomeric enhancers, and results in reduced expression in some mesoderm-derived adult tissues causing intrauterine growth retardation, short stature, lactation failure, and insulin resistance with altered fat distribution. The authors concluded that her phenotype resulted from disruption of her paternally derived *IGF2* gene because her daughter who inherited the identical translocation had normal birth weight (0.01 SDS at 29 weeks gestation).

IGF2 has been shown to play an important role in the regulation of intrauterine growth in animal studies. *IGF2* gene expression is regulated by a complex system of enhancers and promoters that determine tissue-specific and development-specific transcription. The gene is also imprinted so that in utero and in most tissues post-natally, only the paternal allele is expressed. To date, no human mutations in the *IGF2* gene have been described. However, maternal demethylation of the region containing the *IGF2* gene is associated with overgrowth as part of the Beckwith-Wiedemann syndrome, whereas paternal demethylation of the IGF2 gene regulatory region is associated with intra-uterine growth restriction and short stature in some cases of Silver-Russell syndrome. In this article, the authors describe a chromosomal translocation that would separate the *IGF2* gene from its enhancers and is associated with the phenotype of IUGR and diabetes mellitus, which does not fit within either the type 1 or type 2 disease categories. This interesting paper highlights the critical role of IGF2 in pre- rather than postnatal growth in humans, and also highlights its potential role in the regulation of insulin secretion. The authors comment that the diabetes is probably a combination of insulin insensitivity due to altered body fat distribution as well as probable β-cell failure.

New mutations – without imprinting issues

Growth hormone deficiency and splicing fidelity: two serine/arginine-rich proteins, ASF/SF2 and SC35, act antagonistically

Solis AS, Peng R, Crawford JB, Phillips JA 3rd, Patton JG
Department of Biological Sciences, Vanderbilt University, Nashville, Tenn., USA
james.g.patton@vanderbilt.edu

J Biol Chem 2008;283:23619–23626

Background: The majority of mutations that cause isolated growth hormone deficiency type II are the result of aberrant splicing of transcripts encoding human growth hormone, leading to skipping of exon 3 with the production of a 17.5-kDa protein that acts as a dominant negative to block secretion of the full-length 22-kDa form of hGH generated from unaffected alleles. The most frequent mutations include those at the donor splice site of IVS3, as well as mutations in a purine-rich sequence at the beginning of exon 3 known as an exonic splice enhancer (ESE)1 and an intronic splice enhancer in IVS3. The authors had previously identified a splicing regulatory element in exon 3 [exonic splicing enhancer 2 (ESE2)], but the molecular mechanism by which this element prevents exon skipping is unknown. The aim of this study was to better understand the molecular mechanisms underlying correct splicing of the *GH1* gene, and to therefore understand the pathogenesis of a mutation in ESE2 (A1338G) that is associated with IGHD II.

Methods: Plasmid constructs of the wild-type *GH1*, A1338G *GH1*, and exon 3 deletion mutants were constructed and in vivo splicing assays performed using GH3 (rat somatotroph) cells. In vitro splicing assays were performed. Baculovirus-expressed ASF/SF2, SC35, and SRp20 were purified from infected Sf9 cells. RNA affinity chromatography was performed.

Results: The authors showed that two members of the serine/arginine-rich (SR) protein superfamily (ASF/SF2 and SC35) bind to ESE2 and act antagonistically to regulate exon 3 splicing. ASF/SF2 activates exon 3 inclusion, but SC35, acting through a region just downstream of ESE2, can block such activation. These findings explain the disease-causing mechanism of a patient's mutation in ESE2 that creates a functional SC35-binding site that then acts synergistically with the downstream SC35 site to produce pathological levels of exon 3 skipping.

Conclusion: Although the precedent for SR proteins acting as repressors is established, this is the first example of a patient mutation that creates a site through which an SR protein represses splicing.

IGHD Type II is due to dominant negative mutations in the GH1 gene. Mutations in the donor splice site of IVS3 have been identified at IVS3 +1, 2, 3, 5, 6, and are the most frequent cause of the condition. Mutations in an exonic splice enhancer at the beginning of exon 3 (ESE1) have also been associated with IGHD II, as have mutations in an intronic splice enhancer. Additionally, a number of mis-sense mutations have been associated with the phenotype, and these include R77C, R183H, P89L and V110F. This paper describes the molecular mechanisms underlying splicing. Two members of the serine/arginine (SR) protein superfamily (ASF/SF2 and SC35) bind to ESE2 and act antagonistically to regulate exon 3 splicing. Through some elegant in vitro and in vivo studies, the authors have demonstrated that a heterozygous mutation previously described in the *GH1* gene ESE2 (A1338G) is associated with the creation of a binding site for SC35 that then acts synergistically with the downstream SC35-binding site to repress normal splicing.

The –202 A allele of insulin-like growth factor binding protein-3 (IGFBP3) promoter polymorphism is associated with higher IGFBP-3 serum levels and better growth response to growth hormone treatment in patients with severe growth hormone deficiency

Costalonga EF, Antonini SR, Guerra-Junior G, Mendonca BB, Arnhold IJ, Jorge AA

Unidade de Endocrinologia do Desenvolvimento, Laboratorio de Hormonios e Genetica Molecular, Faculdade de Medicina da Universidade de São Paulo, São Paulo, Brazil

alexj@usp.br

J Clin Endocrinol Metab 2009;94:588–595

Background: The response to recombinant human GH (rhGH) therapy in patients with a variety of disorders including GH deficiency (GHD), Turner syndrome and SGA remains highly variable. Genetic factors that influence the response to rhGH remain mostly unknown, although recent studies have suggested that a polymorphic variant of the gene encoding the GH receptor gene can influence the responsiveness to rhGH. A single-nucleotide polymorphism (SNP) in the IGFBP3 gene promoter (–202 A/C), believed to control basal IGFBP3 promoter activity, has been correlated to circulating concentrations of IGFBP3 in healthy adults, with the AA genotype being associated with highest concentrations of IGFBP3 and the CC genotype being associated with lower IGFBP3 concentrations. The aim of the study was to assess the influence of the polymorphism on circulating IGFBP-3 concentrations and growth response to rhGH therapy in children with GHD.

Methods: –202 A/C IGFBP3 genotyping (rs2854744) was performed using PCR amplification followed by restriction digest and was correlated with data of 71 children with severe GHD who remained prepubertal during the first year of rhGH treatment. Of these, 36 had attained adult height after a mean period of rhGH treatment of 8±3 years. IGFBP-3 concentrations were measured at the start and near the end of the first year of treatment and first year growth velocity (GV) calculated during rhGH treatment.

Results: The distribution of patients among the different –202 *IGFBP3* genotypes was 21% AA, 54% AC, and 25% CC. Clinical and laboratory data at the start of treatment were indistinguishable among patients with different –202 A/C IGFBP3 genotypes, although patients with one or two copies of the –202 C IGFBP3 allele had a tendency to lower IGFBP3 concentrations, but this did not reach statistical significance. Despite similar rhGH doses, AA patients had higher IGFBP3 concentrations and higher mean GV in the first year of rhGH treatment than patients with AC or CC genotypes (first year GV, AA = 13.0 ± 2.1 cm/year, AC = 11.4 ± 2.5 cm/year, and CC = 10.8 ± 1.9 cm/year; p = 0.016). Multiple linear regression analyses demonstrated that the influence of –202 A/C IGFBP3 genotype on IGFBP-3 concentrations and GV during the first year of rhGH treatment was independent of other variables. There was a tendency for better final height outcomes in patients with the AA –202 IGFBP3 genotype, although the difference did not reach statistical significance.

Conclusion: The –202 A allele of IGFBP3 promoter region is associated with increased IGFBP-3 concentrations and GV during rhGH treatment in prepubertal GHD children. Patients with at least one C allele had a mean GV that was 1.9cm/year lower than that of patients homozygous for the A allele. Although there was a tendency to improved final height in AA patients, this effect did not reach statistical significance.

The last few years have focused on the pharmacogenomics of rhGH treatment, with considerable debate generated with respect to the effect of a polymorphic variant of the GH receptor (d3-GHR) that results in deletion of exon 3, on the growth response to rhGH treatment. A number of papers have been published that show an improved growth velocity in patients who carry either a single or both d3-GHR alleles [9–11], whereas other studies fail to confirm these observations [12, 13]. The effects on growth velocity are generally small (e.g. 1.7 cm/year). It would appear likely that other genetic variants may also contribute to the marked variability in growth rate. GH promotes growth mainly via IGF-I; transport of the latter in serum is mediated mostly by IGF-binding protein-3 (IGFBP-3) and acid labile subunit. IGFBP-3 can also modulate the bioactivity of IGF-I. Twin studies have indicated that approximately 60% of the inter-individual variability in circulating levels of IGFBP-3 is genetically determined. Deal et al. [14] have identified a number of SNPs in the promoter region of *IGFBP3*. Of these the most relevant is a SNP (A–C nucleotide change) located at –202, upstream of the transcription start site. The AA genotype is associated with higher mean IGFBP-3 concentrations, and the latter decline with the presence of the C allele. In vitro studies have confirmed the higher promoter activity of the A allele in comparison to the C allele. In this article, the authors reveal that the

A allele is associated with an improved response with respect to both IGFBP3 and growth velocity during the first year of GH treatment in a cohort of prepubertal children with severe GHD. It will be important to investigate whether this finding holds true in other GHD cohorts, as well as children with Turner syndrome and SGA. In such children, slight differences in GH sensitivity are likely to be counterbalanced by a corresponding increase in GH secretion. Additionally, it would be important to follow these cohorts up with a view to obtaining longer-term data – in particular, does the presence of the A allele lead to an taller final height?

An agonist-induced conformational change in the growth hormone receptor determines the choice of signalling pathway

Rowlinson SW, Yoshizato H, Barclay JL, Brooks AJ, Behncken SN, Kerr LM, Millard K, Palethorpe K, Nielsen K, Clyde-Smith J, Hancock JF, Waters MJ
Institute for Molecular Bioscience and School of Biomedical Sciences, University of Queensland, Brisbane, Australia
mwaters@imb.uq.edu.au
Nat Cell Biol 2008;10:740–747

Background: The growth and metabolic actions of growth hormone (GH) are believed to be mediated through the GH receptor (GHR) by JAK2 activation. The GHR exists as a constitutive homodimer, with signal transduction by ligand-induced realignment of receptor subunits.
Methods and Results: Based on the crystal structures, the authors identified a conformational change in the F'G' loop of the lower cytokine module, which results from binding of hGH but not the G120R hGH antagonist. Mutations disabling this conformational change cause impairment of ERK but not JAK2 and STAT5 activation by the GHR in FDC-P1 cells. This results from the use of two associated tyrosine kinases by the GHR, with JAK2 activating STAT5, and Lyn activating ERK1/2. The authors provide evidence that Lyn signals through phospholipase C', leading to activation of Ras. Accordingly, mice with mutations in the JAK2 association motif respond to GH with activation of hepatic Src and ERK1/2, but not JAK2/STAT5.
Conclusions: These data suggest that F'G' loop movement alters the signaling choice between JAK2 and a Src family kinase by regulating transmembrane domain realignment. This could explain attenuated ERK but not STAT5 signaling in some GH-resistant patients and suggest pathway-specific cytokine agonists.

The group of Mike Waters has once again performed an impressive piece of work that sheds novel insights into the function of the GHR. They suggest that separate tyrosine kinases associated with the GHR, namely Lyn and JAK2, are activated by different subunit alignments of the GHR dependent on the involvement of the F'G' loop within the GHR. They showed several years ago that GHR activation is initiated by a twist of the transmembrane domains of the 2 dimerized GHR molecules, brought about by GH binding [15]. This is believed to bring two GHR-associated JAK molecules in closer proximity, which results in activation of their kinase activity and subsequent further activation of the JAK-STAT5 pathway. Although it is known that GH can also activate other signaling pathways (MAPK-ERK1/2-RAS and PI3K pathways), it is unclear what triggers the activation of these other pathways and whether the pathways can be activated independently.

In this work, Rowlinson et al. compared GHR bound to hGH or to the G120R-hGH antagonist Pegvisomant which we know is unable to activate GHR signaling, and found a difference in the 3D structure in a 6 amino acid loop (F'G') of the ligand-GHR complexes. They continued to show that GHR F'G' loop mutations result in impaired ERK signaling, and a slightly impaired proliferation rate, but do not affect JAK-Stat signaling. Using siRNA they showed that the kinase involved in this pathway is not JAK2 but Lyn. Box 1 in the GHR is necessary for association of JAK2 with the GHR and mice with a mutated Box1 were therefore generated. These mice are indeed unable to activate the JAK-STAT pathway but able to activate ERK1/2, and no doubt we will soon hear about the growth phenotype of these mice.

This work suggests that the choice of multiple kinases (JAK, Lyn) facilitates a choice of signaling pathways. The ratio of Lyn and JAK may determine signaling, and this may be a means to allow for cell type-specific signaling. It also suggests that GH-induced MAP-ERK signaling plays a role in cell proliferation. For clinical medicine, this offers not only an explanation for cases of short stature with impaired ERK signaling but normal JAK-STAT signaling [16] but also opens the door to develop signaling pathway-specific drugs.

New concepts

IGFBP-4 is an inhibitor of canonical Wnt signalling required for cardiogenesis

Zhu W, Shiojima I, Ito Y, Li Z, Ikeda H, Yoshida M, Naito AT, Nishi J, Ueno H, Umezawa A, Minamino T, Nagai T, Kikuchi A, Asashima M, Komuro I
Department of Cardiovascular Science and Medicine, Chiba University Graduate School of Medicine, Chiba, Japan
komuro-tky@umin.ac.jp
Nature 2008;454:345–349

Background: Some of the actions of IGFBPs have been reported to be independent of IGFs, but the precise mechanisms of IGF-independent actions of IGFBPs are largely unknown. A previously unknown function for IGFBP-4 as a cardiogenic growth factor is reported.
Methods and Results: IGFBP-4 enhanced cardiomyocyte differentiation in vitro and knockdown of *Igfbp4* attenuated cardiomyogenesis both in vitro and in vivo. The cardiogenic effect of IGFBP-4 was independent of its IGF-binding activity but was mediated by the inhibitory effect on canonical Wnt signaling. IGFBP-4 physically interacted with a Wnt receptor, Frizzled 8 (Frz8), and a Wnt co-receptor, low-density lipoprotein receptor-related protein 6 (LRP6), and inhibited the binding of Wnt3A to Frz8 and LRP6. Although IGF-independent, the cardiogenic effect of IGFBP-4 was attenuated by IGFs through IGFBP-4 sequestration.
Conclusions: IGFBP-4 is an inhibitor of the canonical Wnt signaling pathway required for cardiogenesis and provides a molecular link between IGF signaling and Wnt signaling.

This work set out to identify factors required for cardiogenesis. The experimental approach was extremely elegant, the experiments starting out to test conditioned cell media from various cell types for cardiomyocyte induction in a cardiomyocyte progenitor cell line in vitro. To then identify the cardiogenic factor, cDNA clones from the cell line were isolated and tested for their cardiomyocyte induction and thus IGFBP4 was identified.

The heart is the first organ to form during embryogenesis and abnormalities in this process result in congenital heart defects. The authors gave overwhelming evidence that IGFBP4 is involved in heart formation by inhibiting Wnt signaling. It does so after secretion, by physical direct binding to LRP6 and Frizzled-8, cell surface receptors for Wnt. Knockdown of *Igfbp4* in Xenopus embryos revealed the impact of IGFBP4 since 70% of the embryos had a small heart or no heart at all. Interestingly, IGFBP4 is expressed in the embryonic liver, just adjacent to the heart and likely affects the heart in a paracrine fashion. Conversely, the heart secretes factors that affect the liver in a paracrine fashion. IGFBP1, 2 and 6 had a similar, but more modest effect on Wnt inhibition. This suggests genetic redundancy and may account for the fact that Igfbp4-null mice lack a cardiac phenotype. The identification of IGFBP4 as a secreted modulator of heart development shows once again that IGFBPs have a life of their own, and will pave the way for further research into potential applications of IGFBPs.

Neurofibromin regulates somatic growth through the hypothalamic-pituitary axis

Hegedus B, Yeh TH, Lee da Y, Emnett RJ, Li J, Gutmann DH
Department of Neurology, Washington University School of Medicine, St Louis, Mo., USA
gutmannd@neuro.wustl.edu
Hum Mol Genet 2008;17:2956–2966

Background: Neurofibromatosis type 1 (NF1) is associated with short stature in 13–18% of patients. A significant proportion of patients have associated growth hormone deficiency (GHD). The mechanism whereby the condition leads to short stature remains unknown. Neurofibromin is thought to primarily regulate cell growth by modulating Ras activity.
Methods: To study the role of the neurofibromatosis-1 (*NF1*) gene in mammalian brain development, the authors generated mice in which *Nf1* gene inactivation occurs in neuroglial progenitor cells using the brain lipid-binding protein (BLBP) promoter.
Results: Nf1(BLBP)CKO mice exhibit significant reductions in body weight and anterior pituitary gland size. The authors further demonstrate that the small anterior pituitary size reflects loss of neurofibromin expression in the hypothalamus rather than the pituitary, leading to reduced growth hormone-releasing hormone, pituitary growth hormone (GH) and liver insulin-like growth factor-1 (IGF1) production, with a reduction in the number of proliferating cells within the anterior pituitary. Since neurofibromin both negatively regulates Ras activity and positively modulates cAMP levels, the authors examined the signaling pathway responsible for these abnormalities. BLBP-mediated expression of an activated Ras molecule did not recapitulate the body weight and hypothalamic/pituitary defects, and conditional expression of the Ras regulatory GAP domain of neurofibromin did not rescue the growth phenotype of Nf1(BLBP)CKO mice, suggesting that the hypothalamo-pituitary abnormalities associated with neurofibromin loss in the brain are not Ras-dependent. There was a 50% reduction in the levels of cAMP in Nf1(BLBP)CKO hypothalamic homogenates compared with littermate controls. Rolipram, a specific phosphodiesterase-4 inhibitor that elevates CREB activation in the brain and increases cAMP levels, resulted in a partial restoration of the body weight phenotype.
Conclusion: These data demonstrate a critical role for neurofibromin in hypothalamic-pituitary axis function, in part via the modulation of intracellular cAMP levels, and provide further insights into the short stature and GH deficits seen in children with NF1.

Short stature is a relatively common complication of NF1. In the largest study of pituitary function in children with NF1 and short stature, nearly 80% (15/19) of the children were found to have growth hormone deficiency in the absence of suprasellar abnormalities on neuroimaging. The NF1 gene, termed neurofibromin, functions as a negative regulator of Ras. Loss of *Nf1* activity results in increased Ras activity and downstream MAPK/Akt signaling. In this study, the authors show that neurofibromin regulates the function of the hypothalamo-pituitary axis, and that loss of *Nf1* in the brain leads to decreased GHRH, GH and IGF1 levels with anterior pituitary hypoplasia. It would appear that the growth retardation observed in *Nf1* mutant mice may be the result of a primary neuronal defect, since inactivation of the *Nf1* gene in embryonic neural stem/progenitor cells within the developing CNS was associated with a growth defect and anterior pituitary hypoplasia. Additionally, the reduction in cAMP levels in mice deficient in neurofibromin may in part account for the GH deficiency, as both cAMP and CREB are major regulators of hypothalamic development. cAMP is critical for hypothalamic neuronal maturation whereas brain-specific loss of CREB results in hypopituitarism and dwarfism. Hence this paper has identified for the first time a role for neurofibromin in the regulation of hypothalamic function and pituitary development in the mammalian CNS by modulating intracellular cAMP levels. Interestingly, despite the reduced body weights and organ sizes, the brain weights of Nf1 KO mice were unchanged. These disproportionate changes result in relative megalencephaly, similar to what has been reported for children with NF1. This could reflect increased numbers of glial precursors, oligodendrocytes or astrocytes. In support of this hypothesis, magnetic resonance imaging studies have found increases in both grey and white matter volumes in the brains of children with neurofibromatosis type 1.

Glutamate acting on N-methyl-D-aspartate receptors attenuates insulin-like growth factor-1 receptor tyrosine phosphorylation and its survival signaling properties in rat hippocampal neurons

Zheng WH, Quirion R

Department of Psychiatry, Douglas Mental Health University Institute, McGill University, Montreal, Que., Canada
remi.quirion@douglas.mcgill.ca
J Biol Chem 2009;284:855–861

Background: Excess glutamate may play an important role in neurodegenerative processes and neuronal survival. However, the underlying mechanism is unclear.

Methods and Results: Using hippocampal neuronal cell culture, the authors show that glutamate treatment or pretreatment attenuates the tyrosine phosphorylation of the insulin-like growth factor-1 (IGF-1) receptor and adapter proteins (IRS-1 and Shc) and the survival effect of IGF-1. The effect of glutamate was also evident on other molecules in the IGF1 signaling pathway like PI3K and Akt, as well as down-stream targets GSK3β and FOXO3a. The N-methyl-D-aspartate (NMDA) receptor, one of several glutamate receptors, was involved in this process, since the effect was blocked by antagonists of the NMDA receptor, but not by blockers of ionotropic or metabotropic glutamate receptors. In addition, treatment with NMDA inhibited the activation and phosphorylation of IGF-1 receptors and downstream targets induced by IGF-1.

Conclusions: Glutamate can block the effect of IGF-1 by decreasing IGF-1 receptor signaling and responsiveness, hence attenuating the survival properties of this trophic factor in neuronal cells. The results suggest a novel mechanism by which glutamate can reduce cell viability and induce neurotoxicity.

These experiments link two pathways involved in neuronal death and survival. Glutamate is a neurotransmittor involved in multiple neuronal processes in the developing and adult brain, like neurogenesis, synaptogenesis and neurite outgrowth. It plays a major role in several neurodegenerative diseases as well as in hypoxic-ischemic neuronal death and is believed to impair neuron survival. In contrast, IGF1 has an established role in cell survival and is suggested to have neuroprotective effects. The experiments in this paper are straightforward and indeed show that glutamate, through the NMDA receptor rather than other glutamate receptors, impairs the activation of IGF-R signaling pathway and neuron survival in vitro, without affecting the number of IGF1-R. This offers a piece for the mechanistic puzzle of the actions of glutamate on neuron survival. However, the experiments do suggest that IGF1 treatment does not overcome glutamate-induced cell death. Current efforts to improve clinical outcome of brain injury focus on reducing glutamate exposure to injured neurons [17] as well as on manipulating the IGF1 pathway [18], and that approach seems justified.

The circadian clock components CRY1 and CRY2 are necessary to sustain sex dimorphism in mouse liver metabolism

Bur IM, Cohen-Solal AM, Carmignac D, Abecassis PY, Chauvet N, Martin AO, van der Horst GT, Robinson IC, Maurel P, Mollard P, Bonnefont X

CNRS, UMR 5203, Institut de Génomique Fonctionnelle and INSERM, U661 and Université Montpellier, Montpellier, France
Bonnefont@igf.cnrs.fr
J Biol Chem 2009;284:9066–9073

Background: Hepatic enzyme activity is sexually dimorphic in mice and many other mammals including humans and is responsible for, e.g., sexually dimorphic steroid synthesis and drug metabolism. Hepatic enzyme activity however is also a noticeable target of circadian timekeeping. Whether the circadian clock itself contributes to sex-biased metabolism has remained unknown.

Methods: Mice with a deletion of the circadian regulators Cryptochromes Cry1 and Cry2 (Cry1/2–/– mice) were used to study growth, growth hormone production and downstream effects of GH.

Results: Dimorphic liver metabolism is altered in double mutant Cry1/2–/– male mice that lack a functional circadian clock. Expression of a number of sex-specific liver products, including several cytochrome P450 enzymes, are at levels close to those measured in normal females. In addition, body growth of Cry1/2-deficient mice is impaired, also in a sex-biased manner, and this phenotype goes along with an altered pattern of circulating growth hormone (GH) in mutant males, specifically. Hormonal injections that mimic male GH pulses reverse the feminized gene expression profile in the liver of Cry1/2–/– males.

Conclusions: This work suggests that the 24-hour clock paces the dimorphic ultradian pulsatility of GH that is responsible for sex-dependent liver activity. Circadian timing, sex dimorphism, and liver metabolism are thus finely interconnected.

Many physiological processes have a circadian rhythm and are regulated by our body clock. This body clock has a central master circadian pacemaker, residing in the suprachiasmatic nucleus, and a peripheral component, located in peripheral cells like adipocytes, myocytes and hepatocytes and dictates a circadian rhythm in these cells. As a result, transcription of genes involved in processes like gluconeogenesis, nitrogen metabolism and drug metabolism are circadian, and this probably allows anticipation of, for example, nutrient availability. The timing mechanism of both the central and peripheral clocks consists of a transcriptional/translational feedback mechanism of 'clock genes' consisting of the negative regulators Period (Per) and Cryptochrome (Cry), and the positive regulators Clock and Bmal.

Hepatic enzyme activity is sexually dimorphic in mice and humans and the sexual dimorphism is partly dependent on sexually dimorphic GH-secretory patterns and JAK-STAT signaling.

The central and peripheral clocks are disturbed in Cry1/2 null mice and the authors therefore used this model to establish whether the circadian rhythm and GH secretion interact in the regulation of sexually dimorphic hepatic metabolism. Interestingly, they found that indeed interference in the circadian clock disturbs sexually dimorphic hepatic P450 cytochrome enzyme expression but also GH secretion pattern and body growth. Reintroduction of a pulsatile (male) GH secretory pattern re-masculinized some of the hepatic enzyme expression. This suggests that the circadian rhythm is a major regulator of GH secretory patterns thereby affecting growth and hepatic metabolism. For more on peripheral circadian clock, see *Editors' choice.*

Important for clinical practice – tall tales and more imprinting

Treatment of pituitary gigantism with the growth hormone receptor antagonist pegvisomant

Goldenberg N, Racine MS, Thomas P, Degnan B, Chandler W, Barkan A
University of Michigan Medical Center, Division of MEND, Department of Internal Medicine, Ann Arbor, Mich., USA
abarkan@umich.edu
J Clin Endocrinol Metab 2008;93:2953–2956

Background: Pituitary gigantism is a rare disorder characterized by excessive secretion of GH from a somatotroph pituitary tumor. Treatment of pituitary gigantism is complex, entailing the use of surgery, radiotherapy and medical therapy in the form of somatostatin analogs or dopamine agonists, and the results are usually unsatisfactory. The authors of the study describe the results of therapy of 3 children with pituitary gigantism by a GH receptor antagonist, pegvisomant.

Methods: This was a descriptive case series of up to 3.5 years duration at a university hospital. Patients included 3 children (1 female, 2 males) with pituitary gigantism whose GH hypersecretion was incompletely controlled by surgery, somatostatin analog, and dopamine agonist, and who were then treated by the administration of pegvisomant. Plasma IGF-I and growth velocity were measured on the pegvisomant.

Results: In all 3 children, pegvisomant rapidly decreased plasma IGF-I concentrations and growth velocity. Statural growth fell into lower growth percentiles and acromegalic features resolved. Pituitary tumor size did not change in 2 children but increased in 1 boy despite concomitant therapy with a somatostatin analog.

Conclusions: Pegvisomant may be an effective modality for the therapy of pituitary gigantism in children. Titration of the dose is necessary for optimal efficacy, and regular surveillance of tumor size is mandatory.

\This important study adds another therapeutic agent that can be used to treat a rare but potentially devastating disorder, namely pituitary gigantism. Pituitary gigantism can be extremely difficult to treat, often necessitating a combination of surgery, radiotherapy and medical treatment in the form of somatostatin analogs. This study describes the use of a GH antagonist, pegvisomant, in 3 children with pituitary gigantism in whom surgery had failed to cure the excess GH secretion. Initiation of pegvisomant therapy led to a reduction in height velocity with a concomitant reduction in IGF-I concentrations, along with improvement in clinical features such as soft tissue hypertrophy and acromegaloid features. In 2 of the 3 patients, the tumor size remained stable whereas in the 3rd patient it increased, but then stabilized following the cessation of pegvisomant. Pegvisomant binds to the GH receptor and prevents dimerization and subsequent receptor-mediated activity, thus reducing GH-dependent IGF-I generation. One of the drawbacks is an elevation in GH concentrations due to removal of IGF-I-mediated negative feedback. Additionally, an increase in tumor size may ensue on pegvisomant treatment, necessitating the combined use of a somatostatin analog. Hence, although the prompt and sustained improvement in clinical features makes pegvisomant therapy attractive, tumor size must be carefully monitored on therapy.

Clinically distinct epigenetic subgroups in Silver-Russell syndrome: the degree of H19 hypomethylation associates with phenotype severity and genital and skeletal anomalies

Bruce S, Hannula-Jouppi K, Peltonen J, Kere J, Lipsanen-Nyman M
Department of Biosciences and Nutrition, Karolinska Institutet, Huddinge, Sweden
Marita.Lipsanen@hus.fi
J Clin Endocrinol Metab 2009;94:579–587

Background: Silver-Russell syndrome (SRS) is characterized by severe fetal onset growth restriction and variable dysmorphism including relative macrocephaly, triangular facies, skeletal asymmetry and hemihypertrophy, and clinodactyly. Maternal uniparental disomy of chromosome 7 (matUPD7) has been identified in 5–10% of SRS patients. Recently, the H19 imprinting control region (ICR), located on chromosome 11p15.5, has been reported to be hypomethylated in 20–65% of SRS patients.

Methods: The authors investigated the methylation status of 11p15.5 ICRs (H19 and KCNQ1OT1) in 42 SRS patients including 7 matUPD7 patients, and 90 small-for-gestational age (SGA) children without SRS to clarify the relationship between phenotype and H19 methylation status. Clinical data were evaluated from patient records, and 7 hypomethylated patients were clinically and radiologically reexamined.

Results: Hypomethylation of H19 ICR was found in 62% of SRS patients but in no SGA children. A clinical severity score demonstrated strong correlation between the hypomethylation level and phenotype severity. Hypomethylation related to a more severe SRS phenotype, in which asymmetry and micrognathia were especially more common. Extremely hypomethylated patients (<9%) had severe pre- and postnatal growth retardation, relative macrocephaly, asymmetry and 5th finger clinodactyly. Additionally, genital abnormalities were present in the majority: congenital aplasia of the uterus and upper vagina, equivalent to the Mayer-Rokitansky-Küster-Hauser syndrome in females, and cryptorchidism and testicular agenesis in males. In the moderately H19 hypomethylated individuals (9–35%), although many of the classical features were present, the patients were not significantly smaller at birth or 2 years, although they tended to be thinner and shorter at 2 years. Skeletal abnormalities such as abnormally high lumbar vertebrae, lumbar hypomobility, elbow subluxations, and distinct hand and foot anomalies, were more likely in the more severely hypomethylated patients. On the other hand, none of the matUPD7 patients showed a triangular face, and they had a lower incidence of asymmetry, 5th finger clino- and brachydactyly, cryptorchidism, toe syndactyly, muscle hypotonia, crowded teeth and a high arched palate. However, matUPD7 patients presented more frequently with speech delay, feeding difficulties, a high-pitched voice, low set/abnormal ears and excessive sweating.

Conclusions: This study reports a dose-response relationship between the degree of *H19* hypomethylation and phenotype severity in SRS, suggesting that 35% of the variation in clinical severity was explained by the degree of *H19* hypomethylation. The authors report for the first time the association of specific anomalies of the spine, elbows, hands and feet, and genital defects in SRS with severe *H19* hypomethylation. Classical SRS features were found in *H19* hypomethylation and milder symptoms in maternal uniparental disomy of chromosome 7, thus distinguishing two separate clinical and etiological subgroups.

It is now clear that Silver-Russell syndrome is a highly heterogeneous condition. This and previous studies [19] have revealed possible (epi)genotype-phenotype correlations. H19 ICR hypomethylation appears to be the most frequent genetic abnormality identified in patients with SRS, and is associated with a more severe phenotype than matUPD7. Within the hypomethylation cohort, the degree of methylation seemed to correlate with the phenotype, the most severe degree of hypomethylation being associated with the asymmetry, skeletal and urogenital abnormalities. It remains to be established whether long-term outlook will also correlate with the genotype of these patients, and only careful long-term follow-up will allow us to answer such questions.

New hope – inhibition of IGF1 signaling

Characterization of inhibitory anti-insulin-like growth factor receptor antibodies with different epitope specificity and ligand-blocking properties: implications for mechanism of action in vivo

Doern A, Cao X, Sereno A, Reyes CL, Altshuler A, Huang F, Hession C, Flavier A, Favis M, Tran H, Ailor E, Levesque M, Murphy T, Berquist L, Tamraz S, Snipas T, Garber E, Shestowsky WS, Rennard R, Graff CP, Wu X, Snyder W, Cole L, Gregson D, Shields M, Ho SN, Reff ME, Glaser SM, Dong J, Demarest SJ, Hariharan K
Biogen Idec, San Diego, Calif., USA and Applied Photophysics Limited, Leatherhead, Surrey, UK
stephen.demarest@biogenidec.com
J Biol Chem 2009;284:10254–10267

Background: Antibodies directed against the type 1 insulin-like growth factor receptor (IGF-1R) have recently gained significant momentum because of their potential use in cancer treatment. These antibodies inhibit ligand-mediated activation of IGF-1R and the resulting down-stream signaling cascade.
Methods and Results: The authors generated a panel of antibodies against IGF-1R and screened them for their ability to block the binding of IGF-1 or IGF-2. Four distinct inhibitory classes were found as follows: (1) allosteric IGF-1 blockers, (2) allosteric IGF-2 blockers, (3) allosteric IGF-1 and IGF-2 blockers, and (4) competitive IGF-1 and IGF-2 blockers. The epitopes of representative antibodies from each of these classes were mapped using a purified IGF-1R library containing 64 mutations. Most of these antibodies bound overlapping surfaces on the cysteine-rich repeat and L2 domains. One class of allosteric IGF-1 and IGF-2 blockers was identified that bound a separate epitope on the outer surface of the FnIII-1 domain. The dual IGF blockers inhibited ligand binding using a spectrum of mechanisms ranging from highly allosteric to purely competitive. The data also suggest that IGF-1R uses disorder/order within its polypeptide sequence to regulate its activity. The activity of representative allosteric and competitive inhibitors on H322M tumor cell growth in vitro was reflective of their individual ligand-blocking properties.
Conclusions: Many of the clinically used antibodies likely adopt one of the inhibitory mechanisms described, and the outcome of future clinical studies may reveal whether a particular inhibitory mechanism leads to optimal clinical efficacy.

Apart from regulating normal growth, IGF1 and IGF2 play a role in tumor formation, at least partly due to their actions on proliferation, cell survival and angiogenesis through IGF1R. Expression of IGF1/IGF2 or IGF1R is increased in many human malignancies, for example in tumors of the breast, lung, gastrointestinal tract, prostate and bladder [20]. Antibody-mediated inhibition of IGF1-R activity may therefore offer a new therapeutic strategy, and this idea has been taken forward in trials. However, activity and toxicity of antibodies differ, likely due to their specific inhibitory effect on the IGF1/IGF2–IGF1R interaction. This study has evaluated the mechanism of action for a large number of antibodies. Four different classes of action were found: allosteric inhibition of IGF1 binding, allosteric inhibition of IGF2 binding, allosteric inhibiton of both IGF1 and IGF2 binding and competitive inhibition of IGF1 and IGF2 binding. Allosteric inhibition refers to a decreased affinity of a ligand due to action on a site different from the ligand-binding site, and is likely due to a conformational change of the IGF1R but does not block IGF1 or IGF2 action completely. Competitive inhibition however can block action completely and differentiation between these categories is therefore relevant. The authors showed that the in vitro inhibition of tumor growth indeed reflected the individual ligand-blocking properties for some antibodies tested. Using a panel of 64 mutated IGF1-R molecules, binding domains of many antibodies were determined.

This work offers a range of new well-characterized IGF1-R antibodies. It also offers a platform to determine the molecular action of IGF-R antibodies and suggest that most antibodies will fit in one of the four classes. Determining the molecular action of an antibody may allow for the prediction of their clinical actions and this work may therefore help to advance the field of cancer treatment.

New mechanism – for an old question

Growth hormone-releasing hormone as an agonist of the ghrelin receptor GHS-R1a

Casanueva FF, Camiña JP, Carreira MC, Pazos Y, Varga JL, Schally AV
Laboratory of Molecular and Cellular Endocrinology, Research Area, Complejo Hospitalario Universitario de Santiago, Santiago de Compostela, Spain
felipe.casanueva@usc.es

Proc Natl Acad Sci USA 2008;105:20452–20457

Background: Ghrelin synergizes with growth hormone-releasing hormone (GHRH) to potentiate growth hormone (GH) response through a mechanism not yet fully characterized. Additionally, ghrelin is implicated in energy homeostasis, and may contribute to the metabolic syndrome. This study was conducted to analyze the role of GHRH as a potential ligand of the ghrelin receptor, GHS-R1a.

Methods: HEK293 cells were stably transfected with GHS-R1a (HEK-GHSR1a) conjugated with enhanced green fluorescent protein fluorophore. Membrane-binding assays were performed using HEK-293 and HEK-GHSR1a cells. Measurement of intracellular cAMP and inositol phosphate and chemical cross-linking assays were performed.

Results: hGHRH(1–29)NH(2) (GHRH) induces a dose-dependent calcium mobilization in HEK293 cells stably transfected with GHS-R1a, an effect not observed in wild-type HEK293 cells. This calcium rise is also observed using the GHRH receptor agonists JI-34 and JI-36. HEK-GHSR1a membranes showed a higher binding capacity of ^{125}I-GHRH that was displaced by unlabelled GHRH, as well as ghrelin. The presence of increasing amounts of GHRH cooperatively exerted a significant and dose-dependent increase in the ^{125}I-ghrelin-binding capacity in HEK-GHSR1a cells. Radioligand binding and cross-linking studies revealed that the calcium response to GHRH is mediated by the ghrelin receptor GHS-R1a. GHRH activates the signaling route of inositol phosphate and potentiates the maximal response to ghrelin measured in inositol phosphate turnover. In addition, confocal microscopy in CHO cells transfected with GHS-R1a tagged with enhanced green fluorescent protein shows that GHRH activates GHS-R1a endocytosis. Furthermore, the selective GHRH-R antagonists, JV-1-42 and JMR-132, act also as antagonists of the ghrelin receptor GHS-R1a.

Conclusion: The study findings suggest that GHRH interacts with the ghrelin receptor GHS-R1a and, in consequence, modifies the ghrelin-associated intracellular signaling pathway. This interaction may represent a form of regulation, which could play a putative role in the physiology of GH regulation and appetite control.

From its very early research the GH secretagogs showed synergism with GHRH in the release of GH [21]. This paper describes a possible mechanism whereby GHRH and ghrelin synergistically release GH. GHRH interacts with the ghrelin receptor GHS-R1, and allosterically enhances ghrelin action, displaying positive binding cooperation. Binding of GHRH to GHS-R1 then activates the signaling route of inositol phosphate and this in turn leads to a rise in intracellular calcium. Finally, GHRH leads to endocytosis of GHS-R1. The complete elucidation of this process will aid in understanding the interaction between GHRH and ghrelin and its impact on GH secretion and appetite control, and hence in understanding regulation of growth in terms of both height and weight.

The hormonal action of IGF1 in postnatal mouse growth

Stratikopoulos E, Szabolcs M, Dragatsis I, Klinakis A, Efstratiadis A
Department of Genetics and Development, Columbia University, New York, N.Y., USA
ae4@columbia.edu
Proc Natl Acad Sci USA 2008;105:19378–19383

Background: IGF1 is secreted by the liver and circulates in plasma. However, whether it acts systemically as a classical hormone to stimulate growth has been disputed since a conditional, liver-specific Igf1 gene knockout in mice (LID mice) significantly reduced the level of serum IGF1, but did not affect average body weight. Because alternate interpretations of these negative data are tenable, the Efstratiadis group addressed genetically the question of systemic IGF1 action by using a positive experimental strategy based on the cre/loxP recombination system.
Methods: Bitransgenic mice were generated that carry in an *Igf1* null background a dormant *Igf1* cDNA placed downstream of a transcriptional 'stop' DNA sequence flanked by *loxP* sites ('floxed') and also a *cre* transgene driven by a liver-specific promoter. The *Igf1* cDNA, which was inserted by knock-in into the mutated and inactive *Igf1* locus itself to ensure proper transcriptional regulation, was conditionally expressed from cognate promoters exclusively in the liver after Cre-mediated excision of the floxed block.
Results: 6 different groups of mice were generated. If U = ubiquitous IGF1 expression, L = liver IGF1 expression, and number = number of alleles, groups were 1×U, 2×U, 1×U/1×L, 2×L (=LIP), Null and WT. LIP mice had larger weights and bone size than Null mice from 25 days of age.
Conclusions: The authors conclude that endocrine IGF1 plays a very significant role in mouse growth, as its action contributes approximately 30% of the adult body size and sustains postnatal development, including the reproductive functions of both mouse sexes.

This paper describes an elegantly designed labor-intensive experiment aimed to answer a specific question. The authors generated Igf1 null mice that express Igf1 only in the liver ('LIP' mice for 'Liver IGF1 Producers'), but to ensure that IGF1 was produced in a physiological amount and pattern, they used a genetic approach so that the transgene IGF1 was transcribed under the control of the endogenous IGF1 locus, but in the liver only. As controls, mice were used in which IGF1 should be expressed under its own locus in all tissues. Mice with a gradation of ubiquitous and hepatic IGF1 production (homozygous or heterozygous) were thus available, as well as complete Igf null mice and normal WT mice.

LIP mice were heavier than Null mice from 25 days of age and had larger tibial length at 10 weeks of age. The hierarchy for weight was (% of normal): 2×U 70%, 1×U/1×L 61%, 1×U 54%, LIP 50%, Null 34%, but, as in other experiments, the effect on tibial growth was much smaller (Null 67% of normal). Do the results justify the conclusion that endocrine IGF1 contributes 30% to adult body size though? There are a few unavoidable complications. The efficiency of recombination necessary for *Igf1* transgene expression is beyond control and was low prenatally in LIP mice, so that liver-specific IGF1 production only started postnatally and plasma IGF1 was only 44% of normal at 10 weeks of age. In 2×U mice, the plasma IGF1 concentration ranged from 30% of normal around birth to 50% in adult life and mice were indeed dwarfed. This low level prenatal IGF1 production makes it difficult to compare the control mice to LIP mice or normal mice. High perinatal mortality in LIP and Null mice (90%) meant that only very few mice were available for growth assessment (n = 3/group), and these mice also lost weight after weaning possibly due to feeding difficulties. Interpretation of the data is further complicated by testosterone deficiency in the Null mice.

In conclusion, male LIP mice are larger than male IGF Null mice but how much is being contributed by a deficiency of GH, IGF1, testosterone, malnutrition or catch-up growth, or even by altered local IGF1 sensitivity, remains difficult to assess.

Autocrine IGF-1 action in adipocytes controls systemic IGF-1 concentrations and growth

Klöting N, Koch L, Wunderlich T, Kern M, Ruschke K, Krone W, Brüning JC, Blüher M
Department of Medicine, University of Leipzig, Leipzig, Germany
jens.bruening@uni-koeln.de
Diabetes 2008;57:2074–2082

Background: IGF1 and IGF1 receptor (IGF-1R) have been implicated in the regulation of adipocyte differentiation and lipid accumulation in vitro.
Methods: To investigate the role of IGF-1 receptors in vivo, the authors have inactivated the *Igf1r* gene in adipose tissue (IGF1R-aP2Cre mice) using conditional gene targeting strategies.
Results: IGF1R-aP2Cre mice had increased adipose tissue mass with more and larger adipocytes with increased lipid accumulation in epigonadal but not subcutaneous fat pads. The IGF1R-depleted adipocytes showed increased insulin receptor mRNA content but whole body insulin and glucose tolerance was unaffected. Surprisingly, IGF1R-aP2Cre mice exhibited markedly increased somatic growth in the presence of elevated IGF1 serum concentrations and IGF1 mRNA expression in liver and adipose tissue. IGF1 stimulation of wild-type adipocytes significantly decreased IGF1 mRNA expression, as expected, but IGF1 mRNA increased in IGF1R-deficient adipocytes upon IGF1 stimulation.
Conclusions: IGF1R signaling in adipocytes is not crucial for the development and differentiation of adipose tissue in vivo. The authors concluded that a negative IGF-1R-mediated feedback mechanism of IGF1 on its own gene expression exists in adipocytes, indicating an unexpected role for adipose tissue IGF1 signaling in the regulation of IGF1 serum concentrations in control of somatic growth. Bartke and Kopchick [22], however suggest, in a letter to the editor, the involvement of altered GH secretion.

This group has taken the reverse strategy to the Efstratiadis group to study the role of IGF1 and created mice that have a tissue-specific deletion of IGF1R. Surprisingly, the adipocyte IGF1R–/– mice showed, apart from increased size of epigonadal fat pads, increased growth. IGF1 mRNA was almost doubled in adipose tissue and liver, systemic IGF1 and IGFBP3 concentrations were increased (20%), and a late onset increase in weight and length (15%) was noted. Since adipocyte IGF1 content was increased, the authors hypothesized that adipose IGF1 signaling regulates serum IGF1 concentration and growth. However, the increase in growth, IGF1 and IGFBP3 production may well reflect increased GH secretion. This is the first of a few models with tissue-specific IGF1R deletion [23, 24] that shows such a marked effect on growth and systemic IGF1 concentrations. This mouse model therefore may not give as much insight as hoped in the (endocrine) effect of IGF1 on adipocytes, but, given the known adverse effect of obesity on GH secretion, may be of great importance in studying the role of adipose tissue in the feedback control of GH secretion.

Brain IGF-1 receptors control mammalian growth and lifespan through a neuroendocrine mechanism

Kappeler L, De Magalhaes Filho CM, Dupont J, Leneuve P, Cervera P, Périn L, Loudes C, Blaise A, Klein R, Epelbaum J, Le Bouc Y, Holzenberger M
Inserm U893, Hôpital Saint-Antoine, Paris, France
martin.holzenberger@ inserm.fr
PLoS Biol 2008;6:e254

Background: Mutations that decrease insulin-like growth factor (IGF) and growth hormone signaling limit body size and prolong lifespan in mice. In vertebrates, the GH-IGF1 axis is controlled by neuroendocrine hormones. Hormone-like regulations discovered in nematodes and flies suggest that IGF signals in the nervous system can determine lifespan, but it is unclear whether this applies to higher organisms.
Methods: Using conditional mutagenesis in the mouse and a Nestin-Cre promoter to target the brain but not pituitary, mice with a brain-specific *Igf1r* deletion were created.
Results: Partial inactivation of *Igf1r* in the embryonic brain selectively inhibited GH and IGF-I pathways after birth. This caused growth retardation, smaller adult size and metabolic alterations, and led to delayed mortality and longer mean lifespan.
Conclusions: Brain IGF1R regulates somatotropic development. Early changes in neuroendocrine development can durably modify the life trajectory in mammals. The underlying mechanism appears to be an

adaptive plasticity of somatotropic functions allowing organisms to decelerate growth and preserve resources, and thereby improve fitness in challenging environments. The results also suggest that tonic somatotropic signaling entails the risk of shortened lifespan.

Kappeler et al. aimed to study the neuronal control of aging through insulin-like signals, and therefore created brain-specific IGF1R null mice. In Yearbook 2008 we discussed the relation between reduced activity of the GH/IGF1 pathway and increased lifespan in a range of species as well as an extensive study of a cohort of centenarians that may suggest a reduced IGF1 action in some of these individuals [1, 25]. Interestingly, brain Igf1r–/– mice are born small but have a similar phenotype as described for the adipose tissue-specific Igf1r deletion: increased (30–40%) serum IGF1 concentrations from the age of 4 weeks and late onset (4 months) increased growth. However, lifespan was unaffected in these homozygous mice and the authors therefore chose to focus on the heterozygous mice that, indeed, on average have an increased lifespan (approx. 10%). They have a mild growth defect (10%) from the age of 3 weeks. The authors showed very nicely that this was due to a specific hypothalamic-pituitary somatotropic dysfunction and that the mice had low hypothalamic GHRH, low Pit1 expression, small pituitaries with low GH content and low systemic IGF1 and ALS concentrations as well as the metabolic consequences of GH deficiency; enlarged adipose tissue and impaired glucose tolerance. The increased average lifespan was mostly due to a lower mortality rate at middle age, but mortality rate at higher age and maximum age reached was not different from controls. These mice show that the IGF1 (feedback) action in the brain regulates the GHRH-GH-IGF axis and suggest that deficient IGF1 action results in protection from death at an early age, at least in mice. Whether the downstream GH/IGF1 deficiency or the neuroendocrine environment is responsible for this protection remains a question. Relative IGF1 deficiency/resistance has been suggested to underlie the regulation of lifespan in some other species and is indeed the common factor between these mice and some centenarians. The question as to why GH deficiency in humans does not seem to enhance lifespan remains unanswered [26]. In the mean time, these mice add nicely to the collection of models for GH deficiency.

Review – going up and down the slopes

Motivations and methods for analyzing pulsatile hormone secretion

Veldhuis JD, Keenan DM, Pincus SM
Endocrine Research Unit, Department of Internal Medicine, Mayo Medical School, Mayo Clinic, Rochester, Minn., USA
Veldhuis.Johannes@mayo.edu

Endocr Rev 2008;29:823–864

Overview: Endocrine glands communicate with remote target cells via a mixture of signal exchange both continuous and intermittent. Continuous signaling allows slowly varying control, whereas intermittency permits large rapid adjustments. The control systems that mediate such homeostatic corrections operate in a species-, gender-, age-, and context-selective fashion. Mechanisms of adaptive interglandular signaling in vivo are becoming more clear. Principal goals are to understand the physiological origins, significance, and mechanisms of pulsatile hormone secretion. Key issues for analysis of pulsatile secretion are: (1) to quantify the number, size, shape, and uniformity of pulses, nonpulsatile (basal) secretion, and elimination kinetics; (2) to evaluate regulation of the axis as a whole, and (3) to reconstruct dose-response interactions without disrupting hormone connections.
Conclusion: This review focuses on the motivations driving and the methodologies used for such analyses but also reviews the knowledge of pulsatile endocrine systems.

This is an in-depth review from the leaders in the field, and is a must for those involved in pulse analysis, but of interest for anyone who would like to broaden their understanding of the mechanisms and consequences of pulsatile hormone secretion and the potentials and pitfalls of methods analyzing secretion. It discusses not only the classical intermittently secreted hormones like GH and

LH/FSH but also hormones that are secreted in a shorter timeframe like oxytocin, glucagon, insulin and PTH. Mechanisms of pulse generation, implications of pulsatile signals and altered pulsatility in pathology are discussed. Methodologies for pulse analysis, including their application and pitfalls are then described in great detail. The concept of Approximate Entropy (ApEn) analysis, which assesses orderliness of secretion, and its advantages (for example the small amount of data required) are discussed as well as methods to assess synchrony of hormone secretion. By putting emphasis on the application of the analytical methods, this review gives great insight into the regulation of the pulsatile secretion of multiple hormones.

Maternal caffeine intake during pregnancy and risk of fetal growth restriction: a large prospective observational study

CARE Study Group. Collaborators: Boylan S, Cade JE, Dolby VA, Greenwood DC, Hay AW, Kirk SF, Shires S, Simpson N, Thomas JD, Walker J, White KL, Wild CP, Potdar N, Konje JC, Taub N, Charvill J, Chipps KC, Kassam S, Ghandi C, Cooke MS, Konje JC, Cooke M, Cade J, Gott D, Thatcher N, Creton S, Tahourdin C, Gibson G, Greenwood D, Taub N, Gay C, Potdar N, Konje JC, Simpson N, Walker J, Dolby V, Ong H, Kassam S, Chipps K, Boyland S, Kirk S, Cade J, White K, Shires S, Hay A, Wild C, Cooke M, Thomas J, Hill E, Charvill J, Ghandi C
Department of Cancer Studies and Molecular Medicine, University of Leicester, Leicester, UK
jck4@le.ac.uk
BMJ 2008;337:a2332

Background: There is evidence that excessive caffeine intake is associated with lower birth weight, but previous studies have been inconclusive. Maternal caffeine intake is difficult to assess and confounders such as smoking often exist.

Methods: A prospective longitudinal observational study including 2,635 low-risk pregnant women in the UK. Total caffeine intake from 4 weeks before conception and throughout pregnancy was quantified with a validated caffeine assessment tool. Caffeine half-life was determined by measuring caffeine in saliva after a caffeine challenge. Smoking was assessed by measuring salivary cotinine concentrations.

Results: Caffeine consumption throughout pregnancy was associated with an increased risk of fetal growth restriction (odds ratios 1.2 (95% CI 0.9–1.6) for 100–199 mg/day, 1.5 (1.1–2.1) for 200–299 mg/day, and 1.4 (1.0–2.0) for >300 mg/day compared with <100 mg/day; test for trend p < 0.001). Mean caffeine consumption decreased in the first trimester and increased in the third. The association between caffeine and fetal growth restriction was stronger in women with a faster compared to a slower caffeine clearance (test for interaction, p = 0.06).

Conclusion: Caffeine consumption during pregnancy was associated with an increased risk of fetal growth restriction and this association continued throughout pregnancy. It would be sensible to advise to reduce caffeine intake before conception and throughout pregnancy.

In 2001, the Committee on Toxicity of Chemicals in Food in the UK concluded that caffeine intake >300 mg/day may be associated with low birth weight and spontaneous miscarriage, but that the evidence was inconclusive. That caffeine has an effect on the placenta is clear though – ingestion of 200 mg caffeine (approx. 2 cups of coffee) reduces placental blood flow by 25%. The current study aimed to study the effect of caffeine during pregnancy in more detail, and found a relation between caffeine intake and growth restriction (birth weight <10th centile), and is interesting for several reasons. Firstly, the authors claim to have estimated caffeine intake more accurately by taking brand, portion size, mode of preparation and caffeine intake through all dietary sources into account. Sixty-five percent of caffeine intake was from tea and the remainder from coffee, cola and chocolate. Secondly, a 'caffeine challenge test' was performed, and caffeine half-life was calculated. Thirdly, approximately half of the participants reduced their coffee intake spontaneously to <100 mg/day from the first trimester.

After adjustment for smoking, the effect of maternal caffeine intake (>200 mg/day) equaled a 60- to 70-gram reduction in birth weight. The presence of a dose-response relation and an effect of efficiency of caffeine clearance support the authors' conclusion that caffeine intake increases the risk of fetal growth restriction. One double-blind study showed that reducing caffeine intake of regular coffee drinkers did not affect fetal birth weight, but the CARE study group argues that this intervention may have been too late in pregnancy to result in an effect.

Certainly, the last word on caffeine consumption during pregnancy has not been said but as the authors suggest it may be sensible to avoid excessive caffeine intake during pregnancy, as half of pregnant women do already.

Temperature regulates limb length in homeotherms by directly modulating cartilage growth

Serrat MA, King D, Lovejoy CO
Department of Anthropology and School of Biomedical Sciences, Kent State University, Kent, Ohio, USA
Maria.a.serrat@gmail.com

Proc Natl Acad Sci USA 2008;105:19348–19353

Background: Allen's Rule documents a century-old biological observation that strong positive correlations exist among latitude, ambient temperature, and limb length in mammals. Although genetic selection for thermoregulatory adaptation is frequently presumed to be the primary basis of this phenomenon, research has shown that appendage outgrowth is also markedly influenced by environmental temperature. Appendages (ears, limbs and tails) of animals living in cold geographical regions are consistently shorter than those of closely related counterparts occupying warmer climes. Alteration of limb blood flow via vasoconstriction/vasodilation is the current default hypothesis for this growth plasticity.

Methods: Outbred mice were housed continuously at cold (7°C), control-intermediate (21°C) or warm (27°C) ambient temperatures from weaning through maturity (3.5–12 weeks age). Two intermediate end points were evaluated (4.5 and 6.5 weeks) to assess temperature effects during ontogeny. Regional organ and bone perfusion was quantified by measuring relative bone blood flow (BBF) to the hindlimb bones and tail base of juvenile mice using fluorescent microspheres. Additionally, the authors evaluated the growth of neonatal mouse metatarsals in culture maintained at cold (32°C), control (37°C), or warm (39°C) temperatures, holding all other factors constant.

Results: The authors show that the ears, limbs and tails of warm-reared mice were significantly longer than those of siblings raised in the cold, but without any change in body mass. The authors show that tissue perfusion does not fully account for differences in extremity elongation in mice. Mice raised at the coldest temperature had reduced femur, tibia and hindpaw BBF at 4.5 weeks of age, and reduced tibia, paw and tail BBF at 6.5 weeks. However, although the highest growth rates were found in the warmest reared animals, these animals did not also exhibit the correspondingly highest predicted BBF. They show that peripheral tissue temperature closely reflects housing temperature in vivo, and they demonstrate that chondrocyte proliferation and extracellular matrix volume strongly correlate with tissue temperature in metatarsals cultured without vasculature in vitro. Warm metatarsals showed significantly greater growth.

Conclusions: The data suggest that environmental temperature may modulate extremity growth by inducing physiological responses in peripheral tissue temperature, rather than by affecting vascular nutrient delivery. Such temperature lability may then impact extremity size via its direct effect on cell proliferation and matrix production in cartilage. Taken together, these data suggest that vasomotor changes likely modulate extremity growth indirectly, via their effects on appendage temperature, rather than vascular nutrient delivery. When combined with classic evolutionary theory, especially genetic assimilation, these results may substantially impact our understanding of phenotypic variation in living and extinct mammals, including humans.

This fascinating paper raises important questions. The genetic contribution to growth is undisputed, yet poorly understood. Although the role of the environment in regulating growth is unclear, certain environmental factors have been associated with poor growth. These factors include exposure of a fetus to smoking and alcohol, and postnatal child abuse or neglect. This study now proposes a role for environmental temperature in determining extremity growth. Mice reared in warmer conditions had significantly longer ears, limbs and tails than those raised in the cold, and this effect was also observed in neonatal mouse metatarsals grown in culture. These effects were largely due to increased chondrocyte proliferation and matrix volume in warmer conditions. These data may explain the disproportionately shortened long bones in cold-dwelling humans such as Neanderthals, and the relative reduction in tibial length as compared with femoral length that is observed in decreasing environmental temperatures. The contribution of genotype to this process, and its interaction with the environmental temperature, remains to be established.

References
 1. Gevers EF, Dattani MT. Growth and growth factors; in Carel JC, Hochberg Z (eds): Yearbook of Pediatric Endocrinology 2008. Basel, Karger, 2008, pp 43–62.
 2. Weedon MN, Lango H, Lindgren CM, Wallace C, Evans DM, Mangino M, et al: Genome-wide association analysis identifies 20 loci that influence adult height. Nat Genet 2008;40:575–583.
 3. Sanna S, Jackson AU, Nagaraja R, Willer CJ, Chen WM, Bonnycastle LL, et al: Common variants in the GDF5-UQCC region are associated with variation in human height. Nat Genet 2008;40:198–203.
 4. Lettre G, Jackson AU, Gieger C, Schumacher FR, Berndt SI, Sanna S, et al: Identification of ten loci associated with height highlights new biological pathways in human growth. Nat Genet 2008;40:584–591.
 5. Gudbjartsson DF, Walters GB, Thorleifsson G, Stefansson H, Halldorsson BV, Zusmanovich P, et al: Many sequence variants affecting diversity of adult human height. Nat Genet 2008;40:609–615.
 6. Jaubert J, Jaubert F, Martin N, Washburn LL, Lee BK, Eicher EM, et al:Three new allelic mouse mutations that cause skeletal overgrowth involve the natriuretic peptide receptor C gene (Npr3). Proc Natl Acad Sci USA 1999;96:10278–10283.
 7. Peters J: Prader-Willi and snoRNAs. Nat Genet 2008;40:688–689.
 8. Murdoch S, Djuric U, Mazhar B, Seoud M, Khan R, Kuick R, et al: Mutations in NALP7 cause recurrent hydatidiform moles and reproductive wastage in humans. Nat Genet 2006;38:300–302.
 9. Dos Santos C, Essioux L, Teinturier C, Tauber M, Goffin V, Bougneres P: A common polymorphism of the growth hormone receptor is associated with increased responsiveness to growth hormone. Nat Genet 2004;36:720–724.
10. Jorge AA, Marchisotti FG, Montenegro LR, Carvalho LR, Mendonca BB, Arnhold IJ: Growth hormone (GH) pharmacogenetics: influence of GH receptor exon 3 retention or deletion on first-year growth response and final height in patients with severe GH deficiency. J Clin Endocrinol Metab 2006;91:1076–1080.
11. Binder G, Baur F, Schweizer R, Ranke MB: The d3-growth hormone (GH) receptor polymorphism is associated with increased responsiveness to GH in Turner syndrome and short small-for-gestational-age children. J Clin Endocrinol Metab 2006;91:659–664.
12. Blum WF, Machinis K, Shavrikova EP, Keller A, Stobbe H, Pfaeffle RW, et al: The growth response to growth hormone (GH) treatment in children with isolated GH deficiency is independent of the presence of the exon 3-minus isoform of the GH receptor. J Clin Endocrinol Metab 2006;91:4171–4174.
13. Raz B, Janner M, Petkovic V, Lochmatter D, Eble A, Dattani MT, et al: Influence of growth hormone (GH) receptor deletion of exon 3 and full-length isoforms on GH response and final height in patients with severe GH deficiency. J Clin Endocrinol Metab 2008;93:974–980.
14. Deal C, Ma J, Wilkin F, Paquette J, Rozen F, Ge B, et al: Novel promoter polymorphism in insulin-like growth factor-binding protein-3: correlation with serum levels and interaction with known regulators. J Clin Endocrinol Metab 2001;86:1274–1280.
15. Brown RJ, Adams JJ, Pelekanos RA, Wan Y, McKinstry WJ, Palethorpe K, et al: Model for growth hormone receptor activation based on subunit rotation within a receptor dimer. Nat Struct Mol Biol 2005;12:814–821.
16. Lewis MD, Horan M, Millar DS, Newsway V, Easter TE, Fryklund L, et al: A novel dysfunctional growth hormone variant (Ile179Met) exhibits a decreased ability to activate the extracellular signal-regulated kinase pathway. J Clin Endocrinol Metab 2004;89:1068–1075.
17. Gielen M, Retchless BS, Mony L, Johnson JW, Paoletti P: Mechanism of differential control of NMDA receptor activity by NR2 subunits. Nature 2009;459:703–707.
18. Guan J, Gluckman PD: IGF-1 derived small neuropeptides and analogues: a novel strategy for the development of pharmaceuticals for neurological conditions. Br J Pharmacol 2009 [Epub ahead of print]. DOI 10.1111/j.1476-5381.2009.00256.x.
19. Netchine I, Rossignol S, Dufourg MN, Azzi S, Rousseau A, Perin L, et al: 11p15 imprinting center region 1 loss of methylation is a common and specific cause of typical Russell-Silver syndrome: clinical scoring system and epigenetic-phenotypic correlations. J Clin Endocrinol Metab 2007;92:3148–3154.
20. Clemmons DR: Modifying IGF1 activity: an approach to treat endocrine disorders, atherosclerosis and cancer. Nat Rev Drug Discov 2007;6:821–833.
21. Bowers CY, Reynolds GA, Durham D, Barrera CM, Pezzoli SS, Thorner MO: Growth hormone (GH)-releasing peptide stimulates GH release in normal men and acts synergistically with GH-releasing hormone. J Clin Endocrinol Metab 1990;70:975–982.
22. Bartke A, Kopchick J: Comment on: Kloting et al. (2008) Autocrine IGF-1 action in adipocytes controls systemic IGF-1 concentrations and growth: Diabetes 57:2074–2082. Diabetes 2009;58:e3; author reply e4.
23. Zhang M, Xuan S, Bouxsein ML, von Stechow D, Akeno N, Faugere MC, et al: Osteoblast-specific knockout of the insulin-like growth factor (IGF) receptor gene reveals an essential role of IGF signaling in bone matrix mineralization. J Biol Chem 2002;277:44005–44012.
24. Kulkarni RN, Holzenberger M, Shih DQ, Ozcan U, Stoffel M, Magnuson MA, et al: Beta-cell-specific deletion of the Igf1 receptor leads to hyperinsulinemia and glucose intolerance but does not alter beta-cell mass. Nat Genet 2002;31:111–115.
25. Suh Y, Atzmon G, Cho MO, Hwang D, Liu B, Leahy DJ, et al: Functionally significant insulin-like growth factor I receptor mutations in centenarians. Proc Natl Acad Sci USA 2008;105:3438–3442.
26. Besson A, Salemi S, Gallati S, Jenal A, Horn R, Mullis PS, et al: Reduced longevity in untreated patients with isolated growth hormone deficiency. J Clin Endocrinol Metab 2003;88:3664–3667.

Growth Plate, Bone and Calcium

Terhi Heino[a], Dov Tiosano[b], and Lars Sävendahl[c]

[a]Orthopaedic Research Unit, University of Turku, Finland
[b]Pediatric Endocrinology, Rambam Medical Center, Haifa, Israel
[c]Pediatric Endocrinology Unit, Department of Woman and Child Health, Karolinska Institutet, Stockholm, Sweden

Studies of bone biology have been complicated by the highly organized structures and complex cellular biology. Thanks to new models and technologies, our view and understanding of the biological importance of the skeleton has expanded dramatically in the last years. We first take the opportunity to highlight a few papers discussed in this chapter. The possibility of using C-type natriuretic peptide as a novel therapeutic strategy for skeletal dysplasias gives new hope for the treatment of achondroplasia. Two papers demonstrating that oxytocin is a bone-anabolic hormone represent a new paradigm. The recent discovery of the extracellular calcium-sensing receptor as a critical modulator of skeletal development was chosen as the mechanism of the year. Other new mechanisms include the demonstration of prolactin as a regulator of bone metabolism and the discovery of a new estrogen receptor involved in the regulation of bone growth. An important observation for clinical practice is the finding that late menarcheal age can be considered as a risk factor for osteoporosis. We also included a preclinical study indicating that osteocytes are target cells to increase bone mass, a finding which may lead to new treatment options in patients with osteoporosis. Clinical trials are represented by 2 papers that potentially could open up a new therapy of hypoparathyroidism in children and another paper demonstrating that the effectiveness of vitamin D supplementation is independent of the dosing regimen. A concept revised is represented by a paper showing a new player involved in hypophosphatemic rickets. New anti-cancer and anti-inflammatory drugs are reported to interfere with bone growth representing new concerns. Giving some food for thought is a paper suggesting that aspirin might have the capacity to prevent osteoporosis. Finally we chose two reviews: one nicely summarizing the experiences of the use of bisphosphonates in the treatment of osteogenesis imperfecta, and another proposing a new way of classifying rickets based on the etiology of the underlying hypophosphatemia.

New hope: one step further towards an effective treatment of achondroplasia

Systemic administration of C-type natriuretic peptide as a novel therapeutic strategy for skeletal dysplasias

Yasoda A, Kitamura H, Fujii T, Kondo E, Murao N, Miura M, Kanamoto N, Komatsu Y, Arai H, Nakao K
Department of Medicine and Clinical Science, Kyoto University Graduate School of Medicine, Kyoto, Fuji-Gotemba Research Laboratories, Chugai Pharmaceutical Co., Ltd., Shizuoka, Japan
yasoda@kuhp.kyoto-u.ac.jp and nakao@kuhp.kyoto-u.ac.jp
Endocrinology 2009; DOI: 10.1210/en.2008-1676

Background: C-type natriuretic peptide (CNP), a member of the natriuretic peptide family, is a potent stimulator of endochondral bone growth. Targeted overexpression of a CNP transgene in the growth plate has been shown to rescue the impaired bone growth observed in mouse model of achondroplasia (Ach), the most frequent form of human skeletal dysplasias.

Methods: To elucidate whether or not the systemic administration of CNP is a novel drug therapy for skeletal dysplasias, the authors investigated the effects of plasma CNP on impaired bone growth in Ach mice that specifically overexpress CNP in the liver under the control of human serum amyloid P component promoter, or in those treated with a continuous CNP infusion system.

Results: The data show that increased plasma CNP from the liver or by intravenous administration of synthetic CNP-22 rescued the impaired bone growth phenotype of Ach mice without significant adverse effects.

Conclusion: Treatment with systemic CNP could be a potential therapeutic strategy for skeletal dysplasias, including achondroplasia in humans.

Achondroplasia is caused by constitutive active mutation of FGF receptor 3 (FGFR3), which results in disturbed proliferation and differentiation of growth plate chondrocytes followed by impaired endochondral bone growth [1]. Growth hormone has been shown to have only a minimal effect in patients with achondroplasia [2] and today there is no effective treatment available. As discussed in Yearbook 2008, C-type natriuretic peptide (CNP) is a potent stimulator of endochondral bone growth [3]. Mice with targeted overexpression of CNP in cartilage exhibit prominent skeletal overgrowth [4] while mice depleted with CNP are dwarf due to impaired endochondral bone growth [5]. The authors of this paper have previously demonstrated that cartilage-specific overexpression of a CNP transgene rescues the impaired endochondral bone growth in a mouse model of achondroplasia with targeted expression of constitutive active FGFR3 in cartilage (Ach mice), by restoring the decreased matrix production in Ach growth plates through inhibition of FGFR3-mediated MAPK signaling pathway [4]. In this paper, the same authors investigated the effects of plasma CNP on impaired bone growth in Ach mice that specifically overexpress CNP in the liver and in those treated with a continuous CNP-22 infusion system. The data convincingly show that increased plasma CNP from the liver or by intravenous administration of synthetic CNP-22 rescued the impaired bone growth phenotype of Ach mice without significant adverse effects. Nevertheless, safety issues with CNP need further study, as only short-term potential toxicity has been examined in the current study. It is also important to point out that continuous subcutaneous infusion of similar doses of CNP-22 was ineffective which may be due to subcutaneous degradation of CNP-22. As CNP could successfully stimulate the endochondral bone growth of wild-type mice; it could potentially be used for skeletal dysplasias other than achondroplasia. However, it is important to point out that the animals were treated as of their weaning age of 3 weeks and we therefore do not yet know whether this is a requirement for successful therapy. Although further research is needed, systemic administration of CNP or CNP analogs provides a novel promising therapeutic strategy for human skeletal dysplasias, including achondroplasia.

New paradigms: oxytocin is a bone-anabolic hormone

Oxytocin controls differentiation of human mesenchymal stem cells and reverses osteoporosis

Elabd C, Basillais A, Beaupied H, Breuil V, Wagner N, Scheideler M, Zaragosi LE, Massiera F, Lemichez E, Trajanoski Z, Carle G, Euller-Ziegler L, Ailhaud G, Benhamou CL, Dani C, Amri EZ
ISBDC, Université de Nice Sophia-Antipolis, CNRS, Nice, France
amri@unice.fr
Stem Cells 2008;26:2399–2407

Background: Osteoporotic bone loss constitutes a major worldwide public health burden characterized by enhanced skeletal fragility. Whereas an increase in bone resorption is considered as the main contributor to bone loss, the process is also accompanied by increased bone marrow adiposity. Osteoblasts and adipocytes share the same precursor cell and an inverse relationship exists between the two lineages. To develop new therapeutic treatments, it is important to identify signaling pathways that stimulate the osteogenesis of mesenchymal stem cells (MSCs) at the expense of adipogenesis.

Methods: The authors identified the oxytocin receptor pathway as a potential regulator of the osteoblast/adipocyte balance of human multipotent adipose-derived stem cells by transcriptomic analysis. The effects of oxytocin on the osteoblast/adipocyte balance in vitro and the potential of oxytocin to prevent ovariectomy (OVX)-induced bone loss in vivo were tested. In addition, levels of circulating oxytocin were measured in OVX rats and postmenopausal women.

Results: Both oxytocin and carbetocin (a stable oxytocin analog) negatively modulated adipogenesis while promoting osteogenesis in both human multipotent adipose-derived stem cells and human bone marrow MSCs. Consistent with these observations, OVX mice and rats, which become osteoporotic and exhibit disequilibrium of this balance, had significantly decreased oxytocin levels compared to sham-operated controls. Subcutaneous oxytocin injection reversed bone loss and reduced marrow adiposity in OVX mice. Clinically, plasma oxytocin levels were significantly lower in postmenopausal women developing osteoporosis than in their healthy counterparts.

Conclusion: These results suggest that plasma oxytocin levels represent a novel diagnostic marker for osteoporosis and that oxytocin administration could be a potential therapy to prevent bone loss.

Oxytocin is an anabolic bone hormone

Tamma R, Colaianni G, Zhu LL, DiBenedetto A, Greco G, Montemurro G, Patano N, Strippoli M, Vergari R, Mancini L, Colucci S, Grano M, Faccio R, Liu X, Li J, Usmani S, Bachar M, Bab I, Nishimori K, Young LJ, Buettner C, Iqbal J, Sun L, Zaidi M, Zallone A

Department of Human Anatomy and Histology, University of Bari, Bari, Italy
mone.zaidi@mssm.edu or a.zallone@anatomia.uniba.it
Proc Natl Acad Sci USA 2009;106:7149–7154

Background: Oxytocin, a primitive neurohypophyseal hormone, has so far been thought to only modulate lactation and social bonding. Here, the authors attempted to determine whether oxytocin directly affects bone remodeling.

Methods: The skeletal phenotype of oxytocin and oxytocin receptor knockout mice was analyzed by histomorphometry and µCT. The effects of local and peripheral injections of oxytocin on bone parameters were studied. Furthermore, in vitro cultures of murine and human osteoblasts and osteoclasts were performed.

Results: The authors demonstrated that oxytocin is a direct regulator of bone mass. Deletion of oxytocin or the oxytocin receptor in male or female mice caused osteoporosis, which resulted from reduced bone formation. Consistent with low bone formation, oxytocin was shown to stimulate the differentiation of osteoblasts to a mineralizing phenotype. The molecular mechanism involved the upregulation of BMP-2, which in turn controlled Schnurri-2 and 3, Osterix, and ATF-4 expression. In contrast, oxytocin had dual effects on the osteoclast. It stimulated osteoclast formation both directly and indirectly. On the other hand, oxytocin inhibited bone resorption by mature osteoclasts by triggering cytosolic calcium release and nitric oxide synthesis.

Conclusion: The complementary genetic and pharmacologic approaches presented in this paper revealed oxytocin as a novel anabolic regulator of bone mass, with potential implications for osteoporosis therapy.

The mammalian peptide hormone oxytocin is most well known for its roles in bonding, attachment and female reproduction: it is released after distension of the cervix and vagina during labor and after stimulation of the nipples, thus respectively facilitating birth and breastfeeding. These two papers describe a new potential role for oxytocin as an anabolic regulator of bone mass. Elabd et al. were looking for factors that are differentially regulated during the adipogenic and osteogenic differentiation of mesenchymal stem cells (MSCs) and found the oxytocin receptor gene as a potential candidate. They showed that oxytocin modulates the osteoblast/adipocyte balance of MSCs in vitro and prevents ovariectomy (OVX)-induced bone loss in mice in vivo. In addition, serum and plasma oxytocin levels were decreased both in OVX rats and in postmenopausal women developing bone loss. An important question raised by their findings was whether the effect of oxytocin on the skeleton is direct or central? This was recently addressed in the paper by Tamma et al. who, in knockout mouse models, showed that peripheral oxytocin has a direct and dominant action on the skeleton. The effect was mainly mediated through the stimulation of osteoblast formation, with variable effects on osteoclasts. These data indeed lead to the speculation that oxytocin could potentially be used as a new bone-anabolic therapy. Nevertheless, further experimental studies are needed to verify whether this concept is feasible. Like oxytocin, parathyroid hormone-related protein (PTHrP), another peptide affecting the breast, displays both pro-resorptive and anabolic actions. PTHrP secreted from the breast causes, at least in part, the bone loss that accompanies pregnancy and lactation. Another primitive neuropeptide, calcitonin, which is also increased during pregnancy and lactation, is likely to counteract the stimulatory effects of oxytocin.

Evidence for direct effects of prolactin on human osteoblasts: inhibition of cell growth and mineralization

Seriwatanachai D, Krishnamra N, van Leeuwen JP
Faculty of Science, Department of Physiology, Mahidol University, Bangkok, Thailand
j.vanleeuwen@erasmusmc.nl
J Cell Biochem 2009; DOI: 10.1002/jcb.22161

Background: Hyperprolactinemia is one of the risk factors decreasing bone mass which has been believed to be mediated by hypogonadism. However, the demonstration of prolactin receptors in a human osteosarcoma cell line and primary bone cell cultures from mouse calvariae supported the hypothesis of a direct prolactin (PRL) action on bone cells. The aim of this study was to investigate the role of PRL and its signal transduction pathway in the regulation of bone metabolism via osteoblast differentiation.

Methods: Human pre-osteoblasts (SV-HFO) that differentiate in a 3-week period from proliferating pre-osteoblasts (days 2–7) to extracellular matrix-producing cells (days 7–14), which are eventually mineralized (days 14–21), were used. The concentration of PRL mimicking a lactating period (100 ng/ml) was used to incubate SV-HFO for 21 days in estrogenic medium. The human PRL receptor mRNA and protein are expressed in SV-HFO.

Results: PRL significantly decreased osteoblast number (DNA content) which was due to a decrease in proliferation. PRL increased osteogenic markers, RUNX2 and ALP, in the early stage of osteoblast differentiation while decreasing it later, suggesting a bidirectional effect. Calcium measurement and Alizarin red staining showed a reduction in mineralization by PRL while having no effect on osteoblast activity or RANKL/OPG mRNA ratio. PRL action on mineralization was not via the PI-3 kinase pathway.

Conclusions: The present study provides evidence of a direct effect of PRL on osteoblast differentiation and in vitro mineralization.

Bone loss occurring during lactation is due to accelerated bone resorption. The trigger for bone resorption is the combination of increased circulating levels of PTHrP, oxytocin from the previous

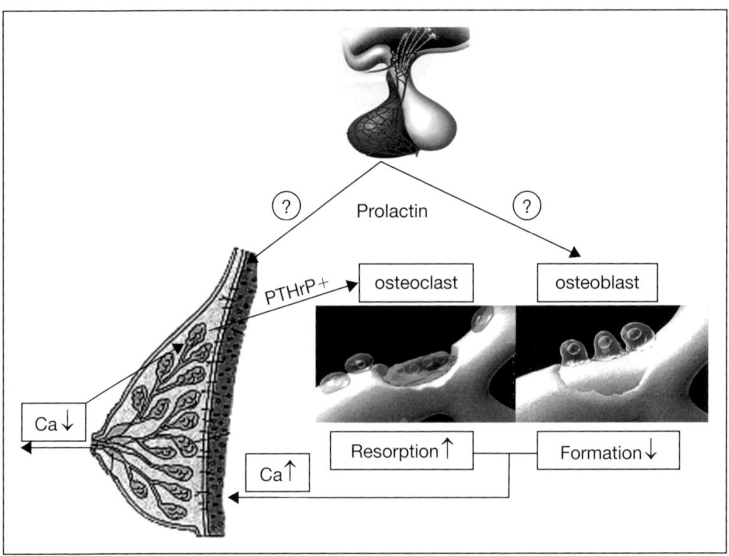

Fig. 1. Hypocalcemia reduces overall production and calcium content in milk. The lactating mammary gland can sense the extracellular calcium through a calcium-sensing receptor and adjust its secretion to the milk and increases PTHrP secretion from the mammary epithelial cells. The combination of low estrogens and high PTHrP during lactation enhances bone resorption. This was one side of the circle, now we learn that prolactin, the most important hormone during lactation, also suppresses osteoblast differentiation and maturation and by that inhibits bone remodeling and calcium deposition in bone.

comment, decreased circulating levels of estrogen, and a negative calcium balance [6]. When calcium becomes limited, calcium restriction decreases the calcium content of milk, increases milk osmolality and protein concentration, and decreases overall milk production. In order to prevent this cascade, PTHrP is secreted from the mammary gland to act on the maternal bone, the physiological calcium reservoir to enhance calcium release [7]. From this paper, we have now learned that prolactin, the most important hormone for lactation, also plays a physiological role to decrease osteoblast proliferation which leads to a reduction of new bone formation (fig. 1).

Mechanism of the year: now we know how calcium modulates skeletal development

The extracellular calcium-sensing receptor (CaSR) is a critical modulator of skeletal development

Chang W, Tu C, Chen TH, Bikle D, Shoback D
Endocrine Research Unit, Department of Veterans Affairs Medical Center, Department of Medicine, University of California, San Francisco, Calif., USA
wenhan.chang@ucsf.edu
Sci Signal 2008;1:ra1

Background: The extracellular Ca^{2+}-sensing receptor (CaSR) is well known to play an important role in the functions of the parathyroid gland and the kidney. Severe hyperparathyroidism, premature death, and incomplete gene excision in $Casr^{-/-}$ mice have precluded the assessment of CaSR function in other tissues.
Methods: The authors generated mice with tissue-specific deletion of $Casr$ in the parathyroid gland, bone, or cartilage.
Results: Deletion of $Casr$ in the parathyroid gland or bone was found to result in profound bone defects, whereas deletion of $Casr$ in chondrocytes resulted in death before embryonic day 13 (E13). Mice in which chondrocyte-specific deletion of $Casr$ was induced between E16 and E18 were viable but showed delayed growth plate development.
Conclusion: The data show a critical role for the CaSR in early embryogenesis and skeletal development.

Heterozygous and homozygous inactivating mutations in *Casr* cause familial benign hypocalciuric hypercalcemia (FBHH) and neonatal severe hyperparathyroidism (NSHPT), respectively [8]. Patients with NSHPT have severe skeletal demineralization at birth, which is thought to be due to severe hyperparathyroidism. The presence of CaSRs in bone and cartilage has, however, raised the question of whether defective signaling of CaSRs in bone cells, chondrocytes, or both may contribute to the skeletal phenotype in NSHPT. The authors unexpectedly observed a marked reduction in the abundance of the CaSR in the bones of mice with tissue-specific *Casr* deletion in the parathyroid gland, which suggests that loss of CaSR signaling in that tissue may also contribute to skeletal pathology. This study provides the first evidence supporting yet another level of coordination between the parathyroid gland and bone, which is mediated by CaSR, and the direct involvement of CaSR signaling in the differentiation of osteoblasts and growth plate chondrocytes and skeletal development in vivo. Furthermore, it suggests that inhibition of *Casr* expression in bone in states of hyperparathyroidism may be part of the mechanism underlying the skeletal defects in this disorder. It remains unclear why the expression of CaSR is decreased in bone when *Casr* is specifically knocked out only in the parathyroid gland. The hypercalcemic phenotype might regulate the abundance of *Casr* in bone by a feedback loop.

PTH(1–34) replacement therapy in a child with hypoparathyroidism caused by a sporadic calcium receptor mutation

Theman TA, Collins MT, Dempster DW, Zhou H, Reynolds JC, Brahim JS, Roschger P, Klaushofer K, Winer KK
Craniofacial and Skeletal Diseases Branch, National Institute of Dental and Craniofacial Research, National Institutes of Health, Department of Health and Human Services, Bethesda, Md., USA
mc247k@nih.gov
J Bone Miner Res 2009;24:964–973

Background: Autosomal dominant hypocalcemia (ADH) causes hypoparathyroidism due to activating mutations in the calcium-sensing receptor (CaSR). Treatment with parathyroid hormone, PTH(1–34), may be superior to conventional therapy but is contraindicated in children, and long-term effects on the skeleton are unknown.
Methods: A 20-year-old female with ADH was treated with PTH continuously for 14 years since 6 years and 2 months of age. A bone biopsy was obtained for histomorphometry and quantitative backscattered electron imaging (qBEI). These results were compared with on1e age-, sex-, and length of hypoparathyroidism-matched control not on PTH and 2 sex-matched ADH controls before and after 1 year of PTH.
Results: The patient's growth was normal. Hypercalciuria and hypermagnesuria persisted despite normal or subnormal serum calcium and magnesium levels. Nephrocalcinosis developed by 19 years of age. Cancellous bone volume was dramatically elevated in the patient and in ADH controls after 1 year of PTH. Bone mineral density distribution by qBEI of the patient and ADH controls was strikingly shifted toward lower mineralization compared with the non-ADH control. Moreover, the ADH controls exhibited a further reduction in mineralization after 1 year of PTH. There were no fractures or osteosarcoma.
Conclusions: Long-term PTH replacement in a child with ADH was safe, increased bone mass without negatively impacting mineralization, and improved serum mineral control but did not prevent nephrocalcinosis. These findings imply a role for the CaSR in bone matrix mineralization.

Effects of once versus twice-daily parathyroid hormone 1–34 therapy in children with hypoparathyroidism

Winer KK, Sinaii N, Peterson D, Sainz B Jr, Cutler GB Jr
National Institute of Child Health and Human Development, National Institutes of Health, Bethesda, Md., USA
winerk@mail.nih.gov
J Clin Endocrinol Metab 2008;93:3389–3395

Background: Long-term conventional therapy in hypoparathyroidism with vitamin D and analogs may lead to nephrocalcinosis and renal insufficiency. The aim of the study was to compare the response of once-daily vs. twice-daily PTH(1–34) treatment in children with hypoparathyroidism.
Methods: Fourteen children ages 4–17 years with chronic hypoparathyroidism were studied. In a randomized cross-over trial, lasting 28 weeks, which compared two dose regimens, once-daily vs. twice-daily PTH(1–34). Each 14-week study arm was divided into a 2-week inpatient dose-adjustment phase and a 12-week outpatient phase.
Results: Repeated serum measures over a 24-hour period showed that twice-daily PTH(1–34) increased serum calcium and magnesium levels more effectively than a once-daily dose. This was especially evident during the second half of the day (12–24 h). PTH(1–34) normalized mean 24-hour urine calcium excretion on both treatment schedules. This was achieved with half the PTH(1–34) dose during the twice-daily regimen compared with the once-daily regimen (twice-daily 25 ±15 µg/day vs. once-daily 58 ± 28 µg/day; p < 0.001).
Conclusions: The results showed, as in the previous study of adult patients with hypoparathyroidism, that a twice-daily regimen produced significantly improved metabolic control compared with once-daily PTH(1–34).

Since 2002, recombinant human PTH(1–34) (teriparatide) has been approved for the treatment of postmenopausal osteoporosis. In these 2 papers from the same center it was shown that a twice-daily regimen produced significantly improved metabolic control compared with once-daily PTH(1–34) when given to pediatric patients. As to the long-term effect of recombinant human PTH(1–34) on bone mineral density in patients with a mutated CaSR, it was found that the cancellous bone volume dramatically increased. Based on studies that reported an increased incidence of bone neoplasms in juvenile Fischer 344 rats receiving daily high-dose injections of PTH(1–34) for 2 years (the average lifespan of rats), the US Food and Drug Administration added a 'black-box' warning regarding osteogenic sarcoma in the rat model [9, 10]. Under this 'black-box' warning it should be emphasized that treatment with recombinant human PTH(1–34) should be restricted only to controlled studies during infancy, childhood or puberty.

Clinical trials: effectiveness of vitamin D supplementation is independent of dosing regimen

Treatment of hypovitaminosis D in infants and toddlers

Gordon CM, Williams AL, Feldman HA, May J, Sinclair L, Vasquez A, Cox JE
Divisions of Adolescent Medicine and Endocrinology, Children's Hospital Boston, Boston, Mass., USA
catherine.gordon@childrens.harvard.edu
J Clin Endocrinol Metab 2008;93:2716–2721

Background: Hypovitaminosis D appears to be on the rise in young children, with implications for skeletal and overall health. The objective of the study was to compare the safety and efficacy of vitamin D_2 daily, vitamin D_2 weekly, and vitamin D_3 daily, combined with supplemental calcium, in raising serum 25-hydroxyvitamin D [25(OH)D] and lowering PTH concentrations.
Methods: This was a 6-week randomized controlled trial. Forty otherwise healthy infants and toddlers with hypovitaminosis D [25(OH)D <20 ng/ml] were enrolled. Participants were assigned to 1 of 3 regimens: 2,000 IU oral vitamin D_2 daily, 50,000 IU vitamin D_2 weekly, or 2,000 IU vitamin D_3 daily. Each was also prescribed elemental calcium (50 mg/kg/day). Infants received treatment for 6 weeks.
Results: All treatments approximately tripled the 25(OH)D concentration. Preplanned comparisons were nonsignificant: daily vitamin D_2 vs. weekly vitamin D_2 (12% difference in effect, p = 0.66) and daily D_2 vs. daily D_3 (7%, p = 0.82). The mean serum calcium change was small and similar in the 3 groups. There was no significant difference in PTH suppression.
Conclusions: The short-term vitamin D_2 2,000 IU daily, vitamin D_2 50,000 IU weekly, or vitamin D_3 2,000 IU daily yielded equivalent outcomes in the treatment of hypovitaminosis D among young children. Therefore, pediatric providers can individualize the treatment regimen for a given patient to ensure compliance, given that no difference in efficacy or safety was noted among these 3 common treatment regimens.

Modern lifestyle sustains a high incidence of hypovitaminosis D, which is the most frequent cause for rickets. Although the recommendations for vitamin D supplementation are well known [11], compliance with vitamin D supplementation is often a problem. The aim of the present study was to examine the efficacy of each treatment in raising serum 25(OH)D and lowering PTH concentrations; and the safety and tolerance of each regimen in infants and toddlers treated with either a daily low dose of vitamin D_2, a higher dose of vitamin D_2 once weekly, or a low dose of vitamin D_3 once daily. Sun exposure and fish consumption provide vitamin D_3 as cholecalciferol while vitamin D_2 is a plant-derived form of vitamin D produced through ultraviolet exposure of foods (ergocalciferol). Both vitamin D_2 and vitamin D_3 when ingested undergo metabolism in the liver to form 25-hydroxyvitamin D [25(OH)D; D represents either D_2 or D_3] and in the kidneys to 1,25-dihydroxyvitamin D [12]. The question whether vitamin D_2 is as effective as vitamin D_3 in maintaining 25-hydroxyvitamin D status was investigated and reassured in healthy adults [13]. In this study it was demonstrate that 2,000 IU daily vitamin D_2, 50,000 IU vitamin D_2 weekly, or 2,000 IU daily vitamin D_3 yield equivalent outcomes in the short-term treatment of hypovitaminosis D among otherwise healthy infants and toddlers.

These results indicate that pediatric providers can determine the appropriate method of treatment for a given patient or family to ensure compliance, given that no difference in efficacy or safety was noted.

Concept revisited: longitudinal assessment of the effects of estrogen receptor-α deletion on human bone

Impact on bone of an estrogen receptor-α gene loss of function mutation

Smith EP, Specker B, Bachrach BE, Kimbro KS, Li XJ, Young MF, Fedarko NS, Abuzzahab MJ, Frank GR, Cohen RM, Lubahn DB, Korach KS
Division of Endocrinology, Diabetes and Metabolism, Department of Medicine, University of Cincinnati College of Medicine, Vontz Center for Molecular Studies, Cincinnati, Ohio, USA
smithep@email.uc.edu
J Clin Endocrinol Metab 2008;93:3088–3096

Background: There exists only one kindred with a known instance of a germ line loss of function mutation of estrogen receptor-α (ERα). The aim was to assess the impact of a loss of function mutation in the ERα gene on bone histomorphometry, bone volumetric density, bone geometry and skeletal growth, and to evaluate the effect of ERα heterozygosity on spine density and adult height in an extended pedigree.

Methods: A longitudinal follow-up of the propositus with homozygous loss of function mutation of ERα and a single contact evaluation of the kindred were performed. Iliac crest bone biopsy and peripheral quantitative computed tomography (pQCT) of propositus with serial measures of spine areal bone mineral density (aBMD) by dual-energy X-ray absorptiometry (DXA) and bone age were performed. Members of the pedigree were evaluated for ERα mutation carrier status and spine aBMD.

Results: Bone biopsy revealed marked osteopenia, low trabecular volume, decreased thickness, normal trabecular number, and low activation frequency. Radial periosteal circumference was similar, endosteal circumference larger, and trabecular and cortical volumetric BMD markedly lower than controls. Spine aBMD at age 28.5 years was 0.745 g/cm^2 which decreased to 0.684 g/cm^2 (Z score −3.85) at 35.5 years while bone age advanced from 15.0 to 17.5 years. Kindred analysis revealed that gene carriers had spine aBMD Z scores of <0 (p = 0.003), although no difference was observed between carriers and non-mutant members (−0.84 ± 0.26 vs. −0.64 ± 0.16).

Conclusion: Homozygous ERα disruption markedly affects bone growth, bone mineral content and bone structure but not periosteal circumference. ERα heterozygosity appears to not impair spine aBMD.

Estrogens are known to be important for skeletal maturation. There is only one known human instance of a disruptive mutation in ERα, causing estrogen resistance [14]. When the phenotype of this tall 28-year-old 'Cincinnati man' was first reported, he had masculinized normally in adolescence but had never experienced a growth spurt. At the age of 28 years, he was still growing with a height of 208 cm and bone age of 15 years. He had developed genu valgum and marked axillary acanthosis nigricans. Gonadotropin and estrogen levels were increased and testosterone concentrations were in the adult normal range. In addition, it was shown that bone mineral density as measured by DXA was markedly reduced. In the current paper, Smith et al. have longitudinally assessed the bone phenotype of the propositus and performed ERα mutation carrier analysis of all family members who provided consent. This study provides additional substantial evidence for an important role for ERα in bone metabolism and indicates that there exists a complex contribution of both estrogens and androgens in bone growth, bone mineral content acquisition and structural integrity of the skeleton. A striking finding in his skeleton is marked thinning of the cortex with increased trabecularization. This may shed light on the debate of bone fragility in the estrogen-deficient Turner patients, who have normal BMD, but fragile cortical bones. Interestingly, haploinsufficiency for ERα is not associated with osteopenia or tall stature, indicating that only a major disruption in ERα expression has a clear impact on the skeleton.

The role of the G protein-coupled receptor GPR30 in the effects of estrogen in ovariectomized mice

Windahl SH, Andersson N, Chagin AS, Martensson UE, Carlsten H, Olde B, Swanson C, Moverare-Skrtic S, Sävendahl
L, Lagerquist MK, Leeb-Lundberg LM, Ohlsson C
Institute of Medicine, Sahlgrenska Academy, Göteborg University, Göteborg
Claes.Ohlsson@medic.gu.se
Am J Physiol Endocrinol Metab 2009;296:E490–496

Background: In vitro studies suggest that the membrane G protein-coupled receptor GPR30 is a functional estrogen receptor (ER). The aim of the present study was to determine the possible in vivo role of GPR30 as a functional ER primarily for the regulation of bone mass and longitudinal bone growth, but also for some other well-known estrogen-regulated parameters.

Methods: Three-month-old ovariectomized GPR30-deficient mice ($GPR30^{-/-}$) and wild-type (WT) mice were treated with either vehicle or increasing doses of estradiol (E_2; 0, 30, 70, 160, or 830 ng/mouse/ day). Body composition [bone mineral density (BMD), fat mass, and lean mass] was analyzed by dual-energy-X ray absorptiometry, while the cortical and trabecular bone compartments were analyzed by peripheral quantitative computerized tomography. Quantitative histological analyses were performed in the distal femur growth plate. Bone marrow cellularity and distribution were analyzed using a fluorescence-activated cell sorter.

Results: E_2 treatment reduced longitudinal bone growth, reflected by decreased femur length and distal femur growth plate height, in the WT mice but not in the $GPR30^{-/-}$ mice compared with vehicle-treated mice. On the other hand, the estrogenic responses on all other investigated parameters, including increase in bone mass (total body BMD, spine BMD, trabecular BMD, and cortical bone thickness), increase in uterine weight, thymic atrophy, fat mass reduction, and increase in bone marrow cellularity, were similar for all of the investigated E_2 doses in WT and $GPR30^{-/-}$ mice.

Conclusion: These in vivo findings demonstrate that GPR30 is required for a normal estrogenic response in the growth plate. In contrast, GPR30 is not required for normal estrogenic responses on several major well-known estrogen-regulated parameters.

Estrogens exert a variety of important physiological effects which have been suggested to be mainly mediated via the two known nuclear estrogen receptors (ERs), ERα and ERβ. The 'Cincinnati man' with a point mutation in the ERα had nonfused growth plates and continued to grow after sexual maturation, indicating that ERα is required for the effects of estrogens on the human growth plate [14]. In vitro studies [15] have suggested that the membrane G protein-coupled receptor GPR30 is also a functional ER. Using a newly developed $GPR30^{-/-}$ mouse model, the authors recently demonstrated that GPR30 deletion abolished E_2-stimulated insulin release both in vivo and in vitro [16]. However, the in vivo role of GPR30 as a functional ER for the regulation of skeletal parameters, including bone mass and longitudinal bone growth, has so far been unknown. In the present paper, the same authors present data supporting that GPR30 is required for a normal estrogenic response in the growth plate suggesting that GPR30 may work in concert with the nuclear ERs in mediating estrogenic effects in growth plate cartilage. However, it should be noted that vehicle-treated $GPR30^{-/-}$ mice displayed reduced growth plate height compared with vehicle-treated WT mice and that this was associated with a nonsignificant trend of reduced femur length in the vehicle-treated $GPR30^{-/-}$. Thus, one cannot exclude that the lack of a significant E_2 effect in the growth plates of $GPR30^{-/-}$ mice is a consequence of reduced growth plate activity already existing in vehicle-treated $GPR30^{-/-}$ mice. Nevertheless, a role of GPR30 in the growth plate is supported by recent findings [3] that GPR30 immunoreactivity is present in the human growth plate with the highest expression in the hypertrophic zone. In addition, GPR30 immunoreactivity was demonstrated to decline during pubertal progression, suggesting that GPR30 might be involved in the modulation of longitudinal bone growth [17]. It can be concluded that although GPR30 seems not to be a functional ER in several major ER-responsive tissues, it is mediating E_2-stimulated insulin release and is required for a normal estrogenic response in the growth plate. GPR30 might be a future therapeutic target for the modulation of longitudinal bone growth.

Deleterious effect of late menarche on distal tibia microstructure in healthy 20-year-old and premenopausal middle-aged women

Chevalley T, Bonjour JP, Ferrari S, Rizzoli R
Division of Bone Diseases, Department of Rehabilitation and Geriatrics, Geneva University Hospitals and Faculty of Medicine, Geneva, Switzerland
Thierry.Chevalley@hcuge.ch
J Bone Miner Res 2009;24:144–152

Background: Late menarche is a known risk factor for fragility fractures. The authors hypothesized that pubertal timing-dependent alterations in bone structural components would persist from peak bone mass to menopause, independent of premenopausal bone loss.

Methods: The influence of menarcheal age on femoral neck aBMD by DXA and microstructure of distal tibia by high resolution pQCT were studied in healthy young adult (age 20.4 ± 0.6 [SD] years, n = 124) and premenopausal middle-aged (age 45.8 ± 3.4 years, n = 120) women. Median menarcheal age was 13.0 ± 1.2 and 13.1 ± 1.7 years in young adult and premenopausal middle-aged women, respectively.

Results: In young adults and premenopausal middle-aged women (n = 244), femoral neck aBMD, total volumetric BMD and cortical thickness of distal tibia were inversely correlated to menarcheal age. After segregation by the median menarcheal age in early and late subgroups, the significant influences of both menarcheal age (p = 0.004) and chronological age (p < 0.0001) were observed for femoral neck aBMD and trabecular bone volume fraction of the distal tibia with similar differences in T scores between late and early subgroups in young adults and premenopausal middle-aged women. Cortical thickness was negatively influenced by menarcheal age, whereas trabecular thickness was negatively influenced by chronological age. There was also a striking inverse relationship between cross-sectional area and cortical thickness (R = –0.57, p < 0.001).

Conclusion: The negative influence of late menarcheal age at weight-bearing sites remained unattenuated a few years before menopause and was independent of premenopausal bone loss. Alterations in both bone mineral mass and microstructural components may explain the increased risk of fragility fractures associated with later menarcheal age.

Several factors in women that are related to their reproductive life influence bone health. The age at menarche and variations in pubertal timing are known to influence the risk of fragility fractures [18]. In the current paper, Chevalley et al. aimed to study whether the influence of menarcheal age at the time of peak bone mass attainment was also detectable in a cohort of premenopausal women close to the mean age of menopause onset. The study design allowed testing the hypothesis of whether any deleterious effect of premenopausal bone loss in healthy women would be additive to the persisting negative influence of late menarche. Based on their findings, it appears that pubertal timing in women is an important factor modulating the risk of sustaining a fragility fracture during adulthood. The deficit observed at the age of peak bone mass, which is attributable to late pubertal timing, remained evident and significant even 25 years later at an age close to the onset of menopause. In healthy women, a delay of approximately 2 years in menarcheal age was linked to significant decreases in T scores of the femoral neck aBMD and trabecular density at the distal tibia. The launch of the World Health Organization technical report 'Assessment of osteoporosis at the primary health care level' and the related web-based FRAX® tool (http://www.shef.ac.uk/FRAX/) have been major milestones towards helping health professionals worldwide to improve identification of patients at high risk of fracture. An individual's risk factors such as age, sex, weight, height, and femoral neck BMD (if available) are entered into the website tool, followed by clinical risk factors which include a prior fragility fracture, parental history of hip fracture, current tobacco smoking, long-term use of glucocorticoids, rheumatoid arthritis, other causes of secondary osteoporosis and daily alcohol consumption. Before late menarcheal age can be included as a risk factor for females in the FRAX® tool, the data in this paper must be confirmed in a larger population and the background conditions leading to late menarche need to be better scrutinized.

Sclerostin antibody treatment increases bone formation, bone mass, and bone strength in a rat model of postmenopausal osteoporosis

Li X, Ominsky MS, Warmington KS, Morony S, Gong J, Cao J, Gao Y, Shalhoub V, Tipton B, Haldankar R, Chen Q, Winters A, Boone T, Geng Z, Niu QT, Ke HZ, Kostenuik PJ, Simonet WS, Lacey DL, Paszty C
Department of Metabolic Disorders, Amgen, Thousand Oaks, Calif., USA
cpatzty@amgen.com

J Bone Miner Res 2009;24:578–588

Background: A long-standing goal in the treatment of bone loss conditions, such as osteoporosis, has been the development of bone-rebuilding anabolic agents. The osteocyte-derived secreted protein sclerostin has been shown to be a key negative regulator of bone formation, although the magnitude and extent of sclerostin's role in the aging skeleton is still unclear. The aim was to study sclerostin biology and to assess the pharmacologic effects of sclerostin inhibition.

Methods: The authors used a cell culture model of bone formation to identify a promising sclerostin-neutralizing monoclonal antibody (Scl-AbII), which then was tested in an aged ovariectomized rat model of postmenopausal osteoporosis. Six-month-old female rats were ovariectomized and left untreated for 1 year to allow significant estrogen deficiency-induced bone loss, at which point Scl-AbII was administered for 5 weeks.

Results: Scl-AbII treatment in these animals had robust anabolic effects, with marked increases in bone formation on trabecular, periosteal, endocortical, and intracortical surfaces. This resulted in complete reversal of estrogen deficiency-induced bone loss at several skeletal sites, but also further increased bone mass and bone strength to levels greater than those found in non-ovariectomized control rats.

Conclusion: These preclinical results establish sclerostin's role as a pivotal negative regulator of bone formation in the aging skeleton. In addition, antibody-mediated inhibition of sclerostin represents a promising new therapeutic approach for the anabolic treatment of bone-related disorders.

The vast majority of therapeutics that are being used in the treatment of bone loss conditions are antiresorptive agents (e.g. bisphosphonates) that exert their clinical effect by decreasing the rate of bone loss and achieving a reduction in fracture incidence. However, there has been a long-standing goal to develop bone-rebuilding anabolics. Currently, the only approved bone anabolic is parathyroid hormone which, either in full-length or truncated form, is administered by daily injections. A new possible target for bone anabolic treatment has emerged from the discovery of a protein called sclerostin. The sclerostin gene was originally identified by mutational analyses of an extremely rare genetic disorder, sclerosteosis (Van Buchem's disease), which is an autosomal recessive sclerosing bone dysplasia characterized by massive bone overgrowth [19]. Sclerostin has been demonstrated to block bone formation both in vivo and in vitro. It is produced by mature osteocytes and has not been found in any other cell type, making it very bone-specific and thus an optimal drug candidate. The authors of this elegant article developed, screened and tested a particular sclerostin antibody, which resulted in a complete reversal of estrogen deficiency-induced bone loss. More dramatically, bone mass and strength were further increased to greater levels than in controls. These results indicate that osteocyte-derived sclerostin is a pivotal negative regulator of bone formation, bone mass and bone strength, and has great clinical potential. The osteocyte has long been hypothesized to orchestrate local bone remodeling and the value of this cell type as a drug discovery target is becoming more evident. As reviewed in Yearbook 2008 [3], osteocytes can control physiological functions distant from bone by the production of osteocalcin and FGF-23 but clearly also have local effects on skeletal metabolism via sclerostin. Interestingly, sclerostin was recently also found to play an essential role in mediating bone response to mechanical unloading, an effect which was found to be mediated through Wnt/β-catenin signaling [20]. Wnt/β-catenin signaling plays a key role in controlling bone mass via regulating multiple aspects including osteoblast differentiation and function and its activity has also previously been shown to be enhanced upon mechanical loading [21].

Vitamin D receptor genotype in hypophosphatemic rickets as a predictor of growth and response to treatment

Jehan F, Gaucher C, Nguyen TM, Walrant-Debray O, Lahlou N, Sinding C, Dechaux M, Garabedian M
Institut National de la Santé et de la Recherche Médicale Unit 561, Hôpital Saint Vincent de Paul, Paris, France
frederic.jehan@inserm.fr

J Clin Endocrinol Metab 2008;93:4672–4682

Background: Treatment of X-linked hypophosphatemic rickets improves bone mineralization and bone deformities, but its effect on skeletal growth is highly variable. The aim of the study was to explore whether genetic variants in the promoter region of the vitamin D receptor (VDR) gene may explain the response to treatment.
Methods: The VDR promoter haplotype structure was studied in a large cohort of 91 patients with hypophosphatemic rickets including 62 patients receiving 1α-hydroxyvitamin D_3 derivatives and phosphates from early childhood.
Results: Treatment improved bone deformities and final height, but 39% of treated patients still had short stature at the end of growth (–2 SD score or below). Height was closely associated with VDR promoter Hap1 genotype. Hap1$^-$ patients (35% of the cohort) had severe growth defects. This disadvantageous association of Hap1$^-$ status with height was visible before treatment, under treatment, and on to adulthood. Compared with Hap1$^+$ patients, those who were Hap1$^-$ had a higher urinary calcium response to 1α-hydroxyvitamin D_3 and had significantly lower circulating FGF23 levels.
Conclusions: The VDR promoter genotype can serve as a key predictor of growth under treatment with 1α-hydroxyvitamin D_3 derivatives in patients with hypophosphatemic rickets, including those with established PHEX alterations. The VDR promoter genotype appears to provide valuable information for adjusting treatment and for deciding upon the utility of early GH therapy.

Children with hypophosphatemic rickets grow poorly and have a shorter than expected final height. In this study the authors found that analysis of VDR promoter genotype appears to be a valuable tool for predicting the severity of the growth defect and the risk of developing hypercalciuria. The severe growth defect in Hap1$^-$ patients cannot easily be attributed to a higher sensitivity to vitamin D and was obviously disconnected from the severity of bone deformities and from the biological phenotype. The present data are at odds with that obtained in healthy adolescents, showing that girls with a Hap1$^-$ genotype were taller, not shorter, than girls with a Hap1$^+$ genotype [22]. This suggests a currently unknown local VDR effect on cell proliferation or differentiation in the growth plates of long bones that involves one or more factors altered by mutations of the *Phex* gene. Further studies are needed to conclude whether VDR promoter genotype analysis will play a role in defining an optimal therapeutic strategy that includes GH treatment in hypophosphatemic patients. Genotype-phenotype inconsistencies were puzzling when we used to think of monogenic diseases. In the new era of genome-wide association studies nothing remains monogenic, and VDR polymorphism (certainly not the only one) may contribute to the phenotype variability in Phex gene mutations.

Damaging effects of chronic low-dose methotrexate usage on primary bone formation in young rats and potential protective effects of folinic acid supplementary treatment

Fan C, Cool JC, Scherer MA, Foster BK, Shandala T, Tapp H, Xian CJ
Department of Orthopaedic Surgery, Women's and Children's Hospital, Adelaide, SA, Australia
cory.xian@unisa.edu.au

Bone 2009;44:61–70

Background: Methotrexate (MTX) is an often used anti-metabolite in cancer treatment and is frequently used as an anti-rheumatic drug. While MTX chemotherapy at a high dose is known to cause bone growth defects in growing bones, the effects of its chronic use at a low dose on the growing skeleton remain less clear.

Methods: The authors examined the effects on bone growth of long-term MTX chemotherapy at a low dose in young rats, and potential protective effects of supplementary treatment with the antidote folinic acid (given i.p. at 1 mg/kg 6 h after MTX).

Results: Two cycles of 5 once-daily MTX injections (0.75 mg/kg, 5 days on/9 days off/5 days on) caused a significant reduction in the heights of growth plate and primary spongiosa bone when analyzed on day 22 and compared to controls. In contrast, a similar dosing regimen but at a lower dose (0.4 mg/kg) caused only slight or no reduction in heights of both regions. However, after the induction phase at this 0.4 mg/kg dosing, continued use of MTX at a low dose (once weekly at 0.2 mg/kg) caused a reduction in primary spongiosa height and bone volume in weeks 9 and 14, which was associated with an increased osteoclast formation and decreased osteoblast bone surface density in the primary spongiosa. Folinic acid supplementation prevented the MTX effects in the primary spongiosa.

Conclusion: The data show that acute use of MTX can damage growth plate and primary bone at a high dose, but not at a low dose. However, long-term use of MTX at a low dose can reduce primary bone formation, an effect which is prevented by folic acid supplementation.

The intensive use of chemotherapy with anti-cancer drugs has been commonly associated with bone growth arrest and osteoporosis in survivors, and it has also become apparent that children are showing poor bone growth after chemotherapy has stopped. Methotrexate (MTX), an often used anti-cancer and anti-rheumatic drug, acts as an anti-folate metabolite affecting purine/thymidylate and thus DNA synthesis and cell proliferation. Despite the effectiveness of MTX in both cancer chemotherapy and rheumatoid arthritis management, discontinuation is common due to the occurrence of its adverse side effects. MTX is known to cause bone growth defects in pediatric cancer patients, and fractures in children have been reported during and after chemotherapy treatment [23], which may be due to the accumulation of dose during long-term chemotherapy treatment. The authors hypothesized that the damaging effects of MTX on bone growth and bone formation will be treatment dosage- and duration-dependent and that supplementary folinic acid may provide protective effects during long-term low-dose MTX chemotherapy. Their data show that acute use of MTX can damage growth plate and primary bone at a high dose, but not at a low dose. However, long-term use of MTX at a low dose also reduced primary bone formation, an effect which was prevented by folic acid supplementation. Further studies are needed to characterize the MTX skeletal damaging effects and the underlying mechanisms and to investigate benefits and possible mechanisms of folinic acid action in protecting bone growth during MTX chemotherapy.

Bone growth during rapamycin therapy in young rats

Sanchez CP, He YZ
Department of Pediatrics, University of Wisconsin School of Medicine and Public Health, Madison, Wisc., USA
cpsanchez@pediatrics.wisc.edu
BMC Pediatr 2009;9:3

Background: Rapamycin is an effective immunosuppressant widely used to maintain the renal allograft in pediatric patients. As rapamycin has potent anti-proliferative and anti-angiogenic properties, it was hypothesized that linear growth may be adversely affected if used in growing individuals.

Methods: Weanling 3-week-old rats were given rapamycin (2.5 mg/kg) daily by gavage for 2 or 4 weeks. Serum levels of calcium, phosphate, PTH, urea nitrogen, creatinine and insulin-growth factor I (IGF-I) were analyzed. Histomorphometric analysis of the growth plate cartilage, in situ hybridization experiments and immunohistochemical studies for various proteins were performed.

Results: At the end of the 2 weeks, body and tibia length measurements were shorter after rapamycin therapy associated with an enlargement of the hypertrophic zone and a decrease in chondrocyte proliferation in the growth plate cartilage. The increased number of hypertrophic chondrocytes may be partly explained by reduced expression of parathyroid hormone/parathyroid hormone-related peptide (PTH/PTHrP) and an increase in Indian hedgehog (Ihh). In addition, the number of chondro/osteoclasts declined in the chondro-osseous junction. Although body and tibial length remained short after 4 weeks of rapamycin, changes in the expression of chondrocyte proliferation, chondrocyte differentiation and chondro/osteoclastic resorption, which were significant after 2 weeks of rapamycin, improved at the end of 4 weeks.

Conclusion: When given to young rats, 2 weeks of rapamycin significantly decreased endochondral bone growth. At the end of 4 weeks, no catch-up growth was demonstrated although markers of chondrocyte proliferation and differentiation improved.

Rapamycin is a powerful immunosuppressant widely used in children to maintain the renal allograft. Studies have shown that rapamycin decreases cell proliferation by inhibition of the mammalian target of rapamycin (*mTOR*), a key regulator in cell growth [24]. In addition, rapamycin has been demonstrated to exert anti-angiogenic properties to control tumor growth by reduction in vascular endothelial growth factor (*VEGF*) expression [25]. Since rapamycin is now a standard immunosuppressant used to maintain an organ transplant in children, linear growth may be affected if rapamycin is administered long-term to young and growing patients. The authors aimed to assess the short- and long-term effects of rapamycin on endochondral bone growth in young rats with normal renal function using markers of chondrocyte proliferation, chondrocyte differentiation, chondroclast/osteoclastic resorption and angiogenesis in the tibial growth plate. Their data suggest that rapamycin suppresses bone growth, an effect which may be linked to an observed decline in chondrocyte proliferation, enhancement of chondrocyte maturation, and alterations in cartilage resorption and vascularization. The present study showed a downregulation by rapamycin of *PTH/PTHrP* accompanied by enhancement of *Ihh*, a mechanism that has been reviewed in the Yearbook series several times over. Interestingly, the authors found that the 2-week effects of rapamycin on chondrocyte proliferation, chondrocyte maturation and vascular invasion may improve to near normal if rapamycin is administered continuously as the animal matures although no catch-up growth was demonstrated. Therefore, it is too early to draw any conclusions regarding any long-term effects of rapamycin on longitudinal bone growth. Furthermore, it is important to point out that the rapamycin dose used in this study was higher than the currently prescribed amount in pediatric patients. Clinical studies are needed to assess whether long-term therapy with rapamycin can affect linear growth in young pediatric patients.

Food for thought: could aspirin prevent osteoporosis?

Pharmacologic stem cell based intervention as a new approach to osteoporosis treatment in rodents

Yamaza T, Miura Y, Bi Y, Liu Y, Akiyama K, Sonoyama W, Patel V, Gutkind S, Young M, Gronthos S, Le A, Wang CY, Chen W, Shi S
Center for Craniofacial Molecular Biology, University of Southern California School of Dentistry, Los Angeles, Calif., USA
wchen@mail.nih.gov or songtaos@usc.edu
PLoS ONE 2008;3:e2615

Background: Osteoporosis is the most prevalent skeletal disorder, characterized by a low bone mineral density (BMD) and bone structural deterioration, leading to bone fragility fractures. Accelerated bone resorption by osteoclasts has been established as a principal mechanism in osteoporosis. However, recent experimental evidence suggests that apoptosis of osteoblasts and osteocytes would also account for the imbalance in bone remodeling in osteoporosis. The aim was to examine whether aspirin, which has been reported as an effective drug improving bone mineral density in human epidemiology studies, regulates the balance between bone resorption and bone formation at the level of stem cell differentiation.

Methods: The authors performed multiple in vitro and in vivo experiments on activated T cells and bone marrow mesenchymal stem cells (MSCs). The role of aspirin was evaluated both in vitro and in vivo. The ovariectomy (OVX)-induced osteoporosis model in the mouse was selected to examine the feasibility and mechanisms of aspirin-mediated therapy for osteoporosis.

Results: T-cell-mediated MSC impairment was found to play a crucial role in OVX-induced osteoporosis. Ex vivo mechanistic studies revealed that T-cell-mediated MSC impairment was mainly attributed to the apoptosis of MSCs via the Fas/Fas ligand pathway. Aspirin inhibited T-cell activation and Fas ligand induced MSC apoptosis in vitro. Furthermore, aspirin increased osteogenesis of MSCs and inhibited osteoclast activity in OVX mice, leading to ameliorating bone density.

Conclusion: A novel mechanism for osteoporosis in which activated T cells induce MSC apoptosis via the Fas/Fas ligand pathway was identified. The results suggest that pharmacologic stem cell-based intervention by aspirin to activate osteoblasts and inhibit osteoclasts may be a new alternative in the treatment of osteoporosis.

Have you ever thought of aspirin as a potential medicine to restore bone mineral balance after estrogen-deprivation? This complex study comes from 5 different research centers in the US, Japan and Australia, and states two provocative messages. The first is an extension of prior studies on the role of T cells in the pathogenesis of osteoporosis. Previously, the role of lymphocytes in pathological bone loss has focused on the effects on bone resorption. Here, the authors present an impressive number of in vitro and in vivo experiments demonstrating that activated T cells are also involved in the apoptosis of bone marrow MSCs, suggesting that activated T cells may decrease bone formation. The second message is a new finding that pretreatment with aspirin diminishes bone loss in OVX mice by a T-cell-dependent mechanism. OVX mice were pretreated for 2 months with aspirin before surgery and continued on aspirin for another month after OVX. These aspirin-treated OVX mice were compared with sham-operated and OVX mice without any aspirin treatment. Mice treated with aspirin had less trabecular bone loss compared to OVX only mice. However, since there were no sham-operated controls treated with aspirin, it is not clear whether the effects observed with aspirin treatment are specific to OVX. This work certainly gives some food for thought: it suggests that aspirin has a potential to be used as an anti-osteoporosis drug, although many questions still remain. For example, the direct mechanism of aspirin action was not identified in this study. However, since human epidemiologic studies have suggested an association of aspirin with BMD, and since low dose aspirin is widely used and relatively safe, prospective studies of its effects on the rapid peri- and post-menopausal bone loss would be feasible and of great clinical interest.

Review: bisphosphonates are beneficial in the treatment of pediatric osteogenesis imperfecta patients but long-term effects remain to be clarified

Effects of bisphosphonates in children with osteogenesis imperfecta: an AACPDM systematic review

Castillo H, Samson-Fang L
Cincinnati Children's Hospital Medical Center, Cincinnati, Ohio, USA
Lisa.Samson-Fang@hsc.utah.edu

Dev Med Child Neurol 2009;51:17–29

Background: The American Academy for Cerebral Palsy and Developmental Medicine (AACPDM) has undertaken the development of systematic reviews to summarize the literature about specific interventions to assist children with developmental disabilities.

Methods: This systematic review of the effects of bisphosphonate treatment in children with osteogenesis imperfecta (OI) was conducted using methodology for developing systematic reviews of treatment interventions (Revision 1.1) 2004. The review was limited to studies in which bisphosphonate was the intervention and the participants were children with a defined OI. Literature search for studies published in PubMed, CINAHL, and the Cochrane Database of Systematic Reviews was performed. Of 109 citations, 70 met inclusion criteria. Outcomes were classified based on a level of evidence ranking (http://www.cebm.net/index.aspx?o=1047).

Results: Even though a large number of publications on this topic exist, only 8 studies had a sufficiently high level of internal validity to be truly informative. These studies confirmed the improvement in bone density. Many, but not all, studies demonstrated a reduction in fracture rate and enhanced growth. Only very limited evaluation of broader treatment impacts (e.g. deformity, need for orthopedic surgery, pain, functioning, or quality of life) was available. Short-term side effects were reported as minimal.

Conclusion: The authors conclude that additional research is needed to verify the safe treatment of infants with bisphosphonates. It is not yet clear, which medication and dosing regimen is optimal and how long patients should be treated. The evidence would be strengthened by a larger controlled trial, because many studies lacked adequate power to evaluate stated outcomes. The effects of bisphosphonates in children with milder forms of OI and severe forms that are not due to mutations in the type I pro-collagen gene (e.g. types VII and VIII) are not addressed in the current literature. More studies evaluating especially medication choices, optimal dosing, duration of treatment, post-treatment impacts, and long-term side effects are necessary.

OI is an inherited bone disease with no cure. Gene therapy has been suggested as one possibility but the variety of mutations and the difficulties in controlling gene expression makes this very distant. Current treatment strategy is based on the use of bisphosphonates to prevent fractures and on surgery. This is a systematic review of the current literature, in which intervention studies with any bisphosphonate on OI children (aged < 18 yr at time of treatment) were included. Studies were assigned a level of evidence ranking according to study design and methods. Then, the authors coded each level of evidence outcome by a component of the International Classification of Functioning, Disability and Health. Analysis of the component, where the intervention was expected to work (i.e. body function and structure), showed a consistent finding of improved bone density. Reduction in the fracture rate by 30–60% was demonstrated in 3 of 4 small randomized trials. Statistically significant positive effects on growth were reported in 2 of 5 studies. The authors furthermore evaluated the evidence on the bisphosphonate intervention on other components (e.g. activity, participation) and on the magnitude and nature of medical complications. An encouraging finding was that very few serious short-term side effects were reported in the published literature and that these side effects were generally mild and reversible. Taken together, this review could confirm the improvement in bone density by bisphosphonate intervention in pediatric OI patients. A reduction in fracture rate and enhanced growth were demonstrated in many but not all studies. However, little information was available on how long to treat and what the long-term effects are. To conclude, larger controlled trials are needed, since many studies have so far lacked adequate power to evaluate the stated outcomes. Since the use of bisphosphonates is widespread and with the known benefits it is not ethical to perform a randomized controlled trial with an untreated control group. Ideally, future studies should be performed in homogenous groups and should include information on potential confounders. Perhaps a large multicenter study with patients assigned to different dosing regimens could be considered? It is important to point out that while proven to be effective in OI, bisphosphonate therapy in other pediatric patients remains controversial because of inadequate long-term efficacy and safety data. For this reason, many experts recommend limiting the use of these agents to those children with recurrent extremity fractures, symptomatic vertebral collapse, and reduced bone mass. As recently reviewed [26], current data are inadequate to support the use of bisphosphonates in children to treat reductions in bone mass/density alone. More research is needed to define appropriate indications for bisphosphonate therapy and the optimal agent, dose, and duration of use in pediatric patients.

Review: diagnosing rickets based on the etiology of hypophosphatemia

Hypophosphatemia: the common denominator of all rickets

Tiosano D, Hochberg Z
Meyer Children's Hospital, Rambam Medical Center, Haifa, Israel
d_tiosano@rambam.health.gov.il

J Bone Miner Metab 2009; DOI 10.1007/s00774-009-0079-1

Background: Rickets is a disease of hypertrophic growth plate chondrocytes which is caused by hypophosphatemia that leads to a defect in terminal hypertrophic chondrocyte apoptosis. This highlights the critical role of phosphorous in cartilage and bone metabolism.

Results: This paper gives a broad overview of phosphorous metabolism, transport and function in maintaining phosphorous supply to the growth plate, bone osteoblast and the kidney.

Conclusion: A new classification for the differential diagnosis of rickets is proposed. This is based on the mechanisms leading to hypophosphatemia – high PTH activity, high FGF23 activity or renal phosphaturia.

The common denominator of all rickets is hypophosphatemia. Hypophosphatemia prevents apoptosis in the hypertrophic cells in the growth plate. In the absence of apoptosis, the hypertrophic cells accumulate in the growth plate and form the rachitic bone. Based on these facts, the authors propose that the diagnosis of rickets should be based on the etiologies of hypophosphatemia. The three major entities that can lead to hypophosphatemia are high PTH activity, high FGF23 activity and renal defects that lead to Pi wasting. Hallmarks of high PTH activity are: hypophosphatemia, phosphaturia, disturbance in vitamin D metabolism and low calcium. Hallmarks for high FGF23 activity are hypophosphatemia and phosphaturia with inappropriately low $1,25(OH)_2D$. Hallmarks for renal rickets are hypophosphatemia and phosphaturia with high $1,25(OH)_2D$ that causes hypercalciuria. Besides proposing a new classification of rickets, the review gives an overview of the underlying causes of rickets.

References

1. Rousseau F, Bonaventure J, Legeai-Mallet L, Pelet A, Rozet JM, Maroteaux P, et al: Mutations in the gene encoding fibroblast growth factor receptor-3 in achondroplasia. Nature 1994;371:252–254.
2. Seino Y, Yamanaka Y, Shinohara M, Ikegami S, Koike M, Miyazawa M, et al: Growth hormone therapy in achondroplasia. Horm Res 2000;53(suppl 3):53–56.
3. Chrysis D, Heino T, Sävendahl L: Growth plate, bone and calcium; in Carel J-C, Hochberg Z (eds): Yearbook of Pediatric Endocrinology 2008. Basel, Karger; 2008. pp 63–79.
4. Yasoda A, Komatsu Y, Chusho H, Miyazawa T, Ozasa A, Miura M, et al: Overexpression of CNP in chondrocytes rescues achondroplasia through a MAPK-dependent pathway. Nat Med 2004;10:80–86.
5. Chusho H, Tamura N, Ogawa Y, Yasoda A, Suda M, Miyazawa T, et al: Dwarfism and early death in mice lacking C-type natriuretic peptide. Proc Natl Acad Sci USA 2001;98:4016–4021.
6. VanHouten J, Dann P, McGeoch G, Brown EM, Krapcho K, Neville M, et al: The calcium-sensing receptor regulates mammary gland parathyroid hormone-related protein production and calcium transport. J Clin Invest 2004;113:598–608.
7. VanHouten JN, Dann P, Stewart AF, Watson CJ, Pollak M, Karaplis AC, et al: Mammary-specific deletion of parathyroid hormone-related protein preserves bone mass during lactation. J Clin Invest 2003;112:1429–1436.
8. Brown EM: The calcium-sensing receptor: physiology, pathophysiology and CaR-based therapeutics. Subcell Biochem 2007;45:139–167.
9. Vahle JL, Sato M, Long GG, Young JK, Francis PC, Engelhardt JA, et al: Skeletal changes in rats given daily subcutaneous injections of recombinant human parathyroid hormone (1–34) for 2 years and relevance to human safety. Toxicol Pathol 2002;30:312–321.
10. Vahle JL, Long GG, Sandusky G, Westmore M, Ma YL, Sato M: Bone neoplasms in F344 rats given teriparatide [rhPTH(1–34)] are dependent on duration of treatment and dose. Toxicol Pathol 2004;32:426–438.
11. Wagner CL, Greer FR: Prevention of rickets and vitamin D deficiency in infants, children, and adolescents. Pediatrics 2008;122:1142–1152.
12. Holick MF: Resurrection of vitamin D deficiency and rickets. J Clin Invest 2006;116:2062–2072.
13. Holick MF, Biancuzzo RM, Chen TC, Klein EK, Young A, Bibuld D, et al: Vitamin D2 is as effective as vitamin D3 in maintaining circulating concentrations of 25-hydroxyvitamin D. J Clin Endocrinol Metab 2008;93:677–681.
14. Smith EP, Boyd J, Frank GR, Takahashi H, Cohen RM, Specker B, et al: Estrogen resistance caused by a mutation in the estrogen-receptor gene in a man. N Engl J Med 1994;331:1056–1061.
15. Revankar CM, Cimino DF, Sklar LA, Arterburn JB, Prossnitz ER: A transmembrane intracellular estrogen receptor mediates rapid cell signaling. Science 2005;307:1625–1630.
16. Martensson UE, Salehi SA, Windahl S, Gomez MF, Sward K, Daszkiewicz-Nilsson J, et al: Deletion of the G protein-coupled receptor 30 impairs glucose tolerance, reduces bone growth, increases blood pressure, and eliminates estradiol-stimulated insulin release in female mice. Endocrinology 2009;150:687–698.
17. Chagin AS, Savendahl L: GPR30 estrogen receptor expression in the growth plate declines as puberty progresses. J Clin Endocrinol Metab 2007;92:4873–4877.
18. Roy DK, O'Neill TW, Finn JD, Lunt M, Silman AJ, Felsenberg D, et al: Determinants of incident vertebral fracture in men and women: results from the European Prospective Osteoporosis Study (EPOS). Osteoporos Int 2003;14:19–26.
19. Balemans W, Ebeling M, Patel N, Van Hul E, Olson P, Dioszegi M, et al: Increased bone density in sclerosteosis is due to the deficiency of a novel secreted protein (SOST). Hum Mol Genet 2001;10:537–543.
20. Lin C, Jiang X, Dai Z, Guo X, Weng T, Wang J, et al: Sclerostin mediates bone response to mechanical unloading via antagonizing Wnt/beta-catenin signaling. J Bone Miner Res 2009; DOI: 10.1359/JBMR.090411.
21. Robinson JA, Chatterjee-Kishore M, Yaworsky PJ, Cullen DM, Zhao W, Li C, et al: Wnt/beta-catenin signaling is a normal physiological response to mechanical loading in bone. J Biol Chem 2006;281:31720–31728.
22. d'Alesio A, Garabedian M, Sabatier JP, Guaydier-Souquieres G, Marcelli C, Lemacon A, et al: Two single-nucleotide polymorphisms in the human vitamin D receptor promoter change protein-DNA complex formation and are associated with height and vitamin D status in adolescent girls. Hum Mol Genet 2005;14:3539–3548.
23. Mandel K, Atkinson S, Barr RD, Pencharz P: Skeletal morbidity in childhood acute lymphoblastic leukemia. J Clin Oncol 2004;22:1215–1221.
24. Fingar DC, Blenis J: Target of rapamycin (TOR): an integrator of nutrient and growth factor signals and coordinator of cell growth and cell cycle progression. Oncogene 2004;23:3151–3171.

25. Manegold PC, Paringer C, Kulka U, Krimmel K, Eichhorn ME, Wilkowski R, et al: Antiangiogenic therapy with mammalian target of rapamycin inhibitor RAD001 (Everolimus) increases radiosensitivity in solid cancer. Clin Cancer Res 2008;14:892–900.
26. Bachrach LK, Ward LM: Clinical review 1: Bisphosphonate use in childhood osteoporosis. J Clin Endocrinol Metab 2009;94:400–409.

Reproductive Endocrinology

Olle Söder and Lena Sahlin

Paediatric Endocrinology Unit, Department of Women's and Children's Health, Astrid Lindgren Children's Hospital; Q2:08, Karolinska Institutet and Karolinska University Hospital, Stockholm, Sweden

Reproductive biology and endocrinology is a lively research area attracting considerable attention as the implications concern the everyday life of human beings. Last year's chapter focused somewhat on the rapidly expanding stem cell field which, also this year, has shown continuous high activity, and some contributions adding novel possibilities for fertility preservation have been included. Genetics offers interesting discoveries adding new genes to the scene and revealing novel functions of old friends. Basic cell biology still delivers novel concepts by contributing 3 papers on the role of micro RNAs in reproduction. There is also interesting work linking endocrinology with behavioral sciences. Not everything can be covered and other chapters of this book also deal with subjects linked to reproduction. This chapter aims to present a mix of experimental and clinical papers advancing the field with positive implications for human beings.

New hope
Fertility preservation

Ovary and uterus transplantation

Gosden RG
Center for Reproductive Medicine and Infertility, Weill Medical College of Cornell University, New York, N.Y., USA
rgg2004@med.cornell.edu
Reproduction 2008;136:671–680

Background: The survival rates for children treated for cancer have increased. Therefore a concern for preservation of fertility is an important aspect to consider in the follow-up, when the children enter adolescence and adulthood. In these cases ovarian and uterine transplantation could have potential applications. *Methods:* Cryopreservation of tissue is providing opportunities for banking, e.g., ovaries for indefinite periods before transplanting them back to restore fertility. The natural plasticity of the ovary facilitates grafting to different sites where they can be revascularized and rapidly restore the normal physiology of secretion and ovulation. Uterine transplantation by vascular anastomosis provides potentially longer function but is technically much more demanding and riskier for the recipient. *Results:* In humans, autografts have functioned for up to 3 years before needing replacement. Uterine transplantation has enabled successful pregnancies in several species, but not yet in humans. Neither ovary nor uterus is privileged immunologically and allografts become rapidly rejected except in hosts whose immune system is deficient or suppressed pharmacologically. *Conclusions:* Cryopreservation and uterine transplantation, with their limitations, raise hope for the preservation of fertility in the increasing number of survivors after childhood cancers.

Production of offspring from a germline stem cell line derived from neonatal ovaries

Zou K, Yuan Z, Yang Z, Luo H, Sun K, Zhou L, Xiang J, Shi L, Yu Q, Zhang Y, Hou R, Wu J
School of Life Science and Biotechnology, Shanghai Jiao Tong University, Shanghai, China
Nat Cell Biol 2009;11:631–636

Background: The idea that females of most mammalian species have lost their capacity for oocyte production at birth has recently been challenged by the finding that juvenile and adult mouse ovaries possess mitotically active germ cells. The existence of female germ line stem cells (FGSCs) in postnatal mammalian ovaries is still a controversial issue among reproductive biologists and stem cell researchers.

Methods: In the present study a neonatal mouse FGSC line was established, with normal karyotype and high telomerase activity, by immunomagnetic isolation and cultured for more than 15 months.

Results: FGSCs from adult mice were isolated and cultured for more than 6 months. These FGSCs were infected with GFP virus and transplanted into the ovaries of infertile mice. Transplanted cells underwent oogenesis and the mice produced offspring that had the GFP transgene.

Conclusions: These findings contribute to basic research into oogenesis and stem cell self-renewal and open up new possibilities for use of FGSCs in biotechnology and medicine. Thus, there is a possibility for oocyte renewal after birth!

Long-term spermatogonial survival in cryopreserved and xenografted immature human testicular tissue

Wyns C, Van Langendonckt A, Wese FX, Donnez J, Curaba M

Department of Gynecology, Université Catholique de Louvain, Cliniques, Universitaires Saint-Luc, Brussels, Belgium

Hum Reprod 2008;23:2402–2414

Background: Preservation of the male germ line in prepubertal boys undergoing gonadotoxic treatment is a crucial consideration in terms of their future quality of life. As these patients do not yet produce spermatozoa for freezing, only immature tissue is available for storage.

Methods: The survival, proliferation and differentiation capacity of spermatogonia were studied after cryopreservation and long-term transplantation of immature testicular tissue pieces. Single pieces of testicular tissue (2–8 mm) from prepubertal boys (7–14 years) were cryopreserved, thawed and transplanted into the scrotum of mice for 6 months. Upon removal, histological, immunohistochemical and ultrastructural analyses and testicular sperm extraction (TESE) were used to evaluate the tissue.

Results: Histology showed 55 ± 42% of tubules to be intact. MAGE-A4 immunostaining showed mean spermatogonial recovery to be 3.7 ± 5.5%, with 35% of these cells expressing Ki67, giving evidence of proliferation in tissue from boys <14 years of age. No apoptosis was found, as demonstrated by the absence of active caspase-3 and TUNEL staining. Numerous premeiotic spermatocytes, a few spermatocytes at the pachytene stage and spermatid-like cells were observed. No immunostaining was observed for lactate dehydrogenase C, ACE or proacrosin, indicating that the spermatid-like structures observed by histology did not express the meiotic and post-meiotic markers characteristic of normal spermatids. No ultrastructural alterations of the tissue were encountered.

Conclusions: The present study demonstrates that spermatogonia are able to survive and proliferate after cryopreservation and long-term transplantation. Complete regeneration of normal spermatogenesis was not observed since, beyond the pachytene stage, no adequate characterization of germ cells was obtained. Further studies are thus required to investigate the differentiation potential of cryopreserved germ cells.

The 3 publications above are selected from the rapidly emerging literature opening up new avenues to prevent and treat infertility in both sexes after damage to the reproductive organs. Such adverse events are common in children and young adults undergoing aggressive treatments for cancer. The expanding field of late-effects research aims at helping this growing group of new survivors to a better life after cure, employing novel techniques and tools. New survivors subscribing to endocrine services are found not only among cancer patients but also in children born at an extremely premature gestational age, in those with severe metabolic disorders and congenital malformations, and in other patient groups. The stem cell field holds great promise for these patients and is illustrated by the paper on germ line stem cells isolated from postnatal ovaries. This paper challenges the dogma that females lose their capacity for oocyte production at birth, a concept that has held considerable controversy for some time. The authors show convincingly that a female germ line stem cell line established from the postnatal ovary could produce offspring when transplanted into the ovaries of infertile mice. The review by Gosden extends the discussion beyond ovaries and germ cells by discussing the possibility of uterus transplantation. This may be of interest in cases where uterine tissue has been permanently damaged by irradiation to the pelvis. Although technically demanding such an approach has proven successful in experimental animals, and gives hopes for the future also in humans. Testicular damage to prepubertal males before spermatogenesis is established may result in infertility due to azoospermia. It is now 15 years since Brinster et al. [1] showed a prophylactic cure for such an event by demonstrating that mouse hosts receiving spermatogonial stem cells as transplants into the seminiferous tubules were able to produce donor-derived offspring. This breakthrough has since then been replicated in many species but still not in humans. There are still many technical obstacles to be overcome before such a procedure can be established as a safe method in the clinic. The paper by Wyns et al. deals with such attempts focusing on human testis tissue samples.

Spermatogonia survived cryopreservation and transplantation and the few remaining spermatogonia found in long-term orthotopic xenografts of immature human testicular tissue from boys <14 years of age proliferated, suggesting that some SGSCs could be present in this cell population. However, complete regeneration of normal spermatogenesis was not observed, and spermatogenesis stopped at the pachytene spermatocyte stage. The question arises whether cryopreservation with a view to fertility restoration is appropriate in peripubertal boys.

New paradigms
Reviews on non-genomic effects of progesterone

Non-genomic progesterone actions in female reproduction

Gellersen B, Fernandes MS, Brosens JJ
Endokrinologikum Hamburg, Hamburg, Germany
gellersen@endokrinologikum.com
Hum Reprod Update 2009;15:119–138

Honey, we need to talk about the membrane progestin receptors

Fernandes MS, Brosens JJ, Gellersen B
Institute of Reproductive and Developmental Biology, Imperial College London, Hammersmith Hospital, London, UK
Steroids 2008;73:942–952

Background: Progesterone controls key female reproductive events that range from ovulation to implantation, maintenance of pregnancy and breast development. In addition to activating the 'classical' progesterone receptors (PRs)-A and B, progesterone also elicits a variety of rapid signaling events independent of transcriptional or genomic regulation. The combination of rapid non-genomic events and the slower transcriptional actions is thought to determine the functional response to progesterone in the female reproductive system in a cell-type- and environment-specific manner.

Methods: The first of the 2 reviews covers current knowledge (PubMed up to August 2008) on the mechanisms and relevance of non-genomic progesterone signaling in female reproduction.

Results: Several putative progesterone-binding moieties have been implicated in rapid signaling events, including the nuclear PR and its variants, PR membrane component 1, and the novel family of membrane progestin receptors. Progesterone and its metabolites have also been implicated in regulation of e.g. γ-aminobutyric acid type A, oxytocin and sigma-1 receptors. Identification of the mechanisms and receptors that mediate rapid progesterone signaling is an area of research burdened with difficulties and controversy. The recent discovery of 3 closely related cell surface receptors that bind to progesterone and mediate its actions on various cytoplasmic signaling cascades has been regarded as a major breakthrough. The novel membrane progestin receptors (mPRα, β, γ) are reported to be similar to, and function as, G-protein-coupled receptors. However, studies by these authors failed to confirm that mPRs are expressed on the cell surface. In addition, they were also not able to verify that mPRs mediate rapid progesterone signaling events, not even that they are real progestin-binding moieties.

Conclusions: While the reason for these startling opposing results remains unclear, these critical reviews of existing data can help to shed some light onto the controversial mPRs. The controversy around membrane-bound PR still remains.

The concept of membrane receptors for steroid hormones exerting non-genomic actions by employing rapid cytoplasmatic signaling pathways has been an interesting but controversial subject for many years. All classes of steroid hormones have been implicated within this context but a major focus has been on the sex steroids [2]. For progestins the existence of such receptors is best shown by studies in lower species such as fish [3], but convincing data from higher organisms are sparse. The selected reviews update the field to the current status. The recent identification of the membrane progestin receptor has not provided the long sought after solution to the unresolved issues in the mechanism of rapid non-genomic progestin actions. Rather, it has sparked a new debate as to the function of these novel proteins. The very promising features of these molecules raised hopes that specific agonists and antagonists could be developed, capable of dissecting nuclear from extra-nuclear, slow from rapid, genomic from non-genomic actions. It is unclear at this stage where the journey will lead. This information may be useful for a pediatric endocrinologist, but the feeling is still that more questions than answers are provided.

Food for the eye
Paparazzo of the year

Laparoscopic observation of spontaneous human ovulation

Lousse JC, Donnez J
Department of Gynecology, Université Catholique de Louvain, Brussels, Belgium
Fertil Steril 2008;90:833–834

A surgeon, scheduled to perform a laparoscopic hysterectomy on a woman on day 16 of the menstrual cycle, observed spontaneous ovulation in the left ovary, as illustrated by protrusion of the mature follicle and oocyte release into the peritoneal cavity. The release of an egg was considered a sudden, explosive event, but it took place over a period of at least 15 min [see also New Scientist of June 11, 2008].

Being at the right time at the right place with a camera the surgeon was able to catch human ovulation at the very moment when the egg was released from the ovarian surface. Must be seen! Comments are superfluous.

Mechanisms explained
ERα – a key player both in the female and male reproductive tract

An estrogen receptor-α knock-in mutation provides evidence of ligand-independent signaling and allows modulation of ligand-induced pathways in vivo

Sinkevicius KW, Burdette JE, Woloszyn K, Hewitt SC, Hamilton K, Sugg SL, Temple KA, Wondisford FE, Korach KS, Woodruff TK, Greene GL
Ben May Department for Cancer Research, University of Chicago, Chicago, Ill., USA
Endocrinology 2008;149:2970–2979

Estrogen-dependent and -independent estrogen receptor-α signaling separately regulate male fertility

Sinkevicius KW, Laine M, Lotan TL, Woloszyn K, Richburg JH, Greene GL
Ben May Department for Cancer Research, University of Chicago, Chicago, Ill., USA
Endocrinology 2009;150:2898–2905

Background: Estrogen receptor-α (ERα) plays a critical role in reproductive tract development and fertility. To determine if estrogen-dependent and/or -independent ERα mechanisms are involved in fertility, the authors examined estrogen non-responsive ERα knock-in (ENERKI) mice.

Methods: ENERKI mice were generated to distinguish between ligand-induced and ligand-independent ERα actions in vivo. These mice have a mutation in the ligand-binding domain of ERα, which significantly reduces ERα interaction with and response to endogenous estrogens, whereas not affecting growth factor activation of ligand-independent pathways.

Results: ENERKI mice have hypoplastic uterine tissues and rudimentary mammary gland ductal trees. Females are infertile due to anovulation, and their ovaries contain hemorrhagic cystic follicles because of chronically elevated levels of LH. The ENERKI phenotype confirmed that ligand-induced activation of ERα is crucial in the female reproductive tract and mammary gland development. Growth factor treatments induced uterine epithelial proliferation in ovariectomized ENERKI females, directly demonstrating that ERα ligand-independent pathways were active. The synthetic ERα selective agonist propyl pyrazole triol (PPT) treatment initiated at puberty stimulated ENERKI uterine development, whereas neonatal treatments were needed to restore mammary gland ductal elongation, indicating that neonatal ligand-induced ERα activation may prime mammary ducts to become more responsive to estrogens in adult tissues. In the male reproductive system it was found that ligand-independent ERα signaling is essential for concentrating epididymal sperm via regulation of efferent ductule fluid reabsorption. On the other hand, estrogen-dependent ERα signaling is required for germ cell viability, most likely through support of Sertoli cell function. By treating ENERKI mice with PPT it was discovered that male fertility requires neonatal estrogen-mediated ERα signalling.

Conclusions: These results indicate both estrogen-dependent and -independent pathways to play separable roles in male murine reproductive tract development. Thus, the ENERKI mouse model is a valuable tool to investigate ERα ligand dependent and independent pathways in the reproductive tract of both males and females.

These are interesting novel data on the role of ERα in male (and female) reproduction. There are both estrogen-dependent and independent actions of ERα, the latter exerted by ER activation by growth factors independent of the traditional ligand. The knock-in model was designed to distinguish between these 2 pathways. In the male the importance of ERα for fluid homeostasis in the testis and epididymis was verified and deducted to be an estrogen-independent effect. The importance of estrogen (or ER) for male germ cell survival was also supported, adding to previous data in other species [4, 5]. The data suggest that the role of ERα in human infertility should be examined more closely. Because only 1 human male has been reported to have an inactivating ERα mutation, it is unlikely that mutations leading to ERα deletion account for a significant percentage of human male infertility cases. However, the role of ERα polymorphisms in male infertility remains to be established.

New Mechanisms
Pubertal hormones restructure the brain

Pubertal hormones modulate the addition of new cells to sexually dimorphic brain regions

Ahmed EI, Zehr JL, Schulz KM, Lorenz BH, DonCarlos LL, Sisk CL
Neuroscience Program, Michigan State University, East Lansing, Mich., USA
Nature Neurosci 2008;11:995–997

Background: Structural sexual dimorphism of the brain results in behavioral differences between the sexes that are well recognized. However, the regulation and timing of the establishment of these differences are not well understood.

Methods: Young male and female rats were labeled with BrdU and the number and location of newly formed cells determined in sexually dimorphic brain regions in the presence and absence of sex steroids.

Results: New cells are added to the rat brain during puberty, and sex differences in the number of newly added cells correspond to sex differences in adult volume in each region. Pubertal sex steroids influence the addition of new cells, presumably by promoting cell genesis and/or survival in sexually dimorphic structures in a sex-specific manner.

Conclusions: Hormone-modulated addition of cells to sexually dimorphic brain regions is an active mechanism for maintaining functional sex differences during adolescence and into adulthood.

Testosterone programs adult social behavior before and during, but not after, adolescence

Schulz KM, Zehr JL, Salas-Ramirez KY, Sisk CL
Department of Psychology and Neuroscience Program, Michigan State University, East Lansing, Mich., USA
Endocrinology 2009; Epub ahead of print

Background: The pubertal and adolescent brain is a major target for sex hormones but our understanding of such hormonal influences on adolescent behavioral development is not well understood.
Methods: The authors investigated how variations in the timing of testosterone exposure, relative to adolescence, alters the strength of steroid-sensitive neural circuits underlying social behavior in male Syrian hamsters. Animals were exposed to early, on-time, and late pubertal development by treating gonadectomized males with testosterone implants for 19 days before, during or after adolescence. Effects of preadolescent testosterone treatment on behavior and brain regional volumes within the mating neural circuit of juvenile males were also investigated.
Results: Androgen treatment before or during adolescence, but not after, facilitated mating behavior in adulthood. In addition, pre-adolescent testosterone treatments most effectively increased mating behavior overall, indicating that the timing of exposure to pubertal hormones contributes to individual differences in adult behavior. Pre-adolescent testosterone treatment did not induce reproductive behavior in juvenile males but did increase volumes of the BST, SDN, MePD, and MePV to adult-typical size. In contrast, juvenile MeAD and VMH volumes were not changed by preadolescent testosterone treatment, suggesting that further maturation of these brain regions during adolescence is required for the expression of male reproductive behavior.
Conclusions: Adolescent maturation of social behavior may involve both steroid-independent and steroid-dependent processes, and adolescence marks the end of a postnatal period of sensitivity to steroid-dependent organization of the brain. These results have important translational implications for human pubertal development and are in line with recent data from the same group referred to herein (see above) demonstrating sexually dimorphic additions of new cells in certain brain areas during adolescence.

These papers link exposure to sex steroids, particularly androgens, at appropriate time points of development to sexual dimorphism in brain morphology and behavior. Although the present studies were performed in experimental animals, modern brain imaging techniques associated with metabolic and functional elements now available in human medicine [6] may soon be used to ask similar questions in pediatric and adolescent patient groups. Results to come are expected to add important implications for our management of children with DSD, pubertal and behavioral disorders, and other conditions. One wonders about brain organization in children with early virilization, and whether the timing of pubertal onset affects such organization. Although this research did not directly model a psychiatric disease state, the finding that adult behaviors vary depending on the timing of hormone exposure across the adolescent period speaks for the possibility that direct hormone–brain interactions moderate the effects of pubertal timing on many behaviors, even in humans.

Association studies of common variants in 10 hypogonadotropic hypogonadism genes with age at menarche

Gajdos ZK, Butler JL, Henderson KD, He C, Supelak PJ, Egyud M, Price A, Reich D, Clayton PE, Le Marchand L, Hunter DJ, Henderson BE, Palmert MR, Hirschhorn JN
Program in Genomics and Division of Endocrinology, Children's Hospital, and Department of Genetics, Harvard Medical School, Boston, Mass., USA
J Clin Endocrinol Metab 2008;93:4290–4298

Background: Although the timing of puberty is a highly heritable trait, little is known about the genes that regulate pubertal timing in the general population. Several genes have been identified that, when mutated, cause disorders of delayed or absent puberty such as hypogonadotropic hypogonadism (HH). Because severe variants in HH-related genes cause a severe puberty phenotype, we hypothesized that common subtle variation in these genes could contribute to the population variation in pubertal timing.

Methods: The common genetic variation in 10 HH-related genes in 1,801 women from the Hawaii and Los Angeles Multiethnic Cohort with either early (age <11 years) or late (age >14 years) menarche and in other replication samples was assessed. In addition to these common variants, the most frequently reported HH mutations were also determined to assess their role in the population variation in pubertal timing. Within the general community, 1,801 women from the Hawaii and Los Angeles Multiethnic Cohort participated. The association of genetic variation with age at menarche was assessed.

Results: No significant association between any of the variants tested and age at menarche was detected; although it cannot be ruled out that a modest effect of these variants or of other variants may operate at long distances from the coding region. In several self-reported racial/ethnic groups represented in the study, an association between estimated genetic ancestry and age at menarche was observed.

Conclusions: The results suggest that common variants near 10 HH-related loci do not play a substantial role in the regulation of age at menarche in the general population.

The nature and function of the 'pubertal clock' regulating the onset of puberty in humans is not well understood, although this timing is highly heritable. Contrary to expectations, the laborious approach taken by these authors did not pay off since none of the tested HH-related genes was found to be associated with the age at menarche in a large cohort of women. This underlines the complexity of this issue and the need for a more genome-wide approach to make progress in this important research. Such efforts are underway in ongoing studies by other investigators [see also the selected paper by Ong et al. below], but negative results over a decade seem to indicate that the timing of puberty is not in the gene sequence, but rather in their expression.

Female mice delay reproductive aging in males

Schmidt JA, Oatley JM, Brinster RL
Department of Animal Biology, University of Pennsylvania, Philadelphia, Pa., USA
Biol Reprod 2009;80:1009–1014

Background: Reproductive aging of the male is characterized by decreasing reproductive function and fertility but factors that protect against this process in the aging male are largely unknown. Previous work has demonstrated that both female presence and aging have a dramatic effect on fertility in the male; yet, the effect of female presence on fertility in the aging male mouse is unknown. The objective of this work was to determine the effect of long-term isolation or cohabitation with females on fertility in aged male mice.

Methods: Male mice were housed with or without females until between 16 and 32 months of age. Males were subjected to fertility tests at specific ages, after which serum and testes were isolated for radioimmunoassay and histological analysis.

Results: Male mice continuously housed with females remain fertile longer (approximately 20% of the reproductive lifespan) than male mice housed alone. Fertility became significantly reduced 6 months sooner for males housed alone compared with males housed with females; however, the rate of decline was the same for males housed with or without females once fertility began to decrease. Testis weight decreased as the mice aged, and a nearly significant positive effect of female presence was observed. Additionally, histological analysis indicated that abnormal spermatogenesis occurred sooner in isolated males, suggesting that defects in spermatogenesis may play a role in the greater decrease in fertility in isolated males.

Conclusions: These results have significant implications for the maintenance of male fertility in wildlife, livestock, and human populations.

These are fascinating and provocative data demonstrating that the physical presence of females delays reproductive aging in males. Although the evidence comes from mice, the possible translation of these results into human biology has obvious and important societal and psychosocial implications. In evolutionary terms, where fitness is measured in fecundity, this makes a lot of sense: for a species longevity increases fitness only if a reproductive partner is around. However whether this 'mechanism' works both ways, i.e. females vs. males, as demonstrated here, and vice versa males vs. females, remains to be established. The findings may have particular relevance in societies with increasing ageing populations, with demands for maintained high quality of life. Exactly how the medical profession will adapt and transform these novel findings into medical advice and practice will be interesting to follow.

Genetics
New gene and novel functions of old friends

Ovaries and female phenotype in a girl with 46,XY karyotype and mutations in the CBX2 gene

Biason-Lauber A, Konrad D, Meyer M, DeBeaufort C, Schoenle EJ
Division of Endocrinology/Diabetology, University Children's Hospital, Zurich, Switzerland
anna.lauber@kispi.uzh.ch
Am J Hum Genet 2009;84:658–663

Background: A specific molecular diagnosis is identified in only 20% of disorders of sex development cases. SRY alone is insufficient to induce testicular development and several other components of the male pathway have been identified, including Sox9, Dmrt1, Fgf9, Dhh, Sox8, and Dax1. WNT4 appears to be essential for sexual differentiation in women. Mice with targeted ablation of M33, an ortholog of *Drosophila* polycomb, show male-to-female sex reversal. Apart from sterility, most M33 knockout Sry-positive mice were phenotypically perfect females. A human counterpart of murine M33 deletion has so far not been identified.

Methods: A girl with a prenatal 46,XY karyotype was born with a completely normal female phenotype, including uterus and histologically normal ovaries. The human homolog of M33, Chromobox homolog 2 (CBX2), was analyzed.

Results: A loss-of-function mutation of CBX2 was found, identifying the present case as a human counterpart of the murine model.

Conclusions: By placing CBX2 upstream of SRY, an additional component of the still incomplete cascade of factors regulating human sex development has been added.

Mutations in CHD7, encoding a chromatin-remodeling protein, cause idiopathic hypogonadotropic hypogonadism and Kallmann syndrome

Kim HG, Kurth I, Lan F, Meliciani I, Wenzel W, Eom SH, Kang GB, Rosenberger G, Tekin M, Ozata M, Bick DP, Sherins RJ, Walker SL, Shi Y, Gusella JF, Layman LC
Molecular Neurogenetics Unit, Center for Human Genetic Research, Massachusetts, General Hospital, and Department of Genetics, Harvard Medical School, Boston, Mass., USA
Am J Hum Genet 2008;83:511–519

Background: CHARGE syndrome and Kallmann syndrome (KS) are two distinct developmental disorders sharing overlapping features of impaired olfaction and hypogonadism. KS is a genetically heterogeneous disorder consisting of idiopathic hypogonadotropic hypogonadism (IHH) and anosmia, and is most commonly due to KAL1 or FGFR1 mutations. CHARGE syndrome, a multisystem autosomal-dominant disorder, is caused by CHD7 mutations. The authors hypothesized that CHD7 would be involved in the pathogenesis of IHH and KS (IHH/KS) without the CHARGE phenotype and that IHH/KS represents a milder allelic variant of CHARGE syndrome.
Methods: Mutation screening of the 37 protein-coding exons of CHD7 was performed in 101 IHH/KS patients without a CHARGE phenotype. In an additional 96 IHH/KS patients, exons 6–10, encoding the conserved chromodomains, were sequenced. RT-PCR, SIFT, protein-structure analysis, and in situ hybridization were performed for additional supportive evidence.
Results: Seven heterozygous mutations, 2 splice and 5 missense, which were absent in 180 or more controls, were identified in 3 sporadic KS and 4 sporadic normosmic IHH patients. Three mutations affect chromodomains critical for proper CHD7 function in chromatin remodeling and transcriptional regulation, whereas the other 4 affect conserved residues, suggesting that they are deleterious. CHD7's role is further corroborated by specific expression in IHH/KS-relevant tissues and appropriate developmental expression. Sporadic CHD7 mutations occur in 6% of IHH/KS patients.
Conclusions: CHD7 represents the first identified chromatin-remodeling protein with a role in human puberty and the second gene to cause both normosmic IHH and KS in humans. The findings indicate that both normosmic IHH and KS are mild allelic variants of CHARGE syndrome and are caused by CHD7 mutations.

Mutations in NR5A1 associated with ovarian insufficiency

Lourenço D, Brauner R, Lin L, De Perdigo A, Weryha G, Muresan M, Boudjenah R, Guerra-Junior G, Maciel-Guerra AT, Achermann JC, McElreavey K, Bashamboo A
Human Developmental Genetics, Institut Pasteur, Paris, France
N Engl J Med 2009;360:1200–1210

Background: The genetic causes of nonsyndromic ovarian insufficiency are largely unknown. A nuclear receptor, NR5A1 (better known as SF1), is a key transcriptional regulator of genes involved in the hypothalamic-pituitary-steroidogenic axis. Mutation of NR5A1 causes 46,XY disorders of sex development, with or without adrenal failure, but growing experimental evidence from studies in mice suggests a key role for this factor in ovarian development and function as well.
Methods: To test the hypothesis that mutations in NR5A1 cause disorders of ovarian development and function, the authors sequenced NR5A1 in four families with histories of both 46,XY disorders of sex development and 46,XX primary ovarian insufficiency and in 25 subjects with sporadic ovarian insufficiency. None of the affected subjects had clinical signs of adrenal insufficiency.
Results: Members of each of the 4 families and 2 of the 25 subjects with isolated ovarian insufficiency carried mutations in the NR5A1 gene. In-frame deletions and frameshift and missense mutations were detected. Functional studies indicated that these mutations substantially impaired NR5A1 transactivational activity. Mutations were associated with a range of ovarian anomalies, including 46,XX gonadal dysgenesis and 46,XX primary ovarian insufficiency. These mutations were not observed in more than 700 control alleles.
Conclusions: NR5A1 mutations are associated with 46,XX primary ovarian insufficiency and 46,XY disorders of sex development.

These 3 papers reveal novel genetic contributions to DSD and pubertal disorders. The first human case (XY sex reversal) with a mutation of the CBX2 gene, a homolog of the murine M33 gene, was described by Biason-Lauber et al. The human phenotype matches that of the M33 knockout mouse adding an interesting contribution to the array of genes involved in mammalian sex differentiation. The CBX2 gene is believed to be located upstream of SRY. CDH7 is a chromatin remodeling protein which, when mutated, is known to cause CHARGE syndrome. When analyzing a large group of IHH/Kallmann patients without genetic diagnosis, CDH7 was shown to be involved in 3–5% of cases thus representing a milder phenotype of CHARGE. Even if its precise function is uncertain, CHD7 appears to be important in GnRH and olfactory neuron migration to their embryologic destination in the hypothalamus. Although providing proof-of-concept the paper shows that genes other than CDHT7 must be involved in the pathogenesis of IHH/Kallmann in most cases.

Important work by Lourenço et al. demonstrated that the NR5A1 gene (SF1) is linked to primary ovarian failure and DSD in several independent familial cases without adrenal involvement. This is a major contribution since the background to most cases of such ovarian insufficiency is unknown.

Important for Clinical Practice

Consensus statement on the use of gonadotropin-releasing hormone analogs in children

Carel JC, Eugster EA, Rogol A, Ghizzoni L, Palmert MR; ESPE-LWPES GnRH Analogs, Consensus Conference Group, Antoniazzi F, Berenbaum S, Bourguignon JP, Chrousos, GP, Coste J, Deal S, de Vries L, Foster C, Heger S, Holland J, Jahnukainen K, Juul A, Kaplowitz P, Lahlou N, Lee MM, Lee P, Merke DP, Neely EK, Oostdijk W, Phillip M, Rosenfield RL, Shulman D, Styne D, Tauber M, Wit JM
Department of Pediatric Endocrinology and Diabetes, INSERM U690, Robert Debré Hospital and University Paris, Paris, France
jean-claude.carel@inserm.fr
Pediatrics 2009;123:e752–762

Background: Gonadotropin-releasing hormone analogs revolutionized the treatment of central precocious puberty. However, questions remain regarding their optimal use in central precocious puberty and other conditions.

Methods: The Lawson Wilkins Pediatric Endocrine Society and the European Society for Pediatric Endocrinology convened a consensus conference to review the clinical use of gonadotropin-releasing hormone analogs in children and adolescents.

Participants: When selecting the 30 participants, consideration was given to equal representation from North America (United States and Canada) and Europe, an equal male/female ratio, and a balanced spectrum of professional seniority and expertise. Preference was given to articles written in English with long-term outcome data. The US Public Health grading system was used to grade evidence and rate the strength of conclusions. When evidence was insufficient, conclusions were based on expert opinion. Participants were put into working groups with assigned topics and specific questions. Written materials were prepared and distributed before the conference, revised on the basis of input during the meeting, and presented to the full assembly for final review. If consensus could not be reached, conclusions were based on majority vote. All participants approved the final statement.

Results and Conclusions: The efficacy of gonadotropin-releasing hormone analogs in increasing adult height is undisputed only in early-onset (girls <6 years old) central precocious puberty. Other key areas, such as the psychosocial effects of central precocious puberty and their alteration by gonadotropin-releasing hormone analogs, need additional study. Few controlled prospective studies have been performed with gonadotropin-releasing hormone analogs in children, and many conclusions rely in part on collective expert opinion. The conference did not endorse commonly voiced concerns regarding the use of gonadotropin-releasing hormone analogs, such as promotion of weight gain or long-term diminution of bone mineral density. Use of gonadotropin-releasing hormone analogs for conditions other than central precocious puberty requires additional investigation and cannot be suggested routinely.

Puberty, contraception, and hormonal management for young people with disabilities

Zacharin MR
Department of Endocrinology and Diabetes, Royal Children's Hospital, Melbourne, Vic., Australia
Clin Pediatr (Phila) 2009;48:149–155

Background: Assessment and management of a young person with a severe disability is multifaceted and complex. Variations of puberty can cause major concerns for parents and carers, with fears of imminent menstruation, peer and personal differences, concern for height outcome, as well as grief for a loss of childhood. Addressing physical, emotional, and social issues assists in optimizing outcomes.
Methods and Results: This article outlines specific evaluation and detailed management strategies for female and male pubertal problems in the context of disability, including treatments for extreme pubertal delay or acceleration, menstrual management at different ages, contraceptive issues, and sexual function and choices for both sexes.
Conclusions: This paper gives valuable advice and recommendations for the management of this important and difficult subject in young people.

Two papers contributing to good clinical practice were selected. Although the use of gonadotropin-releasing hormone analogs to treat children with hypergonadotropic precocious puberty is daily routine for every pediatric endocrinologist there are still unresolved questions concerning optimal protocols, combination with growth hormone treatment and other issues. The consensus statement by LWPES/ESPE on this topic after a well-structured conference is therefore much warranted and recommended as evidence base.

The 2nd paper gives valuable advice on how to manage problems with puberty, contraception and sexual function in adolescents with disabilities. This is a sensitive and not much discussed topic in adults with a handicap and even more so in the present age group. The paper is recommended to all colleagues seeing such patients in their clinics including pediatric endocrinologists, pediatricians gynecologists, general practitioners and others.

New paradigms
Big roles for small RNAs

Deletion of Dicer in somatic cells of the female reproductive tract causes sterility

Nagaraja AK, Andreu-Vieyra C, Franco HL, Ma L, Chen R, Han DY, Zhu H, Agno JE, Gunaratne PH, DeMayo FJ, Matzuk MM
Department of Pathology, Baylor College of Medicine, Houston, Tex., USA
Mol Endocrinol 2008;22:2336–2352

Background: Dicer is a ribonuclease enzyme necessary for microRNA (miRNA) processing and the synthesis of siRNAs from long double-stranded RNA. Dicer plays important roles in the mammalian germ line and early embryogenesis but its functions in somatic cells of the female reproductive tract are largely unknown.
Methods: Employing conditional knockout technology mice were made deficient in Dicer1 in the mesenchyme of the developing Müllerian ducts and postnatally in ovarian granulosa cells and mesenchyme-derived cells of the oviducts and uterus.
Results: Deletion of Dicer in these cell types results in female sterility and multiple reproductive defects including decreased ovulation rates, compromised oocyte and embryo integrity, and other structural changes. Sequencing of small RNAs in the oviduct revealed downregulation of specific miRNAs in Dicer conditional knockout females compared with wild-type. These miRNAs are predicted to mainly regulate genes important for Müllerian duct differentiation and mesenchyme-derived structures, several of which were significantly upregulated upon conditional deletion of Dicer1.
Conclusions: Dicer and its miRNA products have critical roles in the development and function of the female reproductive tract.

Dicer1 is required for differentiation of the mouse male germline

Maatouk DM, Loveland KL, McManus MT, Moore K, Harfe BD
Department of Microbiology and Immunology, University of California, Diabetes Center, San Francisco, Calif., USA
Biol Reprod 2008;79:696–703

Background: MicroRNAs (miRNAs) are small noncoding RNAs that posttranscriptionally regulate gene expression. A great number of miRNAs are expressed in mammals but their specific functions are yet to be uncovered. The enzyme Dicer1 is required for miRNA processing, and mouse knockouts of Dicer1 are embryonic lethal before 7.5 days postcoitus.
Methods: The function of miRNAs was examined specifically in the germ line using a conditional knockout of Dicer1 in a mouse model.
Results: Removal of Dicer1 from germ cells resulted in male infertility. Germ cells were present in adult testes, but few tubules contained elongating spermatids. Germ cells that did differentiate to elongating spermatids exhibited abnormal morphology and motility. Rarely, sperm lacking Dicer1 could fertilize wild-type eggs to generate viable offspring.
Conclusions: Dicer1 and miRNAs are essential for proper differentiation of the male germ line. The results point to novel potential mechanisms behind male infertility.

Genetic variation in LIN28B is associated with the timing of puberty

Ong KK, Elks CE, Li S, Zhao JH, Luan J, Andersen LB, Bingham SA, Brage S, Smith GD, Ekelund U, Gillson CJ, Glaser B, Golding J, Hardy R, Khaw KT, Kuh D, Luben R, Marcus M, McGeehin MA, Ness AR, Northstone K, Ring SM, Rubin C, Sims MA, Song K, Strachan DP, Vollenweider P, Waeber G, Waterworth DM, Wong A, Deloukas P, Barroso I, Mooser V, Loos RJ, Wareham NJ
Medical Research Council (MRC) Epidemiology Unit, and Institute of Metabolic Science, Addenbrooke's Hospital, and Department of Paediatrics, University of Cambridge, Cambridge, UK
Nat Genet 2009:41;729–733

Background: The timing of puberty is highly variable but the genetic background of this phenomenon is largely unknown.
Methods: The authors carried out a genome-wide association study for age at menarche in 4,714 women.
Results: An association in LIN28B on chromosome 6 was reported. In independent replication studies in 16,373 women, each major allele was associated with 0.12 years earlier menarche. This allele was also associated with earlier breast development in girls; earlier voice breaking and more advanced pubic hair development in boys; a faster tempo of height growth in girls and boys, and shorter adult height in women and men in keeping with earlier growth cessation. All associations mentioned were highly statistically significant.
Conclusions: These studies identify variation in LIN28B, a potent and specific regulator of microRNA processing, as the first genetic determinant regulating the timing of human pubertal growth and development.

MicroRNAs are small species of non-coding RNA molecules actively produced and processed by the cell to control gene expression at the posttranscriptional level. This intrinsic control system has recently become a hot topic in many areas of human biology. Experimental manipulation of miRNA expression and processing at the systemic level results in severe phenotypes and embryonic lethality. Tissue-specific deletions cause various disturbances dependent on the affected organ system. The dependence of an intact miRNA system for proper development of the male and female reproductive systems is illustrated here by 2 papers selected from the recent literature. Tissue-specific deletion of Dicer1, a key enzyme in miRNA processing, in cells of male and female reproductive organs results in maldifferentiation and infertility as reported by Nagaraja et al. for females and by Maatouk et al. for males.

The importance of miRNA for reproduction is further strengthened by the recent paper by Ong et al. (>40 authors) searching for a genetic background to the timing of puberty. By employing a genome-wide approach with high power, the authors unexpectedly identified a highly significant association in LIN28B on human chromosome 6 with the timing of human pubertal growth and development. LIN28B is a marker of embryonic stem cells and an important regulator of miRNA processing [7] involved in the regulation of IGF-2 expression. A recent genome-wide association study for adult height identified another LIN28B polymorphic mark as 1 of 10 loci with robust association. Different LIN28B isoforms could therefore contribute to the heritability of the timing of growth and development.

Recent decline in age at breast development: the Copenhagen Puberty Study

Aksglaede L, Sørensen K, Petersen JH, Skakkebaek NE, Juul A
Rigshospitalet, Department of Growth and Reproduction, Copenhagen, Denmark
Pediatrics 2009;123:e932–939

Background: Recent publications showing unexpectedly early breast development in American girls have created debate worldwide. However, secular trend analyses are often limited by poor data comparability among studies performed by different researchers in different time periods and populations.

Methods: The authors present new European data systematically collected from the same region and by 1 research group at the beginning and end of the recent 15-year period. Girls (n = 2,095) aged 5.6–20.0 years were studied in 1991–1993 (1991 cohort; n = 1,100) and 2006–2008 (2006 cohort; n = 995). All girls were evaluated by palpation of glandular breast, measurement of height and weight, and blood sampling (for estradiol, luteinizing hormone, and follicle-stimulating hormone). Age distribution at entering pubertal breast stages 2–5, pubic hair stages 2–5, and menarche was estimated for the 2 cohorts.

Results: Onset of puberty, defined as mean estimated age at attainment of glandular breast tissue (Tanner breast stage 2+), occurred significantly earlier in the 2006 cohort (estimated mean age 9.86 years) when compared with the 1991 cohort (estimated mean age 10.88 years). The difference remained significant after adjustment for BMI. Estimated ages at menarche were 13.42 and 13.13 years in the 1991 and 2006 cohorts, respectively. Serum follicle-stimulating hormone and luteinizing hormone did not differ between the 2 cohorts at any age interval, whereas significantly lower estradiol levels were found in 8- to 10-year-old girls from the 2006 cohort compared with similarly aged girls from the 1991 cohort.

Conclusions: The authors found significantly earlier breast development among girls born more recently. Alterations in reproductive hormones and BMI did not explain these marked changes, which suggests that other factors yet to be identified may be involved.

Studies from the US have convincingly demonstrated an earlier start of puberty in girls, particularly in certain ethnic groups. This recent trend, adding an additional component to the secular trend that has been operating for centuries, coincides with the obesity explosion in the US, also mainly affecting the same ethnic groups. Direct correlations between higher BMI and earlier breast development have also been demonstrated in these groups. Despite considerable search, similar trends have been difficult to demonstrate in Europe, which has been suggested to be due to a later onset and less severe obesity trend than that in the US. It is therefore of concern to read the report by Aksglaede et al. on 2 Danish cohorts of girls, one investigated recently and the other 15 years earlier, by the same research group. The authors demonstrate a recent earlier breast development in girls but fail to show a correlation with BMI and the levels of reproductive hormones. Yet, the age at menarche was little affected. In fact, it is surprising that as late as 2006, the average age at menarche was 13.13 years; we thought it was earlier in northern Europe. This points to an influence of environmental factors, the nature of which are still to be determined.

Maternal levels of perfluorinated chemicals and subfecundity

Fei C, McLaughlin JK, Lipworth L, Olsen J
Department of Epidemiology, School of Public Health, University of California, Los Angeles, Calif., USA
Hum Reprod 2009;24:1200–1205

Background: The flame retardants perfluorooctanoate (PFOA) and perfluorooctane sulfonate (PFOS) are ubiquitous manmade compounds that are possible hormonal disruptors. These chemicals are used, e.g., in impregnation of clothes and household fabrics, like carpets.
Methods: In this study the authors examined whether exposure to these compounds may decrease fecundity in humans. Plasma levels of PFOS and PFOA were measured at weeks 4–14 of pregnancy in 1,240 women. For this pregnancy, women were asked to report time to pregnancy (TTP) in five categories (<1, 1–2, 3–5, 6–12 and >12 months). Infertility was defined as having a TTP of >12 months or receiving infertility treatment to establish pregnancy.
Results: Longer TTP was associated with higher maternal levels of PFOA and PFOS. Compared with women in the lowest exposure quartile, the adjusted odds of infertility increased among women in the higher three quartiles of perfluorinated compound levels. Fecundity odds ratios (FORs) were also estimated. The adjusted FORs were virtually identical for women in the 3 highest exposure groups of PFOS compared with the lowest quartile.
Conclusions: The findings from the study suggest that PFOA and PFOS exposure at plasma levels seen in the general population may reduce fecundity. Such results deserve attention, since these substances are all around us and might not only affect us but also generations to come.

Endocrine disruptors (EDs) are manmade chemicals in the environment reported to affect hormonal actions at various levels in the organism. Most convincing data of such effects are from wildlife and proof-of-concept studies in experimental animals. Direct correlation studies in humans are sparse, and causative effects nonexistent. The selected paper demonstrates a correlation between plasma levels of two flame retardants known as EDs and decreased fertility in women. These findings have to be substantiated by more data and confirmation by other groups but still need attention as exposure to these and similar compounds is not easy to avoid in a modern society. Precautionary principles must therefore rule!

References
1. Brinster RL, Avarbock MR: Germline transmission of donor haplotype following spermatogonial transplantation. Proc Natl Acad Sci USA 1994;91:11303–11307.
2. Boonyaratanakornkit V, Edwards DP: Receptor mechanisms mediating non-genomic actions of sex steroids. Semin Reprod Med 2007;25:139–153.
3. Thomas P, Dressing G, Pang Y, Berg H, Tubbs C, Benninghoff A, Doughty K: Progestin, estrogen and androgen G-protein coupled receptors in fish gonads. Steroids 2006;71:310–316.
4. Pentikäinen V, Erkkilä K, Suomalainen L, Parvinen M, Dunkel L: Estradiol acts as a germ cell survival factor in the human testis in vitro. J Clin Endocrinol Metab 2000;85:2057–2067.
5. Wahlgren A, Svechnikov K, Strand ML, Jahnukainen K, Parvinen M, Gustafsson JA, Söder O: Estrogen receptor beta selective ligand 5alpha-androstane-3beta, 17beta-diol stimulates spermatogonial deoxyribonucleic acid synthesis in rat seminiferous epithelium in vitro. Endocrinology 2008;149:2917–2922.
6. Ciumas C, Lindén Hirschberg A, Savic I: High fetal testosterone and sexually dimorphic cerebral networks in females. Cereb Cortex 2009;19:1167–1174.
7. Viswanathan SR, Daley GQ, Gregory RI: Selective blockade of microRNA processing by Lin28. Science 2008;320:97–100.

Adrenals

Bruno Ferraz-de-Souza, Lin Lin and John C Achermann

Developmental Endocrinology Research Group, UCL Institute of Child Health, University College London, London, UK

This year's search of 'adrenal' and 'steroidogenesis' in PubMed yielded more than 6,000 hits from which we have selected the following collection of articles. Whenever possible we have avoided subjects which have been discussed in detail in the Yearbook 2008, unless progress in the field has been incremental [1]. Some emerging themes include modulators of steroidogenesis as a cause of variant phenotypes or new monogenic disorders; peripheral circadian regulation within the adrenal itself; DHEA and adrenarche; and potential cancer therapies developed from studying the molecular pathophysiology of adrenal tumor tissues and cells.

Mechanism of the year
Sulfation defects cause adrenal hyperandrogenism

Inactivating PAPSS2 mutations in a patient with premature pubarche

Noordam C, Dhir V, McNelis JC, Schlereth F, Hanley NA, Krone N, Smeitink JA, Smeets R, Sweep FC, Grinten HL, Arlt W

Centre for Endocrinology, Diabetes, and Metabolism, School of Clinical and Experimental Medicine, University of Birmingham, Birmingham, UK
w.arlt@bham.ac.uk

N Engl J Med 2009;360:2310–2318

Background: Dehydroepiandrosterone (DHEA) sulfotransferase, known as SULT2A1, converts the androgen precursor DHEA to its inactive sulfate ester, DHEAS. This conversion is important in preventing the DHEA being converted to more potent androgens. Normal SULT2A1 catalytic activity requires the sulfate donor, 3'-phosphoadenosine-5'-phosphosulfate (PAPS), which is generated by PAPS synthase 2 (PAPSS2). Defects in these systems could result in impaired DHEA sulfation, resulting in increased conversion of DHEA to androgens.
Methods: Mutational analysis of PAPSS2 in a girl with premature pubarche, hyperandrogenic anovulation, very low DHEAS levels, and increased androgen levels.
Results: Compound heterozygous mutations in the gene encoding human PAPSS2 were identified in this individual. These mutations were found to be inactivateded following coincubation of human SULT2A1 with wild-type or mutant PAPSS2 proteins.
Conclusion: PAPSS2 deficiency is a novel monogenic adrenocortical cause of androgen excess.

Although cytochrome P450 and hydroxysteroid dehydrogenase enzymes play a central role in classic steroidogenic pathways, it is becoming increasingly clear that many other cofactors and modulators of steroidogenic activity also play a key role in regulating this process. Disruption of some of these factors has been shown to result in human disease (e.g. P450 oxidoreductase deficiency; variations in hexose-6-phosphate dehydrogenase) [2, 3]. In this recent report, Wiebke Arlt and colleagues hypothesized that the high DHEA levels and undetectable DHEAS levels found in a girl with premature pubarche, hyperandrogenism, and PCOS/secondary amenorrhea could be due to a defect in part of the sulfation pathway. Sulfation of DHEA into the inactive compound DHEAS is important in reducing circulating levels of DHEA and preventing its conversion into more potent androgens such as testosterone. Sulfation of DHEA is primarily regulated by DHEA sulfotransferase (SULT2A1) in the liver and adrenal, which requires the sulfate donor 3'-phopho-adenosine-5'-phosphosulfate (PAPS) for catalytic activity (fig. 1). PAPS is generated by two isoforms of PAPS synthase, PAPSS1 and PAPSS2. Mutational analysis revealed compound (double) heterozygous changes in PAPSS2 in this girl, which

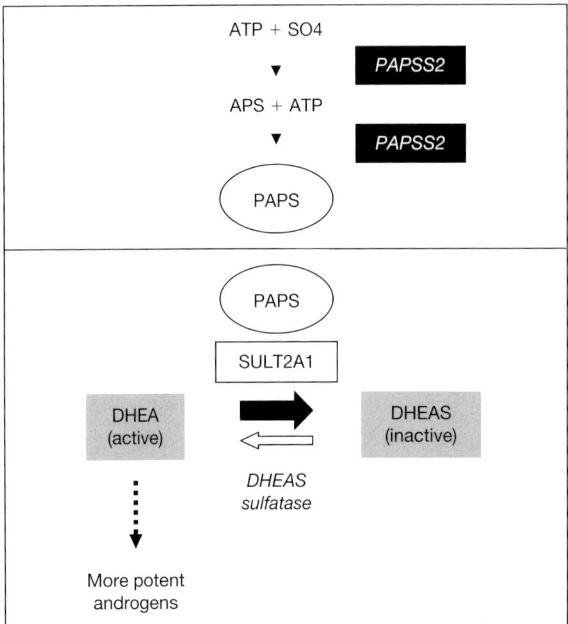

Fig. 1. *Lower panel.* Sulfation of DHEA into the inactive compound DHEAS is important in reducing circulating levels of DHEA and preventing its conversion into more potent androgens such as testosterone. This process is primarily regulated by DHEA sulfotransferase (SULT2A1), which requires interaction with the sulfate donor 3′-phopho-adenosine-5′-phosphosulfate (PAPS) for catalytic activity. *Upper panel.* PAPS synthase 2 (PAPSS2) plays a crucial role in generating PAPS in several tissues. Defects in PAPPS2 have now been shown to cause premature pubarche and hyperandrogenism due to defective DHEA sulfation.

disrupted SULT2A1 activity. Therefore, PAPSS2 deficiency represents a novel regulatory defect of steroidogenesis and a new monogenic cause of adrenal hyperandrogenism. This defect should be considered in children with low or undetectable levels of DHEAS, but with high normal or elevated DHEA and androgens. Of note, loss of PAPSS2 activity has previously been described in one kindred as a cause of spondyloepimetaphyseal dysplasia, Pakistani type (OMIM 603005) [4]. An isoform of PAPSS2 likely plays a key role in proteoglycan sulfation in growth-plate chondrocytes. The girl reported here had advanced bone age, short stature, some vertebral anomalies and shortened tubular bones, which probably reflected a combination of excess androgen exposure together with an underlying bony dysplasia. It remains to be seen how prevalent this condition is, how variable the bony aspects will be, and whether milder disruptions of PAPSS2 or related sulfation factors might be found in more common causes of hyperandrogenism and polycystic ovarian syndrome. On the other hand, DHEAS is a substrate for an activating DHEAS (steroid) sulfatase (fig. 1). This enzyme is expressed in several tissues including adipose tissue and its disruption has been associated with X-linked icthyosis. However, it is quite possible that other clinical and biochemical phenotypes can be associated with disturbances in sulfation systems. You are welcome to guess the phenotypes of these and find such cases.

Programming of hypertension: associations of plasma aldosterone in adult men and women with birthweight, cortisol, and blood pressure

Reynolds RM, Walker BR, Phillips DI, Dennison EM, Fraser R, Mackenzie SM, Davies E, Connell JM
Endocrinology Unit, Centre for Cardiovascular Sciences, Queen's Medical Research Institute, Edinburgh, UK
R.Reynolds@ed.ac.uk
Hypertension 2009;53:932–936

Background: Low birth weight is associated with higher blood pressure in adulthood. Several animal models suggest that this effect may be due to chronic activation of the hypothalamic-pituitary-adrenal or renin-angiotensin-aldosterone axes. In humans, low birth weight has been shown to be associated with elevated plasma cortisol, but associations between birth weight and aldosterone have not been reported.

Methods: Aldosterone was measured in serum samples from 106 women and 205 men from the Hertfordshire cohort (aged 67–78 years) for whom birth weight was recorded. Participants underwent an overnight low-dose (0.25 mg) dexamethasone suppression test and a low-dose (1 µg) ACTH (corticotropin) stimulation test. Genotyping of the −344 C/T polymorphism of the CYP11B2 gene encoding aldosterone synthase was also performed.

Results: Median aldosterone was 6.22 (range 0.15–38.74) ng/dl. This value was higher in men than women (p < 0.0001). Higher aldosterone levels after both dexamethasone and ACTH stimulation were associated with higher blood pressure (r = 0.20, p = 0.001; r = 0.33, p<0.0001, respectively) and with lower birth weight (r = −0.16, p = 0.008; r = −0.21, p = 0.001, respectively). Adjusting for age, gender, obesity, and genotype did not affect the significance of these results.

Conclusion: These findings suggest that, in humans, factors in early life that restrict fetal growth and program activation of the hypothalamic-pituitary-adrenal axis result in increased mineralocorticoid as well as glucocorticoid activity.

Disruption of the Ang II type 1 receptor promotes longevity in mice

Benigni A, Corna D, Zoja C, Sonzogni A, Latini R, Salio M, Conti S, Rottoli D, Longaretti L, Cassis P, Morigi M, Coffman TM, Remuzzi G
Mario Negri Institute for Pharmacological Research, Bergamo, Italy
abenigni@marionegri.it
J Clin Invest 2009;119:524–530

Background: The renin-angiotensin system is a key regulator in the pathogenesis of hypertension and many cardiac and renal diseases in humans. It is likely that angiotensin II (Ang II) regulates this effect through Ang II type 1 receptors (AT$_1$ and AT$_2$) to influence immune responses, inflammation, cell growth and proliferation.

Methods: Generation and characterization of a mouse model with targeted disruption of the Agtr1a gene (encoding AT$_{1A}$).

Results: Agtr1a–/– mice showed marked prolongation of life span compared to wild-types. They developed less cardiac and vascular injury. Multiple organs from these mice displayed less oxidative damage, increased mitochondria and upregulation of the prosurvival genes nicotinamide phosphoribosyltransferase (Nampt) and sirtuin 3 (Sirt3) in the kidney. In cultured tubular epithelial cells, Ang II downregulated Sirt3 mRNA. This effect was inhibited by an AT$_1$ antagonist.

Conclusion: Disruption of AT$_1$ promotes longevity in mice, possibly through the reduction of oxidative stress and overexpression of prosurvival genes. The Ang II/AT$_1$ pathway may be targeted to influence lifespan in mammals.

The association between low birth weight and increased blood pressure and mortality in later life is well established, and a trend towards higher cortisol in children and adults who were smaller at birth has been reported in some studies [5–7]. However, few data exist on the relation between birth weight and the angiotensin-aldosterone axis. In a detailed study of the Hertfordshire cohort (originally investigated by David Barker), John Connell and colleagues show that lower birth weight is associated with higher aldosterone between 67 and 78 years of age, and that aldosterone concentrations were associated with blood pressure measurements. Unfortunately, no measurements of plasma renin activity or aldosterone:renin ratios were reported, and the recorded blood pressures were surprisingly high, potentially reflecting a stress-mediated response. Nevertheless, the fact that recorded aldosterone is higher in later life in individuals born with low birth weight is an important observation. Indeed, the mouse model reported by Benigni et al. shows that disruption of the angiotensin 1A receptor in mice results in quite markedly increased longevity. This is in line with a mouse model of a gain-of-function mutation of AT_1 showing progressive cardiac fibrosis with increased expression of collagen. These studies offer a rationale for exploring the possibility that AT_1 antagonists will prolong life in humans. Indeed, silent activation of the renin-angiotensin system could be a significant factor in programmed excess morbidity and mortality associated with low birth weight.

Extraadrenal 21-hydroxylation by CYP2C19 and CYP3A4: effect on 21-hydroxylase deficiency

Gomes LG, Huang N, Agrawal V, Mendonca BB, Bachega TA, Miller WL
Department of Pediatrics, University of California, San Francisco, Calif., USA
wlmlab@ucsf.edu
J Clin Endocrinol Metab 2009;94:89–95

Background: CYP21A2 gene mutations cause adrenal 21-hydroxylase (P450c21) deficiency (21OHD). CYP21A2 mutations generally correlate well with the 21OHD phenotype, but some children with severe CYP21A2 mutations have residual 21-hydroxylase activity. It is known that progesterone can be 21-hydroxylated by several hepatic P450 enzymes, but the physiological significance of these in modifying 21OHD is not known. Therefore, this study aimed to: (a) determine whether CYP2C19 and CYP3A4 can 21-hydroxylate progesterone and 17-hydroxyprogesterone (17OHP); (b) investigate the potential influence of a common P450 oxidoreductase (POR) variant A503V on these activities, and (c) examine any correlation between CYP2C19 variants and phenotype in patients with 21OHD.
Methods: Human P450c21, CYP2C19, and CYP3A4 were co-expressed in bacteria with wild-type or A503V POR. The 21-hydroxylation of radiolabeled progesterone and 17OHP was assessed, and the maximum velocity (V_{max}) and Michaelis constant (K_m) of the reactions were calculated. CYP2C19 was genotyped in those 21OHD patients where the genotype predicted a severe form of congenital adrenal hyperplasia but in whom the clinical features were milder than expected.
Results: The V_{max}/K_m for 21-hydroxylation of progesterone by CYP2C19 and CYP3A4 were 17 and 10%, respectively, compared to P450c21. Neither CYP2C19 nor CYP3A4 could 21-hydroxylate 17OHP. The A503V variant of POR did not affect this K_m. The CYP2C19 'ultrametabolizer' allele CYP2C19*17 was homozygous in 1 of 5 patients with a 21OHD phenotype that was milder than predicted by the CYP21A2 genotype.
Conclusion: CYP2C19 and CYP3A4 can 21-hydroxylate progesterone but not 17OHP, potentially compensating for mineralocorticoid deficiency, but not for glucocorticoid deficiency. Extraadrenal 21-hydroxylation is likely to reflect the actions of multiple enzymes.

Genotype-phenotype relationships for 21-hydroxylase deficiency are reported to be fairly good, with the severity of the clinical condition usually tracking with the milder defect in compound (double) heterozygote cases. However, it is apparent that some children and adults who are predicted to have severe disease from their genotype status have surprisingly mild biochemical features, and others, with a marked defect in fasciculata glucocorticoid biosynthesis, have normal or mild electrolyte disturbance. The roles of extraadrenal steroid modification is a major area of research, and in this paper Walter Miller and coworkers hypothesize that extraadrenal 21-hydroxylation might play a role in decreasing the severity of CAH in this group of children. Detailed studies of CYP2C19 and CYP3A4 show that these enzymes are able to 21-hydroxylate progesterone but not 17OHP. This effect might reduce the severity of salt loss in some of these patients, especially as mineralocorticoids are normally produced and are active in quantitatively lower concentrations than glucocorticoids in humans. Furthermore, 1 in 5 of patients studied with a milder than expected phenotype was found to be homozygous for the 'ultrametabolizer' CYP2C19 allele. This study focused on two candidate enzymes and also a common variant of P450 oxidoreductase, which was not shown to have a modifying effect [8]. It is possible that other enzymes could play a role in these pathways and that the physiological effects of such changes might be more pronounced in vivo. This paper therefore highlights the importance of extraadrenal steroid modification, which might not only influence patient phenotype but might also influence individual responses to glucocorticoid and mineralocorticoid treatment.

Expression of insulin-like growth factor-II and its receptor in pediatric and adult adrenocortical tumors

Almeida MQ, Fragoso MC, Lotfi CF, Santos MG, Nishi MY, Costa MH, Lerario AM, Maciel CC, Mattos GE, Jorge AA, Mendonca BB, Latronico AC
Unidade de Endocrinologia do Desenvolvimento, Laboratorio de Hormonios e Genetica Molecular/LIM-42 da Disciplina de Endocrinologia do Hospital das Clinicas da Faculdade de Medicina, Universidade de São Paulo, Brasil
madsonalmeida@gmail.com
J Clin Endocrinol Metab 2008;93:3524–3531

Background: Adrenocortical tumors are heterogeneous in nature and their underlying pathogenesis is not well understood. However, studies of adult adrenocortical carcinomas (ACC) have shown that IGF-II overexpression is a frequent feature.
Methods: Expression of IGF-II and its receptor (IGF-IR) was analyzed by quantitative real-time PCR in 57 adrenocortical tumors (37 adenomas and 20 carcinomas; 23 from children, 34 from adults). The effects of a selective IGF-IR kinase inhibitor (NVP-AEW541) on cell proliferation and apoptosis were assessed in NCI H295 cells as well as in a new cell line established from a pediatric adrenocortical adenoma.
Results: Overexpression of IGF-II transcripts was seen in both pediatric ACC and adenomas, and in adult ACC (ACC, 270.5 ± 130.2 vs. adenoma, 16.1 ± 13.3; p = 0.0001). IGF-IR expression was significantly higher in pediatric ACC than adenomas (ACC, 9.1 ± 3.1 vs. adenoma, 2.6 ± 0.3; p = 0.0001), whereas its expression was similar in adult ACC and adenomas. Univariate analysis showed that IGF-IR expression was a predictor of metastases in pediatric ACC (hazard ratio 1.84; 95% confidence interval 1.28–2.66; p = 0.01). The IGF-IR kinase inhibitor, NVP-AEW541, blocked cell proliferation in a time- and dose-dependent manner in both cell lines, primarily through a significant increase in apoptosis.
Conclusion: IGF-IR overexpression appears to be a biomarker of pediatric adrenocortical carcinomas compared to adenomas. A selective IGF-IR kinase inhibitor has antitumor effects in both adult and pediatric adrenocortical tumor cell lines. IGF-IR inhibitors might represent a promising therapy for human adrenocortical carcinoma in the future.

Preclinical targeting of the type I insulin-like growth factor receptor in adrenocortical carcinoma

Barlaskar FM, Spalding AC, Heaton JH, Kuick R, Kim AC, Thomas DG, Giordano TJ, Ben-Josef E, Hammer GD
Department of Internal Medicine-Division of Metabolism, Endocrinology, and Diabetes, University of Michigan Medical School, Ann Arbor, Mich., USA
ghammer@umich.edu
J Clin Endocrinol Metab 2009;94:204–212

Background: Adrenocortical carcinoma (ACC) is a rare and lethal malignancy. Current drug treatment is largely empirical and ineffective. A more effective approach might be to direct new treatments at molecular targets known to be critical in the pathophysiology of ACC.
Methods: Human adrenal tumors and ACC cell lines were profiled by DNA microarray analysis to assess activated IGF signaling. The efficacy of two IGF receptor (IGF-1R) antagonists (NVP-AEW541 and IMC-A12), alone and in combination with mitotane, was assessed in ACC cell lines that display or lack activated IGF signaling and in ACC xenograft tumors in athymic nude mice.
Results: Transcriptional profiling data of human adrenal tumors revealed IGF2 as the single highest upregulated transcript in most carcinomas. The majority of ACC cell lines tested showed constitutive IGF ligand production and activation of downstream effector pathways. Both of the IGF-1R antagonists tested produced significant dose-dependent growth inhibition in ACC cell lines. This growth inhibition was enhanced when mitotane was used in combination with the IGF-1R antagonists. IGF inhibition also markedly reduced ACC xenograft tumor growth greater than that observed with mitotane treatment alone. Combination therapy with mitotane suppressed tumor growth even further.
Conclusion: IGF signaling plays a key role in the pathophysiology of ACC. IGF-1R antagonists provide a rational targeted approach to the treatment of ACC and could form the basis of future clinical trials.

See also:

Inhibition of adrenocortical carcinoma cells proliferation by SF-1 inverse agonists

Doghman M, Cazareth J, Douguet D, Madoux F, Hodder P, Lalli E
Institut de Pharmacologie Moléculaire et Cellulaire, Centre National de la Recherche Scientifique Unité Mixte de Recherche 6097, Valbonne, France
ninino@ipmc.cnrs.fr
J Clin Endocrinol Metab 2009;94:2178–2183

The T cell factor/β-catenin antagonist PKF115-584 inhibits proliferation of adrenocortical carcinoma cells

Doghman M, Cazareth J, Lalli E
Institut de Pharmacologie Moléculaire et Cellulaire, Centre National de la Recherche Scientifique Unité Mixte de Recherche 6097, Valbonne, France
ninino@ipmc.cnrs.fr
J Clin Endocrinol Metab 2008;93:3222–3225

Adrenocortical carcinoma (ACC) can be a difficult tumor to treat and classification and prognostic indices are poor. In recent years, several papers have shown distinct molecular events in these tumors such as overexpression of steroidogenic factor-1 (SF-1), disturbances in inhibin A and β-cateninWNT-4 pathways, and upregulation of insulin-like growth factor signaling [9–11]. These events are often somatic (occurring just within the tumor tissue), and may provide a 'second hit' on top of loss of heterozygosity of a tumor suppressor such as TP53, or dysregulation of imprinting mechanisms in the case of IGF II. Several studies this year are starting to use this information to develop potential novel therapeutic approaches to the treatment of adrenocortical carcinoma. The papers by Almeida et al. and Barlaskar et al. focus on targeting the type 1 insulin-like growth factor receptor and show increased apoptosis of tumor cells in culture and regression of ACC xenograft tumors in nude mice. Furthermore, data from Enzo Lalli's group have shown that inverse agonists of SF-1 or disruption of β-catenin signaling can reduce the growth of adrenal tumor cell lines. Taken together these data suggest that several new therapeutic options may be on the horizon. The difficulty will be targeting these treatments to adrenal or metastatic adrenal carcinoma tissue as, of course, IGF-, β-catenin- and SF-1-mediated pathways are widespread in many different endocrine and metabolic tissues. Nevertheless, these reports do provide good examples of how studying rare events and molecular mechanisms may ultimately translate back into more effective patient treatment.

New concerns: under pressure

Blood pressure in pediatric patients with Cushing syndrome

Lodish MB, Sinaii N, Patronas N, Batista DL, Keil M, Samuel J, Moran J, Verma S, Popovic J, Stratakis CA
Section on Endocrinology Genetics, Program on Developmental Endocrinology Genetics and Pediatric Endocrinology Program, National Institute of Child Health and Human Development, National Institutes of Health, Bethesda, Md., USA
lodishma@mail.nih.gov
J Clin Endocrinol Metab 2009;94:2002–2008

Background: Hypertension (HTN) has been reported in up to 50% of children with Cushing syndrome (CS) but its course, consequences, and relation to different causes of CS are not well documented. *Methods:* Blood pressure (BP) was measured in pediatric patients with CS before and after transphenoidal surgery (TSS; 86 children with Cushing disease, CD) or adrenalectomy (ADX; 27 children with ACTH-independent CS, AICS) to identify the prevalence of residual HTN and consequences of it. *Results:* Patients with CD and AICS had significant HTN before surgery. Higher BP correlated with cortisol levels. Systolic HTN (SHTN) was more frequent in AICS than in CD (74 vs. 44%, p = 0.0077), but the prevalence of diastolic HTN (DHTN) was similar between groups. Significant decreases in SHTN were seen immediately post-TSS and ADX and 1 year later. However, 16 and 4% of the patients with CD, and 21 and 5% of the patients with AICS still had SHTN and DHTN, respectively, at the 1-year follow-up. Two patients suffered serious consequences of hypertension: 1 child had multiple infarcts and another had hypertensive encephalopathy.

Conclusion: Residual HTN can be found in a proportion of children treated for CD despite a significant improvement after surgical cure. HTN appears to correlate with the degree of hypercortisolemia. Serious HTN-related side effects are relatively rare but can occur in the perioperative period.

Hypertension is well established as a presenting feature of Cushing syndrome in children and is extremely important to control in the perioperative period. Although blood pressure usually falls following treatment of the primary cause, this paper shows that a significant proportion of children treated for Cushing disease or ACTH-independent Cushing syndrome have residual hypertension at follow-up 1 year after surgery. This is a difficult group of children to perform well-controlled follow-up studies with as, for example, approximately one third of those treated for Cushing disease were still on steroid replacement therapy at the time of evaluation and 1 of the patients was probably in the early stages of disease recurrence. Furthermore, calculating hypertension based on the 95th percentile adjusted for height, age and gender is complicated by the fact that many of these children had an elevated BMI and their growth patterns are disrupted following their disease. The duration of Cushing or hypertension before diagnosis may be an important prognostic factor, which remains unknown in this cohort, underscoring the importance of early diagnosis of patients with hypercortisolemia and hypertension to prevent late sequelae. Nevertheless, this report does show that residual hypertension may be found in a significant proportion of children treated for Cushing syndrome. As this may be in part due to vascular remodeling or other programmed events, long-term follow-up of blood pressure and morbidity relating to hypertension is essential [12]. A more detailed study of circadian blood pressure in adults who had been treated for Cushing syndrome in childhood or adolescence would be useful in order to get a true reflection of how significant a long-term problem this might be.

Concepts revised: the adrenal's got rhythm

Adrenal peripheral clock controls the autonomous circadian rhythm of glucocorticoid by causing rhythmic steroid production

Son GH, Chung S, Choe HK, Kim HD, Baik SM, Lee H, Lee HW, Choi S, Sun W, Kim H, Cho S, Lee KH, Kim K
Department of Biological Sciences, Seoul National University, Seoul, Korea
kyungjin@snu.ac.kr
Proc Natl Acad Sci USA 2008;105:20970–20975

Background: Adrenal production of glucocorticoids (GC) shows a robust daily oscillation. This circadian rhythm is thought to be controlled by the suprachiasmatic nucleus of the hypothalamus and mediated by the hypothalamic-pituitary-adrenal axis.

Methods: Peripheral clock mechanisms were studied in the adrenal gland itself as well as the effects of an adrenal-specific knockdown of the canonical clock protein BMAL1 in mice.

Results: The adrenal gland has its own peripheral clock that is tightly linked to steroidogenesis by the steroidogenic acute regulatory protein. Mice with adrenal-specific deletion of BMAL1 showed that the adrenal clock machinery is required for circadian GC production. Furthermore, circadian behavioral patterns were disrupted in these animals and altered expression of Period1 was seen in several peripheral organs.

Conclusion: The adrenal has a peripheral clock that plays an essential role in harmonizing mammalian circadian systems by generating a robust circadian GC rhythm.

Circadian rhythms are essential in the hypothalamic pituitary adrenal (HPA) axis. Our traditional view is that the suprachiasmatic nucleus (SCN) of the hypothalamus influences CRF and ACTH release resulting in a peak of GC in the morning and subsequent fall in GC concentrations throughout the day. However, studies more than 30 years ago showed that GC rhythm could be maintained in hypo-physectomized rats given continuous ACTH infusions, suggesting that an inherent circadian rhythm of GC synthesis and release from the adrenal gland could exist [13]. The identification of several molecular and cellular components of oscillatory systems (such as *Clock* and *Period*) has revolution-ized the study of circadian biology. With this has come the realization that many peripheral tissues have their own circadian rhythms. Several recent papers have addressed the role of a potential peripheral clock mechanism in the adrenal gland, which may be regulated through ACTH-independent mechanisms such as melatonin signaling or splanchnic innervation [14–16]. This study by Son and col-leagues goes one step further by generating and characterizing a mouse model with an adrenal-specific knockdown of the clock protein, BMAL1. Using this model, the authors have clearly shown that the adrenal gland has its own clock mechanism regulating steroidogenesis, which is mediated by StAR and disrupted following adrenal specific deletion of BMAL1. The fact that altered patterns of circadian clock proteins were seen in other organs confirms that the adrenal gland itself plays a direct role in regulating the circadian rhythms of other peripheral tissues [17]. This work does not detract from the fact that the hypothalamus plays a key role in synchronizing these systems but the adrenal gland itself is now emerging as an increasingly important regulator of systems chronobiology. Another peripheral clock was reported to tick in the liver, as discussed in the Editors' Choice [p. 240].

Important for clinical practice: reproductive issues in CAH

Clinical and molecular characterization of a cohort of 161 unrelated women with nonclassical congenital adrenal hyperplasia due to 21-hydroxylase deficiency and 330 family members

Bidet M, Bellanne-Chantelot C, Galand-Portier MB, Tardy V, Billaud L, Laborde K, Coussieu C, Morel Y, Vaury C, Golmard JL, Claustre A, Mornet E, Chakhtoura Z, Mowszowicz I, Bachelot A, Touraine P, Kuttenn F
Department of Reproductive Endocrinology, Centre de Références des Maladies Endocriniennes Rares de la Croissance, Assistance Publique-Hôpitaux de Paris Pitié-Salpêtrière, Paris, France
frederique.kuttenn@psl.aphp.fr
J Clin Endocrinol Metab 2009;94:1570–1578

Background: Non-classical congenital adrenal hyperplasia (NC-CAH) due to partial 21OH deficiency is one of the most prevalent autosomal recessive diseases in humans. This study aimed to investigate genotype/phenotype relationship in probands and family members.
Methods: The study group consisted of 161 unrelated women with NC-CAH (diagnosed on account of late-onset symptoms, mainly hirsutism, and a post-ACTH 17-hydroxyprogesterone (17OHP) >10 ng/ml) and 330 of their relatives. Genotyping of CYP21A2 was performed in 124 of the probands.
Results: The most frequent mutation found was V281L. One severe mutation was found in 63.7% of probands and, surprisingly, two severe mutations were found in four probands. Basal and post-ACTH 17OHP concentrations were significantly higher in probands carrying at least one severe mutation than in those with two mild mutations (p < 0.01), but clinical signs, basal testosterone and androstenedione were not significantly different. Among the 330 family members, 51 were homozygotes or compound heterozy-gotes for CYP21A2 changes. Of these, 42 were clinically asymptomatic. A total of 242 were heterozy-gotes and 37 carried no CYP21A2 changes (unaffected). Post-ACTH 21-deoxycortisol (21dF) was significantly higher in heterozygotes than in unaffected, but an overlap existed. In 12 (5%) heterozygotes, post-ACTH 21dF was <0.55 ng/ml, the cutoff value usually accepted for detecting heterozygosity.
Conclusion: NC-CAH has variable expression even within a family, suggesting that modifier factors may modulate phenotype. Post-ACTH 21dF cannot detect heterozygous subjects in all cases. Considering the high frequency of heterozygotes in the general population, it is essential to genotype the partner(s) of the patients with one severe mutation in order to offer genetic counseling.

Nonclassic CAH (NC-CAH) is one of the most common recessively inherited conditions in humans. Extensive studies by New [18] have shown a prevalence of this condition of approximately 1 in 100 of the heterogeneous New York population and 1 in 27 Ashkenazi Jews. However, it is always useful to study conditions in different populations and this paper from a collaborative group in France describes genotype-phenotype relationships in affected individuals and family members in a European cohort of 161 unrelated women with NC-CAH. This study found surprisingly high variability in clinical expression of NC-CAH even within families with the same CYP21A2 genotype suggesting that the modifier factors may modulate the expression of the disease [see paper by Gomes et al. above]. Indeed, 3.2% of patients had a severe mutation detected in both alleles but we are reassured that they have a NC-CAH phenotype, suggesting that other mechanisms are rescuing the phenotype in these cases. Furthermore, more than 60% of the women in this cohort were found to be compound heterozygotes for one mild and one severe CYP21A2 mutation. This is clinically important as these women are at risk of having affected children with classic CAH if their partner carries a severe CYP21A2 change as well, so that genotyping the partner of patients with one severe mutation in order to offer genetic counseling is warranted [19].

Reassessing fecundity in women with classical congenital adrenal hyperplasia (CAH): normal pregnancy rate but reduced fertility rate

Casteras A, De Silva P, Rumsby G, Conway GS
Department of Endocrinology, University College London Hospitals, London, UK
g.conway@ucl.ac.uk

Clin Endocrinol (Oxf) 2009;70:833–837

Background: Although fertility in women with classical congenital adrenal hyperplasia (CAH) is reported to be low, the true pregnancy rate for women trying to conceive with this condition is not known.
Methods: Pregnancy rate (calculated as a proportion achieving pregnancy of those who had attempted conception) and fertility (expressed as live birth rate (LBR) per total population) were calculated in a cohort of 106 women with classical CAH followed in a multidisciplinary service (81 salt-losing (SL) and 25 non-salt-losing (NSL) forms).
Results: Twenty-five (23.6%) women with CAH considered motherhood (16/25 NSL-CAH vs. 9/81 SL-CAH). Of these, 23 had actively tried to conceive and 21 (91.3%) achieved 34 pregnancies. The pregnancy rate was no different from that in the normal population (95%). Pregnancy rates were similar in the SL (88.9%) and NSL (92.9%) subgroups, and optimized glucocorticoid and mineralocorticoid regimen during times of fertility monitoring resulted in spontaneous conception in nearly all of the recent cases. However, the fertility rate was 0.25 live births per woman compared to 1.8 in the UK population (p < 0.001).
Conclusion: This study shows a normal pregnancy rate (91.3%) for women with classical SL and NSL CAH. The fertility rate, however, remains much lower than in general population.

See also:

Fertility and pregnancy outcome in women with congenital adrenal hyperplasia due to 21-hydroxylase deficiency

Hagenfeldt K, Janson PO, Holmdahl G, Falhammar H, Filipsson H, Frisen L, Thoren M, Nordenskjold A
Department of Women and Child Health, Division of Obstetrics and Gynaecology, Karolinska Institutet, Karolinska University Hospital, Stockholm, Sweden
agneta.nordenskjold@ki.se

Hum Reprod 2008;23:1607–1613

Several studies have reported low fertility in women with classic CAH, which has been suggested to reflect poor control or hyperandrogenism/PCOS in many cases. This single center study of fecundity in more than 100 women with CAH considered fertility and pregnancy rates separately. The number of live births per person was considerably below that of women in the general population. However, the pregnancy rate of those trying to get pregnant was around 90%. Similar findings were reported by Hagenfeldt and co-workers. For those women who did not conceive spontaneously within 6 months on routine steroid replacement, follicular phase (day 2–8 of the cycle) progesterone was measured and the dose of prednisolone was increased in three equally divided doses until progesterone was suppressed to less than 2 nmol/l. This approach may have helped optimize fertility by preventing a transient rise in progesterone having an adverse effect on the follicular phase endometrium. The single daily dose of fludrocortisone was also increased if necessary in order to suppress plasma renin activity into the normal range, as poor control of the aldosterone pathway might also give rise to progesterone excess. Whilst these findings are encouraging, the converse side of this study is the high proportion of women (especially those with SL CAH) who did not seek to get pregnant. As the authors state, this probably reflects complex factors including 'less frequent partnerships' and possibly 'gender dysphoria and the after effects of genital surgery'.

Gonadal function, first cases of pregnancy, and child delivery in a woman with lipoid congenital adrenal hyperplasia

Khoury K, Barbar E, Ainmelk Y, Ouellet A, Lehoux JG

Departments of Pediatrics, Faculty of Medicine, University of Sherbrooke, Sherbrooke, Que., Canada

Jean-Guy.LeHoux@USherbrooke.ca

J Clin Endocrinol Metab 2009;94:1333–1337

Background: Mutations in the gene encoding steroidogenic acute regulatory protein (StAR) classically cause lipoid congenital adrenal hyperplasia (LCAH). In this condition, reduced adrenal and gonadal steroid synthesis results in adrenal failure, impaired androgenization in 46,XY individuals, and altered ovarian steroidogenesis in 46,XX girls/women. Pregnancy in LCAH has not yet been reported.

Methods: Data were obtained regarding the gonadal function, pubertal development, and support of pregnancy in a female with a p.L275P mutation in the StAR gene.

Results: The patient (46,XX) presented with LCAH at 4.5 months of age and had developed and grown normally on glucocorticoid and mineralocorticoid replacement. Puberty started at the age of 11 7/12 years and progressed normally with menarche at 14 2/12 years. Regular anovulatory cycles ensued. Following clomiphene stimulation, pregnancy was achieved at 25 years of age but this resulted in a spontaneous abortion at 6 weeks gestation. The second pregnancy (with clomiphene stimulation) occurred a year later. Progesterone therapy was added on the 17th day of the cycle to protect the pregnancy and 2 normal weight boys (dizygotic twins) were born at 30 weeks. Two years later, again with clomiphene stimulation and progesterone treatment, she had a further successful singleton pregnancy and delivered a normal weight female baby at 36 weeks.

Conclusion: Despite dysfunctional StAR, pregnancy is possible in 46,XX women with LCAH using an appropriate therapeutic strategy.

StAR plays an important role in adrenal and gonadal steroidogenesis by regulating the influx of cholesterol into the mitochondrial membrane. The dynamics of this process are complex, as StAR-independent mechanisms exist [20]. Defects in StAR have been proposed to affect steroidogenesis through a 'two-hit mechanism'. In the first hit, impaired StAR activity results in a reduction in steroid production by the adrenal gland or gonads. This results in elevated ACTH or gonadotropin stimulation of the cell which increases lipid uptake and causes accumulation of cholesterol in the cytoplasm. This second hit results in cell toxicity [21]. Girls (46,XX) with classic LCAH usually present with adrenal failure in infancy but show breast development and uterine growth at puberty, possibly because the second hit is less severe in the ovary as gonadotropin stimulation is cyclical, only one follicle is recruited each month, and low-level steroidogenesis may occur [21]. However, cycles are generally believed to be anovulatory, so this report of the induction of 3 pregnancies using clomiphene in a woman with a disruptive StAR mutation offers hope for patients with this rare condition. It is not surprising that progesterone therapy was needed to prevent early fetal loss as the maternal corpus luteum, which also expresses the StAR protein, is the major source of progesterone during the first trimester in humans. Normally, the fetally derived placenta takes over progesterone production in the 2nd and 3rd trimesters and StAR is thought not to play a significant role in placental steroidogenesis. Thus, in both the pregnancies reported here progesterone treatment could be withdrawn at between 17 and 25 weeks gestation. Reports such as this therefore provide interesting insight into the basic regulatory mechanisms of steroidogenesis in humans and important information when counseling families and girls with classic and non-classic forms of LCAH [22].

Effects of dehydroepiandrosterone therapy on pubic hair growth and psychological wellbeing in adolescent girls and young women with central adrenal insufficiency: a double-blind, randomized, placebo-controlled phase III trial

Binder G, Weber S, Ehrismann M, Zaiser N, Meisner C, Ranke MB, Maier L, Wudy SA, Hartmann MF, Heinrich U, Bettendorf M, Doerr HG, Pfaeffle RW, Keller E
Pediatric Endocrinology, University-Children's Hospital, Tübingen, Germany
gerhard.binder@med.uni-tuebingen.de
J Clin Endocrinol Metab 2009;94:1182–1190

Background: The potential benefits of oral dehydroepiandrosterone (DHEA) for hair growth and psychological wellbeing in young females with central adrenal insufficiency are unknown.
Methods: A cohort of 23 young females (mean age 18range 13–25 year) was enrolled in a double-blind randomized placebo-controlled trial of DHEA treatment. All women had: ACTH deficiency plus two or more additional pituitary deficiencies; pubertal stage greater than B2, and a confirmed serum DHEA of <400 ng/ml. Any patients who had had recent tumor (<1 year remission), high-dose (>30 Gy) cranial irradiation, hypothalamic obesity, amaurosis, psychiatric disorders, or poorly controlled hormone replacement were excluded. Patients were randomized to receive 25 mg HPLC-purified DHEA/day (n = 11) or placebo (n = 12) orally for 12 months after stratification into a nontumor (n = 7) and a tumor group (n = 16). Pubic hair stage was assessed at 0, 6, and 12 months (primary endpoint), and psychometric evaluation (Symptom Check-List-90-R and the Centre for Epidemiological Studies-Depression Scale) was performed at 0 and 12 months (secondary endpoint). Androgen levels and safety parameters were measured at 0, 6, and 12 months; 24-hour androgen urinary excretion rates were calculated at 0 and 12 months.
Results: Four of the placebo group dropped out (tumor recurrence; development of type 1 diabetes; change of residence, n = 2), and 1 of the DHEA group dropped out (recurrent anxiety attacks). DHEA substitution normalized DHEA sulfate morning serum levels (2 h after administration; p < 0.006) and 24-hour urinary metabolite levels (androstanediol glucuronide; p < 0.0001). Placebo had no effect. Morning serum levels of androstenedione increased in the DHEA group (p < 0.02) but did not normalize. The DHEA group exhibited significant pubic hair growth (from Tanner stage I–III to II–V; mean +1.5 stages), whereas the placebo group did not (p = 0.0046). Eight of the 10 Symptom Check-List-90-R scores improved in the DHEA group compared to the placebo group, including those for anxiety, depression, interpersonal sensitivity and global severity index (p < 0.048). DHEA was tolerated well.
Conclusion: Daily replacement with 25 mg DHEA orally improved pubic hair growth and psychological wellbeing in a cohort of adolescent girls with hypothalamic-pituitary adrenal insufficiency ('central').

There is currently much debate about the potential benefits of DHEA replacement in women with adrenal disorders. DHEA is produced by the zona reticularis of the adrenal gland following adrenarche and is a major pathway to the generation of androgens in post-pubertal women, which have been implicated in improving libido, cognitive function and mood. Several controlled studies have now been performed in women with Addison's disease and positive benefits of DHEA have been shown in some cases [23]. However, DHEA treatment may also be associated with potential side effects such as hirsutism or adverse lipid profiles, so further detailed properly performed studies in different age groups and conditions are needed [24, 25]. This double-blind randomized placebo-controlled trial of DHEA treatment by Binder and colleagues assessed the benefits of 1 year of DHEA replacement in adolescent girls and young women with secondary adrenal insufficiency. This was a well-structured study but it is complicated by relatively small numbers, heterogeneity in the underlying diagnosis, and relatively high drop out rate for unrelated reasons (e.g. 4 of the 12 girls randomized to receive the placebo did not complete the study). Nevertheless, the authors do report improved hair growth in the treatment group during this period and improved questionnaire-based reports of psychological wellbeing. DHEA probably plays an important role as a neurosteroid, facilitating brain maturation, mood and memory. DHEA treatment is now being recommended on an individual basis for many adult women with primary adrenal insufficiency [26] but relatively few data are available for DHEA replacement in late childhood or adolescence. It would be ideal if several more well-structured and suitably powered studies of DHEA replacement in adolescents could be undertaken before this treatment is offered widely. However, it is quite possible that DHEA treatments will be given to children on an individual basis if randomized control data are not available soon.

MRAP and MRAP2 are bidirectional regulators of the melanocortin receptor family

Chan LF, Webb TR, Chung TT, Meimaridou E, Cooray SN, Guasti L, Chapple JP, Egertova M, Elphick MR, Cheetham ME, Metherell LA, Clark AJ
Queen Mary University of London, Centre for Endocrinology, St. Bartholomew's and Royal London School of Medicine and Dentistry, London, UK
a.j.clark@qmul.ac.uk
Proc Natl Acad Sci USA 2009;106:6146–6151

Background: The melanocortin receptor (MCR) family consists of five G protein-coupled receptors (MC1R-MC5R) with diverse physiologic roles. MC2R (the ACTH receptor) plays a critical role in the hypothalamic-pituitary-adrenal axis. MC3R and MC4R play an important role in regulating energy homeostasis and MC4R mutations are the single most common cause of monogenic obesity currently known. MRAP is an MC2R accessory protein responsible for adrenal MC2R trafficking and function. However, the role of MRAP with other MCRs has not been established.
Methods: This study aimed to identify potential MRAP homologs and to investigate whether MRAP could influence the function of other MCR family members.
Results: A unique homolog of MRAP expressed in brain and the adrenal gland was identified (MRAP2). MRAP and MRAP2 were found to interact with all 5 MCRs. This interaction increased MC2R surface expression and signaling. In contrast, MRAP and MRAP2 reduced MC1R, MC3R, MC4R, and MC5R responsiveness to [Nle4,D-Phe7]α-melanocyte-stimulating hormone (NDP-MSH).
Conclusion: MRAP and MRAP2 are unique bidirectional regulators of the MCR family.

MRAP was first identified in 2005 as the cause of familial glucocorticoid deficiency type II and has been shown to play a key role in trafficking the ACTH receptor (MC2R) to the surface of the adrenal cell to enable interaction with the peptide ligand and initiation of downstream signaling pathways [27, 28]. Currently, there are 5 members of the MCR family. These receptors show unique tissue expression patterns throughout endocrine and metabolic systems but the role of MRAP or its homologs in regulating these other melanocortin receptors is unknown. Here, MRAP and a newly identified homolog termed MRAP2 were confirmed as having major facilitative influences on MC2R surface expression but interacted negatively with other members of the MCR family. Much attention is focusing on the regulation of MC4R as it plays such a central role in regulating appetite, energy homeostasis and obesity. This study supports a role for MRAP and MRAP2 in the regulation of the central melanocortin system, as MRAP/MRAP2 reduced signaling of the MC3R- and MC4R-dependent pathways. This bidirectional regulation of MC2R and MC3R/MC4R may reflect for example a physiologic advantage of switching off appetite at times when a maximal adrenal response is required, such as acute stress. Whether the central effects of MRAP and its homologs could be targeted to alter MC4R expression and influence appetite and weight gain remains to be seen.

Epigenetic regulation of the glucocorticoid receptor in human brain associates with childhood abuse

McGowan PO, Sasaki A, D'Alessio AC, Dymov S, Labonte B, Szyf M, Turecki G, Meaney MJ
Douglas Mental Health University Institute, Montreal, Que., Canada
michael.meaney@mcgill.ca
Nat Neurosci 2009;12:342–348

Background: Hypothalamic-pituitary-adrenal (HPA) function in the rat can be influenced by maternal care through epigenetic programming of glucocorticoid receptor expression. In humans, childhood abuse alters HPA stress responses and increases the risk of suicide.

Methods: Epigenetic regulation of a neuron-specific glucocorticoid receptor (NR3C1) promoter was compared between postmortem hippocampus obtained from: (1) suicide victims with a history of childhood abuse; (2) those from either suicide victims with no childhood abuse, or (3) controls.

Results: Decreased levels of glucocorticoid receptor mRNA were found in the abused suicide group, as well as decreased mRNA transcripts bearing the glucocorticoid receptor 1F splice variant and increased cytosine methylation of an NR3C1 promoter. Decreased NGFI-A transcription factor binding and NGFI-A-inducible gene transcription was seen using patch-methylated NR3C1 promoter constructs that mimicked the methylation state in samples from abused suicide victims.

Conclusion: These findings support data from rats and show that parental care in humans can influence epigenetic regulation of hippocampal glucocorticoid receptor expression.

Sequencing the human genome is undoubtedly one of the greatest achievements so far in the history of mankind. This knowledge has led to extremely important and rapid advances in identifying single-gene disorders, and many loci linked to common population diseases are now being identified. However, it is also likely that not all variations in human biology will be explained by variability at the level of the DNA, so other non-genomic processes need to be considered. This is where the current explosion of interest in epigenetics comes in. Epigenetics can be defined as changes in phenotype or gene expression due to mechanisms that do not involve changes in the underlying DNA sequence. These changes can remain through cell division cycles, sometimes for the lifespan of the organism, and may even be transmitted through generations. The exact mechanisms influencing epigenetic regulation are still being investigated but several processes such as DNA methylation, histone modification (e.g. methylation, acetylation) and RNA interference are likely to be involved. Such modifications can 'silence' or 'activate' expression of key genes with important downstream biological functions. This challenging study from Michael Meaney's group reported glucocorticoid receptor (GR) expression and regulation in the hippocampus of suicide victims and controls. Using a unique resource of banked brains with detailed history and phenotype, the authors showed decreased levels of GR expression only in those adults committing suicide who had been abused in childhood. GR expression was the focus of this work as studies in rats have shown that poor maternal care is associated with decreased hippocampal GR expression and subsequent hyperactivation of the HPA axis in basal and stressed states [29]. Furthermore, childhood abuse has been reported to be associated with altered HPA activity in some studies in humans, although the data are less consistent [30]. The work presented here deals with a sensitive subject and highlights the need to study gene expression changes and regulation in relevant organs, which is not always easy (e.g. the brain). Nevertheless, epigenetic research is set to develop rapidly in the next decade. Hopefully, those from genetic and epigenetic backgrounds will work together to understand regulatory pathways rather than trying to prove one aspect is more important than the other.

Girls with premature adrenarche have accelerated early childhood growth

Utriainen P, Voutilainen R, Jaaskelainen J
Department of Pediatrics, University of Kuopio and Kuopio University Hospital, Kuopio, Finland
pauliina.utriainen@uku.fi
J Pediatr 2009;154:882–887

Background: The relation between premature adrenarche (PA) and early prepubertal growth has not been studied in many different populations.

Methods: Anthropometric data between birth and 7 years of age was reviewed retrospectively for 54 girls with PA and 52 control girls. The growth variables were correlated with concentrations of serum insulin-like growth factor (IGF)-1, dehydroepiandrosterone sulfate and insulin at follow-up (median age 7.6 years).

Results: No significant differences in birth weight or length standard deviation scores (SDSs) occurred between the 2 groups studied. Girls with PA demonstrated a significantly greater length SDS increment during the first 2 years of life (median +1.0 SDS; p < 0.001). Compared with controls, they were taller (median current height 1.2 vs. 0 SDS; p < 0.001) and had gained more weight throughout childhood with differences in weight-for-height becoming significant at a later age. Median serum IGF-1 concentration, adjusted for body mass index and age, was higher in the PA group (24 vs. 19 nmol/l; p < 0.031).

Conclusion: In this population of girls, PA was not associated with small birth size but was associated with increased growth. This increased growth was already evident in early childhood and was not explained by weight gain. Enhanced IGF-1 production may be one factor contributing to the prepubertal growth acceleration in PA.

In several studies, babies born small-for-gestational age have been shown to have an increased incidence of premature adrenarche in childhood, and population-based studies have found an inverse relation between birth weight and DHEA-S [31, 32]. This study, from a North European population, has looked at a cohort of girls with premature adrenarche and not found any significant differences in birth weight amongst them compared to a matched control group. This discrepancy deserves more attention. However, one notable finding was the accelerated growth in infancy and early childhood in the PA group, as well as higher serum IGF-1 concentration. The early growth acceleration supports Ken Ong's findings in a population-based investigation of postnatal growth and DHEA-S [32]. The elevated IGF-1 findings supports data from Silfen et al. [33]. The causes of adrenarche are poorly understood but this study suggests that early events such as growth acceleration and IGF-1 production may be linked with it and could be causative.

Prepubertal healthy children's urinary androstenediol predicts diaphyseal bone strength in late puberty

Remer T, Manz F, Hartmann MF, Schoenau E, Wudy SA
Department of Nutrition and Health, Research Institute of Child Nutrition, Forschungsinstitut für Kinderernährung, Dortmund, Germany
remer@fke-do.de
J Clin Endocrinol Metab 2009;94:575–578

Background: During adrenarche, healthy children secrete increasing amounts of weak androgenic steroids, which can be partly metabolized to potent sex steroids. The relation between adrenarchal androgen release and bone strength in later life is not well documented.

Methods: A cohort of 45 healthy children were studied who had had studies of urine steroid output undertaken at 8 years of age and in whom diaphyseal bone strength was measured at 16 years of age. Prepubertal urinary hormones quantified by gas chromatography-mass spectrometry were: dehydroepiandrosterone, its 16-hydroxylated downstream metabolites, 5-androstene-3β,17β-diol (androstenediol), sums of total androgen and glucocorticoid metabolites, cortisol, and 6β-hydroxycortisol. Proximal forearm bone and muscle area measurements were obtained by peripheral quantitative computed tomography.

Results: Of all the prepubertal hormones analyzed, only sex- and age-specific androstenediol levels were significantly associated with pubertal stage-, height-, and muscularity-adjusted diaphyseal bone modeling (periosteal circumference, β = 0.67 p = 0.002; cortical area, β = 2.15, p = 0.02), bone mineral content (β = 2.2; p = 0.04), and polar strength strain index (β = 12.2; p = 0.002). Androstenediol explained 5–10% of the late-pubertal variability in diaphyseal radius.

Conclusion: Androstenediol is an early predictor of the diaphyseal bone strength in late puberty. This urinary steroid metabolite is produced primarily following peripheral conversion of dehydroepiandrosterone by 17β-hydroxysteroid dehydrogenase.

The biological effects of adrenarche are poorly understood but it is possible that the weak androgenic steroids released from this time are converted to more potent androgens or estrogens at extraadrenal sites, which could have implications for other aspects of endocrine and metabolic function. This study focuses on the urinary metabolite of DHEA , androstenediol. Comparison of pre-pubertal urinary hormones at 8 years of age with markers of bone modeling at 16 years of age showed a correlation between urinary androstenediol and diaphyseal bone strength. Although this only explained 5–10% of the late pubertal variability in diaphyseal radius, this could be a biologically important addition to the accumulation of bone mass during the critical period of late childhood through to early adulthood. This study demonstrates nicely how different data sets at different ages in control populations of children can be integrated over time to start to address some of the important longitudinal interactions in developing endocrine systems.

New genes: another non-classical variant

A novel homozygous mutation in CYP11A1 gene is associated with late-onset adrenal insufficiency and hypospadias in a 46,XY patient

Rubtsov P, Karmanov M, Sverdlova P, Spirin P, Tiulpakov A
Department of Endocrine Genetics, Endocrinology Research Center, Moscow, Russian Federation
ant@endocrincentr.ru
J Clin Endocrinol Metab 2009;94:936–939

Background: The enzyme cytochrome P450 cholesterol side-change cleavage (P450scc, encoded by *CYP11A1*) converts cholesterol to pregnenolone. This reaction is the first and rate-limiting step in the biosynthesis of hormones in all steroidogenic tissues. To date, CYP11A1 mutations have been reported in 6 patients, all of whom had severely under-androgenized external genitalia (Prader stages 1–2) and presented with adrenal insufficiency within the first 4 years of life.
Methods: Mutational analysis of CYP11A1 in a 46,XY patient with mid-shaft hypospadias and cryptorchidism at birth and signs of adrenal failure at 9 years of age.
Results: This boy was found to have a novel homozygous p.L222P mutation in P450scc. His parents were heterozygous carriers for this mutation. Functional studies showed that this p.L222P mutant had approximately 7% functional activity compared with wild-type.
Conclusion: This case represents the mildest phenotype of P450scc deficiency to be described to date. The phenotypic presentation was consistent with partial reduction of P450scc activity with the p.L222P mutant.

The discovery of new genetic causes of endocrine disorders normally focuses on those most severe and predictable phenotypes. With time, it usually emerges that milder or non-classic variants of these conditions exist. Examples of this include the descriptions of non-classical CAH [see Bidet et al., above], non-classic lipoid congenital adrenal hyperplasia [22], late-onset X-linked adrenal hypoplasia congenita and variants of 17α-hydroxylase deficiency associated with only mild genital changes. This case report by Rubtsov et al. describes a novel mutation in P450scc in a boy with hypospadias who developed adrenal insufficiency at 9 years of age. P450scc deficiency was originally thought to be incompatible with survival in humans as this enzyme is essential for progesterone production by the fetally derived placenta from the second trimester onwards, and subsequent maintenance of pregnancy. However 6 cases of P450scc deficiency have now been described [34]. All cases have presented with severe adrenal failure in early childhood and usually under-androgenized external genitalia in 46,XY individuals. The milder case of P450scc deficiency reported here reminds us of the common link between adrenal and gonadal steroidogenesis. Although hypospadias is common, more severe forms of hypospadias associated with cryptorchidism or a small penis may in some cases reflect an underlying steroidogenic defect and in some of these children there may be a risk of adrenal failure later in life. Trying to define those boys at risk is a challenge but it is important not to dismiss potential signs of adrenal failure when a history of hypospadias or undescended testes is present.

Corticotropin tests for hypothalamic-pituitary-adrenal insufficiency: a meta-analysis

Kazlauskaite R, Evans AT, Villabona CV, Abdu TA, Ambrosi B, Atkinson AB, Choi CH, Clayton RN, Courtney CH, Gonc EN, Maghnie M, Rose SR, Soule SG, Tordjman K
John H. Stroger Jr. Hospital of Cook County and Rush Medical College, Chicago, Ill., USA
rasa_kazlauskaite@rush.edu
J Clin Endocrinol Metab 2008;93:424542–424553

Background: The diagnostic value of tests to evaluate hypothalamic-pituitary adrenal insufficiency (HPAI) ('central AI') is controversial. The aim of this meta-analysis was to compare standard-dose and low-dose corticotropin tests for diagnosing HPAI.
Methods: PubMed (1966–2006) was searched for studies reporting the diagnostic value of standard-dose or low-dose corticotropin tests with patient-level data obtained from original investigators. Studies were included if there were more than 10 patients who were being evaluated because of suspected chronic HPAI. Studies were excluded if they used tests with no accepted reference standard for HPAI (insulin hypoglycemia or metyrapone test), if test subjects were in the intensive care unit, or if only normal healthy subjects were used as controls. Receiver operator characteristic (ROC) curves were constructed using patient-level data from each study. Summary ROC curves were generated from these data sets with adjustments for cortisol assay method and study size. The diagnostic value of each test was measured by calculating area under the ROC curve (AUC) and likelihood ratios.
Results: The meta-analysis included patient-level data from 13 of 23 studies (57%; 679 subjects). The AUC were as follows: low-dose corticotropin test, 0.92 (95% CI 0.89–0.94), and standard-dose corticotropin test, 0.79 (95% CI 0.74–0.84). Among patients with paired data (7 studies, 254 subjects), the diagnostic value of the low-dose corticotropin test was superior to that of the standard-dose test (AUC 0.94 and 0.85, respectively; p < 0.001).
Conclusion: The low-dose corticotropin test was superior to standard-dose testing for diagnosing chronic HPAI. However, the low-dose test has technical limitations.

Stimulation tests to assess adrenal function and to diagnose adrenal insufficiency can be challenging to interpret especially in the diagnosis of central hypothalamo-pituitary insufficiency where chronic under-stimulation of the adrenal gland occurs. In such situations, standard doses of corticotropin stimulation, which are massively supraphysiological, may well result in an adequate cortisol response but may not reflect the normal physiological situation at times of stress. With this in mind a low-dose corticotropin stimulation test has been introduced in the past 30–40 years, but very few large series are available that directly compare these two tests in one individual. This meta-analysis of low and standard dose corticotropin tests reviewed literature since 1966 and gathered information where patient-level data were available. Analysis using ROC curves showed that the low dose corticotropin test was better at diagnosing chronic HPAI than standard dose testing. A low-dose test peak of <440 nmol/l best predicted HPAI, whereas a peak of >600 nmol/l best predicted a normal test result. Unfortunately, it is not clear how many of the subjects primarily included in the analysis were children or at least had been treated in childhood or adolescence. Almost half of the cohort had had pituitary macroadenoma, suggesting that the majority of cases were likely to have been treated and tested in adulthood. It would be useful to know if the characteristics of these tests were different in a younger age group. Indeed, a recent study by Maguire et al. [35] of 31 children and adolescents with suspected central adrenal insufficiency and using human corticotropin-releasing hormone testing as the gold-standard for diagnosis (peak <400 nmol/l) suggested that mild cases of HPAI may be missed using a low-dose stimulation test. However, in this study the cortisol peak to diagnose HPAI was set at <267 nmol/l (10th centile for the normal population), which was considerably lower than in the meta-analysis. Nevertheless, both these papers recommend that the low-dose corticotropin stimulation test is useful in those cases of suspected HPAI where an unstressed basal cortisol taken around 9 a.m. falls within an 'intermediate' range (150–390 nmol/l, Kazlauskaite et al., above; 108–381 nmol/l, Maguire et al. [35]). Disadvantages of the low-dose test include: (1) inaccuracies in reconstituting the corticotropin analogue, which requires several dilution steps; (2) adherence of the hormone to plastic tubing, and (3) timing of the cortisol sample (20–30 min after stimulation is recommended by Kazlauskaite et al.). Thus, a greater degree of operator experience and knowledge is required.

Attractive men induce testosterone and cortisol release in women

Lopez HH, Hay AC, Conklin PH
Department of Psychology, Neuroscience Program, Skidmore College, Saratoga Springs, N.Y., USA
hlopez@skidmore.edu
Horm Behav 2009;56:84–92

Background: Recently, studies have demonstrated that men release testosterone and cortisol in response to brief social interactions with young women. The aim of the current study was to determine whether women show a similar endocrine response to physically and behaviorally attractive men.
Methods: The study cohort consisted of 120 women (70 naturally cycling and 50 using hormonal contraceptives) who were shown one of four 20-min video montages extracted from popular films. The following scenarios were depicted: (1) an attractive man courting a young woman (experimental stimulus); (2) a nature documentary (video clip control); (3) an 'unattractive' man courting a woman (male control), and (4) an attractive woman with no men present (female control). Pre- and post-stimulus saliva samples were taken for analysis of testosterone and cortisol by immunoassay.
Results: Naturally cycling women experienced a significant increase in both testosterone and cortisol in response to the experimental stimulus but to none of the control stimuli. Women taking hormonal contraceptives also showed a significant cortisol response to the attractive man.
Conclusion: Women may release adrenal steroid hormones to facilitate courtship interactions with high mate-value men.

The psychology literature is peppered with hypothalamic-pituitary-adrenal axis data of variable quality, but this study is well controlled and interesting. The teleological and physiological significant of the cortisol response is debatable, with one possible effect being 'to mobilize energy reserves for shared activity and possible sexual intercourse'. It is possible that the 'participants enjoyment of the video, independent of whatever attraction they felt to the protagonist, could have mediated hormonal release', although – as the authors state – there is no a priori reason why this should be the case, and there was certainly no response to the interesting selection of control scenarios.

References

1. Ferraz-de-Souza B, Lin L, Achermann JC: Adrenals; in Carel J-C, Hochberg Z (eds) Yearbook of Pediatric Endocrinology 2008. Basel, Karger, 2008, pp 95–108.
2. Fluck CE, Tajima T, Pandey AV, Arlt W, Okuhara K, Verge CF, et al: Mutant P450 oxidoreductase causes disordered steroidogenesis with and without Antley-Bixler syndrome. Nat Genet 2004;36:228–230.
3. Lavery GG, Walker EA, Tiganescu A, Ride JP, Shackleton CH, Tomlinson JW, et al: Steroid biomarkers and genetic studies reveal inactivating mutations in hexose-6-phosphate dehydrogenase in patients with cortisone reductase deficiency. J Clin Endocrinol Metab 2008;93:3827–3832.
4. ul Haque MF, King LM, Krakow D, Cantor RM, Rusiniak ME, Swank RT, et al: Mutations in orthologous genes in human spondyloepimetaphyseal dysplasia and the brachymorphic mouse. Nat Genet 1998;20:157–162.
5. Clark PM, Hindmarsh PC, Shiell AW, Law CM, Honour JW, Barker DJ: Size at birth and adrenocortical function in childhood. Clin Endocrinol (Oxf) 1996;45:721–726.
6. Phillips DI, Walker BR, Reynolds RM, Flanagan DE, Wood PJ, Osmond C, et al: Low birth weight predicts elevated plasma cortisol concentrations in adults from 3 populations. Hypertension 2000;35:1301–1306.
7. Fall CH, Dennison E, Cooper C, Pringle J, Kellingray SD, Hindmarsh P: Does birth weight predict adult serum cortisol concentrations? Twenty-four-hour profiles in the United Kingdom 1920–1930 Hertfordshire Birth Cohort. J Clin Endocrinol Metab 2002;87:2001–2007.
8. Gomes LG, Huang N, Agrawal V, Mendonca BB, Bachega TA, Miller WL: The common P450 oxidoreductase variant A503V is not a modifier gene for 21-hydroxylase deficiency. J Clin Endocrinol Metab 2008;93:2913–2916.
9. Doghman M, Karpova T, Rodrigues GA, Arhatte M, De Moura J, Cavalli LR, et al: Increased steroidogenic factor-1 dosage triggers adrenocortical cell proliferation and cancer. Mol Endocrinol 2007;21:2968–2987.
10. Gaujoux S, Tissier F, Groussin L, Libe R, Ragazzon B, Launay P, et al: Wnt/beta-catenin and 3′,5′-cyclic adenosine 5′-monophosphate/protein kinase A signaling pathways alterations and somatic beta-catenin gene mutations in the progression of adrenocortical tumors. J Clin Endocrinol Metab 2008;93:4135–4140.
11. Kuulasmaa T, Jaaskelainen J, Suppola S, Pietilainen T, Heikkila P, Aaltomaa S, et al: WNT-4 mRNA expression in human adrenocortical tumors and cultured adrenal cells. Horm Metab Res 2008;40:668–673.
12. Nguyen JH, Lodish MB, Patronas NJ, Ugrasbul F, Keil MF, Roberts MD, et al: Extensive and largely reversible ischemic cerebral infarctions in a prepubertal child with hypertension and Cushing disease. J Clin Endocrinol Metab 2009;94:1–2.
13. Meier AH: Daily variation in concentration of plasma corticosteroid in hypophysectomized rats. Endocrinology 1976;98:1475–1479.
14. Wilkinson CW: Circadian clocks: showtime for the adrenal cortex. Endocrinology 2008;149:1451–1453.

15. Valenzuela FJ, Torres-Farfan C, Richter HG, Mendez N, Campino C, Torrealba F, et al: Clock gene expression in adult primate suprachiasmatic nuclei and adrenal: is the adrenal a peripheral clock responsive to melatonin? Endocrinology 2008;149:1454–1461.
16. Ishida A, Mutoh T, Ueyama T, Bando H, Masubuchi S, Nakahara D, et al: Light activates the adrenal gland: timing of gene expression and glucocorticoid release. Cell Metab 2005;2:297–307.
17. Oster H, Damerow S, Kiessling S, Jakubcakova V, Abraham D, Tian J, et al. The circadian rhythm of glucocorticoids is regulated by a gating mechanism residing in the adrenal cortical clock. Cell Metab. 2006 Aug;4(2):163-73.
18. New MI: Extensive clinical experience: nonclassical 21-hydroxylase deficiency. J Clin Endocrinol Metab 2006;91:4205–4214.
19. Moran C, Azziz R, Weintrob N, Witchel SF, Rohmer V, Dewailly D, et al: Reproductive outcome of women with 21-hydroxylase-deficient nonclassic adrenal hyperplasia. J Clin Endocrinol Metab 2006;91:3451–3456.
20. Miller WL: StAR search – what we know about how the steroidogenic acute regulatory protein mediates mitochondrial cholesterol import. Mol Endocrinol 2007;21:589–601.
21. Bose HS, Sugawara T, Strauss JF 3rd, Miller WL: The pathophysiology and genetics of congenital lipoid adrenal hyperplasia. International Congenital Lipoid Adrenal Hyperplasia Consortium. N Engl J Med 1996;335:1870–1878.
22. Baker BY, Lin L, Kim CJ, Raza J, Smith CP, Miller WL, et al: Nonclassic congenital lipoid adrenal hyperplasia: a new disorder of the steroidogenic acute regulatory protein with very late presentation and normal male genitalia. J Clin Endocrinol Metab 2006;91:4781–4785.
23. Arlt W, Callies F, van Vlijmen JC, Koehler I, Reincke M, Bidlingmaier M, et al: Dehydroepiandrosterone replacement in women with adrenal insufficiency. N Engl J Med 1999;341:1013–1020.
24. Srinivasan M, Irving BA, Dhatariya K, Klaus KA, Hartman SJ, McConnell JP, et al: Effect of dehydroepiandrosterone replacement on lipoprotein profile in hypoadrenal women. J Clin Endocrinol Metab 2009;94:761–764.
25. Chang AY, Ghayee HK, Auchus RJ: Dehydroepiandrosterone replacement therapy – panacea, snake oil, or a bit of both? Nat Clin Pract Endocrinol Metab 2008;4:442–443.
26. Arlt W: The approach to the adult with newly diagnosed adrenal insufficiency. J Clin Endocrinol Metab 2009;94:1059–1067.
27. Metherell LA, Chapple JP, Cooray S, David A, Becker C, Ruschendorf F, et al: Mutations in MRAP, encoding a new interacting partner of the ACTH receptor, cause familial glucocorticoid deficiency type 2. Nat Genet 2005;37:166–170.
28. Chung TT, Webb TR, Chan LF, Cooray SN, Metherell LA, King PJ, et al: The majority of adrenocorticotropin receptor (melanocortin 2 receptor) mutations found in familial glucocorticoid deficiency type 1 lead to defective trafficking of the receptor to the cell surface. J Clin Endocrinol Metab 2008;93:4948–4954.
29. Liu D, Diorio J, Tannenbaum B, Caldji C, Francis D, Freedman A, et al: Maternal care, hippocampal glucocorticoid receptors, and hypothalamic-pituitary-adrenal responses to stress. Science 1997;277:1659–1662.
30. Tarullo AR, Gunnar MR: Child maltreatment and the developing HPA axis. Horm Behav 2006;50:632–639.
31. Ibanez L, Potau N, Marcos MV, de Zegher F: Exaggerated adrenarche and hyperinsulinism in adolescent girls born small for gestational age. J Clin Endocrinol Metab 1999;84:4739–4741.
32. Ong KK, Potau N, Petry CJ, Jones R, Ness AR, Honour JW, et al: Opposing influences of prenatal and postnatal weight gain on adrenarche in normal boys and girls. J Clin Endocrinol Metab 2004;89:2647–2651.
33. Silfen ME, Manibo AM, Ferin M, McMahon DJ, Levine LS, Oberfield SE: Elevated free IGF-I levels in prepubertal Hispanic girls with premature adrenarche: relationship with hyperandrogenism and insulin sensitivity. J Clin Endocrinol Metab 2002;87:398–403.
34. Kim CJ, Lin L, Huang N, Quigley CA, AvRuskin TW, Achermann JC, et al: Severe combined adrenal and gonadal deficiency caused by novel mutations in the cholesterol side chain cleavage enzyme, P450scc. J Clin Endocrinol Metab 2008;93:696–702.
35. Maguire AM, Biesheuvel CJ, Ambler GR, Moore B, McLean M, Cowell CT: Evaluation of adrenal function using the human corticotrophin-releasing hormone test, low dose Synacthen test and 9am cortisol level in children and adolescents with central adrenal insufficiency. Clin Endocrinol (Oxf) 2008;68:683–691.

Type 1 Diabetes: Clinical and Experimental

Francesco Chiarelli and Cosimo Giannini

Department of Paediatrics, University of Chieti, Chieti, Italy

Type 1 diabetes mellitus (T1D) is the most common endocrine disease in childhood and adolescence. The increasing worldwide incidence of diabetes highlights the increased need for new means of preventing or retarding the development and progression of diabetes and diabetes-related complications.

In particular, among the several research issues explored, four key fields offer the most promising perspectives: stem cells, offering the clinically opportunity of restoring the autoimmune-related depletion of the β-cells; genomic and proteomic, to define genetic findings as well as biomarkers able to characterize those subjects at increased risk of developing diabetes and diabetes-related complications, and immune-modulation aimed at preventing or reversing the immune-mediated mechanisms involved in diabetes. The continuous progress achieved by these main research areas suggests promising opportunities for better diagnosis and treatment of diabetes in the future.

Mechanism of the year

Curative and β cell regenerative effects of α_1-antitrypsin treatment in autoimmune diabetic NOD mice

Koulmanda M, Bhasin M, Hoffman L, Fan Z, Qipo A, Shi H, Bonner-Weir S, Putheti P, Degauque N, Libermann TA, Auchincloss H Jr, Flier JS, Strom TB
Departments of Surgery and Medicine, Harvard Medical School, Boston, Mass., USA
strom@bidmc.harvard.edu
Proc Natl Acad Sci USA 2008;105:16242–16247

Background: Invasive insulitis represents a destructive T-cell-dependent autoimmune process directed against insulin-producing β cells that is central to the pathogenesis of type 1 diabetes mellitus (T1D) in humans and in a non-obese diabetic (NOD) mouse model. Few therapies have succeeded in restoring long-term, drug-free euglycemia and immune tolerance to β cells in overtly diabetic NOD mice, and none have demonstrably enabled enlargement of the functional β-cell mass. The impact of inflammatory cytokines on the commitment of antigen-activated T cells to various effectors or regulatory T-cell phenotypes and insulin resistance and defective insulin signaling have been emphasized in recent studies.
Methods: In this study Koulmanda et al. tested the hypothesis that inflammatory mechanisms trigger insulitis, insulin resistance, faulty insulin signaling, and the loss of immune tolerance to islets.
Results: In NOD mice, with recent-onset T1D, treatment with α_1-antitrypsin (AAT), an agent that dampens inflammation, does not directly inhibit T-cell activation, ablates invasive insulitis, and restores euglycemia, immune tolerance to β cells, normal insulin signaling, and insulin responsiveness through favorable changes in the inflammation milieu.
Conclusions: These results suggest that the functional mass of β cells expands in AAT-treated diabetic NOD mice.

Several therapeutic approaches for restoring either immune tolerance to β cells as well to the β-cell mass have been investigated during the last decades [1, 2]. Interestingly in this study Koulmanda et al. were able to demonstrate an effective role on autoimmune-induced β-cell loss achieved by treatment with AAT, an acute-phase reactant with serine proteinase inhibitor, and anti-inflammatory and anti-apoptotic effects. In fact in NOD mice with overt new onset T1D, AAT treatment favorably served to dampen expression of proinflammatory, but not anti-inflammatory, cytokines without affecting T cells and the acquisition of an activated phenotype. In addition, AAT therapy was able to decrease the expression of T-helper 1 (Th1)-specific T-bet and Th17-specific retinoic acid-related orphan receptor-γ (ROR-γt) transcription factors as well as mo Foxp3 expression. Therefore, AAT mainly acts by tilting either the balance of expression of proinflammatory to anti-inflammatory cytokines as well the balance of T cell Th1/Th17 effector (dramatically downregulated) to regulatory T-cell genes, sharply toward predominance of anti-inflammatory and regulatory T-cell gene expression. In addition, in the fat tissue of diabetic mice, AAT treatment was able to dampen and restore toward normal three inflammation-related molecules (TNF-α, IL-4, and NF-κB) resulting in a reestablished insulin sensitivity and signaling in peripheral tissues.

These preliminary results open a new encouraging and exciting view on the characterization of the complex network of immune-system activation and cytokine/chemokine-mediated β-cell destruction. In particular, ATT therapy could add further power to previous similar studies (for instance those using anti-CD3 mAb) [3] with the aim of preserving β-cell mass and function. Therefore, further trials are needed in order to completely characterize the effect of ATT in β-cell depletion in young patients with T1D.

In vivo reprogramming of adult pancreatic exocrine cells to β cells

Zhou Q, Brown J, Kanarek A, Rajagopal J, Melton DA
Department of Stem Cell and Regenerative Biology, Howard Hughes Medical Institute, Harvard Stem Cell Institute, Harvard University, Cambridge, Mass., USA
dmelton@harvard.edu
Nature 2008;455:627–632

Background: One goal of regenerative medicine is to instructively convert adult cells into other cell types for tissue repair and regeneration. Although isolated examples of adult cell reprogramming are known, there is no general understanding of how to turn one cell type into another in a controlled manner.
Methods/Results: Using a strategy of reexpressing key developmental regulators in vivo, Zhou et al. identified a specific combination of three transcription factors [Ngn3 (also known as Neurog3), Pdx1 and Mafa] that reprograms differentiated pancreatic exocrine cells in adult mice into cells that closely resemble β cells. Results showed that the induced β cells are indistinguishable from endogenous islet β cells in size, shape and ultrastructure. In addition, these cells expressed genes essential for β-cell function and could ameliorate hyperglycemia by remodeling local vasculature and secreting insulin.
Conclusions: These results provide an example of cellular reprogramming using defined factors in an adult organ and suggest a general paradigm for directing cell reprogramming without reversion to a pluripotent stem cell state.

In this study Zhou et al. have smartly proved the first and relevant step for the future application of regenerative medicine in the treatment of patients with T1D. By starting from the concept of cellular reprogramming or lineage reprogramming [4, 5] (a process characterized by the switching of cells of one type into another type), they investigate the complex and strict step-by-step activation of several transcription factor genes which lead to a mature β cell from a human embryonic stem (hES) cell [6]. After injecting a mixture of adenoviruses into the pancreata of 2-month-old adult mice (that coexpress 9 of the most relevant transcription factors) the investigators were able to demonstrate that the combination of only 3 (*Ngn3, Pdx1* and *Mafa*) of the transcription factors tested were able to reprogram a fully differentiated exocrine cell into cells that closely resemble β cells. In fact, new insulin-positive cells were detected at lower level 3 days after injection, but the intensity of insulin staining increased gradually so that by day 10 the level was comparable to that of endogenous β cells, and still present after 3 months. In addition, surprisingly Zhou et al. showed that the reprogramming of exocrine cells to β cells did not involve multiple rounds of cell proliferation and therefore conversion between exocrine and β cells may require fewer epigenetic changes. Unfortunately, they noticed that the induced β cells did not organize into islet structures and remained as single cells or small clusters. Undoubtedly, this represents a relevant limitation, as the lack of organization impairs their function. In addition, the adjustment of this process for more direct, abundant and easily accessible patient-specific human cells such as fibroblasts, blood cells or adipocytes are needed. Therefore, although it appears clearly evident that further additional studies are needed in order to completely characterize the process and to bypass the related limitations, Zhou et al. have shown the first step in a process that, in the near future, will hopefully enable patient-specific cell therapies by utilizing the cellular reprogramming concept.

CTLs are targeted to kill β cells in patients with type 1 diabetes through recognition of a glucose-regulated preproinsulin epitope

Skowera A, Ellis RJ, Varela-Calviño R, Arif S, Huang GC, Van-Krinks C, Zaremba A, Rackham C, Allen JS, Tree TI, Zhao M, Dayan CM, Sewell AK, Unger W, Drijfhout JW, Ossendorp F, Roep BO, Peakman M
Department of Immunobiology, King's College London, London, UK
mark.peakman@kcl.ac.uk
J Clin Invest 2008;118:3390–3402

Background: The final pathway of β-cell destruction leading to insulin deficiency, hyperglycemia, and clinical T1D is not completely known.

Methods: In this study Skowera et al. showed that circulating CTLs can kill β cells via recognition of a glucose-regulated epitope.

Results: First, 2 naturally processed epitopes from the human preproinsulin signal peptide by elution from HLA-A2 (specifically, the protein encoded by the A*0201 allele) molecules were identified. Processing of these was unconventional, requiring neither the proteasome nor transporter-associated processing (TAP). However, both epitopes were major targets for circulating effector CD8+ T cells from HLA-A2+ patients with T1D. Moreover, cloned preproinsulin signal peptide-specific CD8+ T cells killed human β cells in vitro. Critically, at a high glucose concentration, β-cell presentation of preproinsulin signal epitope increased, as did CTL killing.

Conclusions: This study provides direct evidence that autoreactive CTLs are present in the circulation of patients with T1D and that they can kill human β cells. In addition, these results identify a mechanism of self-antigen presentation that is under pathophysiological regulation and could expose insulin-producing β cells to increasing cytotoxicity at the later stages of the development of clinical diabetes. Therefore, data suggest that autoreactive CTLs are important targets for immune-based interventions in T1D and argue for early, aggressive insulin treatment to preserve remaining β cells.

Skowera et al. add some relevant information on the immune-based mechanisms involved in the β-cell mass destruction and offer a potential explanation for the preservation on β cells achieved by early aggressive insulin therapy [7–9]. First, by creating surrogate β cells expressing a single autoantigen and HLA class I molecules, they were able to investigate their naturally displayed peptide repertoire. In fact, it was shown that surrogate β cells uncovered the signal peptide (SP) as a source of preproinsulin (PPI) epitopes that constitute major targets of CD8+ T cell responses in HLA-A2+ patients with T1D. In addition, in vitro analysis showed that human HLA-A2-expressing β cells are killed by expanded clones of PPI SP-specific CD8+ T cells, especially when β cells are exposed to high glucose concentrations. These findings offer three major novelties. First, these results suggest the possibility of developing CD8+ T-cell-specific strategies to halt β-cell destruction. In addition, in vitro analysis clearly showed that hyperglycemia-induced β-cell stress determines a characteristic and novel pathway through which PPI SP epitopes are expressed. This observation implies that I-CLiPs and ER proteases are critical for CTL epitope presentation. The relevant role of these epitopes in autoimmune destruction of β cells has been demonstrated in an interesting recent study. In fact, Toma et al. [10] were able to define class-I-restricted epitopes located within the leader sequence of human preproinsulin through in vivo (transgenic mice) and ex vivo (diabetic patients) assays, confirming the possible role of preproinsulin-specific CD8+ T cells in human T1D. Targeting these pathways could offer new therapeutic agents for prevention of β-cell destruction. Furthermore, these findings attempt to provide evidence of a mechanism leading β cells, stressed by the need to control blood glucose levels as diabetes develops, to become enhanced targets for the immune system. This observation suggests that an early and aggressive introduction of insulin treatment might be a possible rationale approach that could at least slow the progression of β-cell destruction. Previous studies, albeit on small numbers of subjects, have suggested that preservation of endogenous insulin reserve might benefit from administration of insulin in the pre-diabetic period [11] or from tight metabolic control soon after diagnosis [12, 13]. In contrast, other studies failed to prove a positive effect on diabetes prevention or delay by administering insulin in persons at high risk of diabetes [7, 8]. However, as there is a progressive loss of β-cell mass and function from the initiation of insulitis through diabetes presentation, it could be speculated that the time at which the progression of disease is identified and treated is of practical importance. In fact, the residual cells may represent the source of new β cells and combination agents that are more likely to be effective if there are β cells that can respond. Therefore, based on these findings further studies are needed to completely define the effectiveness of insulin alone or combined agents in the prevention of or slowing the progression of β-cell destruction.

New hope

Urinary proteomics in diabetes and chronic kidney diseases

Rossing K, Mischak H, Dakna M, Zürbig P, Novak J, Julian BA, Good DM, Coon JJ, Tarnow L, Rossing P
Steno Diabetes Center, Gentofte, Denmark
krossing@dadlnet.dk
J Am Soc Nephrol 2008;19:1283–1290

Background: Urinary biomarkers for diabetes, diabetic nephropathy, and non-diabetic proteinuric renal diseases were sought.
Methods: Using high-resolution capillary electrophoresis coupled with electrospray-ionization mass spectrometry, biomarkers were defined and validated in blinded data sets including 305 individuals.
Results: A panel of 40 biomarkers distinguished patients with diabetes from healthy individuals with 89% sensitivity and 91% specificity. In patients with diabetes, 102 urinary biomarkers differed significantly between patients with normo-albuminuria and nephropathy, and a model that included 65 of these correctly identified diabetic nephropathy with 97% sensitivity and specificity. Furthermore, this panel of biomarkers identified patients who had microalbuminuria and diabetes and progressed toward overt diabetic nephropathy over 3 years. Differentiation between diabetic nephropathy and other chronic renal diseases reached 81% sensitivity and 91% specificity. Many of the biomarkers were fragments of collagen type I, and quantities were reduced in patients with diabetes or diabetic nephropathy.
Conclusions: These data clearly show that analysis of the urinary proteome may allow early detection of diabetic nephropathy and may provide prognostic information.

Rossing et al. were able to detect a highly sensitive and specific urinary proteomic pattern distinct for diabetes, diabetic nephropathy, and non-diabetic proteinuric renal diseases. In fact, by analyzing urinary profiles with the online combination of capillary electrophoresis and electrospray mass spectrometry, they investigated whether a single or a combination of polypeptides, present at a frequency of >50%, may characterize patients with diabetes and their risk of developing vascular complications. In particular, after identifying a sequence of 40 identified biomarkers, they showed that 53 of 59 patients with diabetes (patients with diabetes and normo-albuminuria or microalbuminuria or nephropathy) and 32 of 35 healthy control subjects were correctly classified, resulting in 89% sensitivity and 91% specificity. The possibility of proteomic analysis to differentiate the severity of kidney damage (defined as normo- or microalbuminuria and as overt nephropathy) was further proven. In fact, after defining 65 of 102 identified biomarkers by a 'take-one-out' analysis, they showed 97% sensitivity and specificity reached by the linear combination of these polypeptides. In addition, more information was obtained by performing the analysis in 8 of 30 patients with diabetes and microalbuminuria which showed an increase in albuminuria of about 25% or progressed to macroalbuminuria during a 3-year follow-up interval. Thus, biomarkers were useful not only to detect patients with overt nephropathy but also to predict its development in patients with diabetes and microalbuminuria. This study clearly shows the contribution of system biology in the study of diabetes. In fact, a new generation of mass spectrometers will be available, with better sensitivity, mass accuracy and resolution; these new systems could offer new markers of kidney function. In addition, the most striking observation was the decreased excretion of specific collagen fragments in patients with diabetes and healthy controls as well as within patients with diabetes. Nonetheless, Rossing et al. showed several additional collagen fragments which were less common in patients with diabetic nephropathy compared with normo-albuminuric diabetic patients. As these fragments are likely products of specific proteases and are related to the balanced synthesis and activity of protease inhibitors, the complete characterization of the products might give relevant tools for further characterization of the natural history of diabetic nephropathy. In particular, they might serve as indicators of the activity of these enzymes as well as the synthesis of the proteins involved in the morphological kidney changes in diabetic nephropathy.

Tyrosine kinase inhibitors reverse type 1 diabetes in nonobese diabetic mice

Louvet C, Szot GL, Lang J, Lee MR, Martinier N, Bollag G, Zhu S, Weiss A, Bluestone JA
Diabetes Center and the Department of Medicine, University of California, San Francisco, Calif., USA
aweiss@medicine.ucsf.edu

Proc Natl Acad Sci USA 2008;105:18895–18900

Background: The recent development of small-molecule tyrosine kinase inhibitors offers increasing opportunities for the treatment of autoimmune diseases.
Methods: In this study, Louvet et al. attempted to investigate the potential of this new class of drugs to treat and cure T1D in the NOD mouse.
Results: Treatment of pre-diabetic and new onset diabetic mice with imatinib (Gleevec) prevented and reversed T1D. Similar results were observed with sunitinib (Sutent), an additional approved multikinase inhibitor, suggesting that the primary target of imatinib, c-Abl, was not essential in blocking the disease in this model. Additional studies with another tyrosine kinase inhibitor, PLX647 (targeting c-Kit and c-Fms) or an anti-c-Kit mAb showed only marginal efficacy, whereas a soluble form of platelet-derived growth factor receptor (PDGFR), PDGFR-β-Ig, rapidly reversed diabetes. These findings strongly suggest that inhibition of PDGFR is critical for reversing diabetes and highlight the crucial role of inflammation in the development of T1D. These conclusions were supported by the finding that the adaptive immune system was not significantly affected by imatinib treatment. Finally, and most significantly, imatinib treatment led to durable remission after discontinuation of therapy at 10 weeks in a majority of mice.
Conclusions: Long-term efficacy and tolerance is likely to depend on inhibiting a combination of tyrosine kinases supporting the use of selective kinase inhibitors as a new and potentially very attractive approach for the treatment of T1D.

In this promising study, starting from the demonstration of a positive effect of imatinib (an inhibitor of the inactive conformation of Abl protein tyrosine kinases) on several autoimmune diseases [14] and Crohn's disease [15], Louvet et al. investigated whether this drug might be effective in preventing or treating T1D. In particular, by treating the NOD mouse (a model autoimmune diabetes in which the disease occurs spontaneously at about 12–14 weeks and shares many phenotypic and genetic similarities with T1D in human subjects), they were able to demonstrate that tyrosine kinase inhibitors not only prevent the onset of diabetes, given during a pre-diabetic stage, but also reverse the disease when given at the time of diabetes presentation. Surprisingly, Louvet et al. showed that limiting treatment to 8–10 weeks, after the onset of diabetes, was sufficient to reverse the disease and induce long-term remission consistent with reestablishment of immune tolerance. However, it is relevant to stress that imatinib, while preventing clinical disease, diminishes but does not eliminate leukocyte infiltration of the pancreas. These results are consistent with recent studies demonstrating a direct protective effect of imatinib on type 2 diabetes in rodents [16] and suggest that this molecule and other kinase inhibitors (such as sunitinib) have a potential therapeutic effect in patients with T1D. Nevertheless, a complete characterization of the mechanisms by which these drugs act in autoimmune diseases need to be determined; in fact, whether imatinib operates through direct function on B or T cells or both, or indirectly by modulating the expression of INF-γ in T cells or of other chemokines or cytokines involved in β-cell loss is not completely defined. Therefore, newer studies evaluating the underlying mechanisms by which tyrosine kinase inhibitors stably prevent and reverse the immune-mediated response to self-cells are needed. Further findings will possibly make these drugs, or especially newer highly selective kinase inhibitors, realistic new therapeutic tools for clinical treatment of diabetes and other autoimmune diseases.

Young women with type 1 diabetes have lower bone mineral density that persists over time

Mastrandrea LD, Wactawski-Wende J, Donahue RP, Hovey KM, Clark A, Quattrin T
Department of Pediatrics, University at Buffalo, School of Medicine and Biomedical Sciences, Buffalo, N.Y., USA
ldm@buffalo.edu
Diabetes Care 2008;31:1729–1735

Background: Individuals with T1D have decreased bone mineral density (BMD); yet the natural history and pathogenesis of osteopenia are unclear. In a previous study Mastrandrea et al. showed that women with T1D (aged 13–35 years) have lower BMD than community age-matched healthy control subjects. In order to determine the natural history of BMD in young women with and without diabetes, they performed a 2-year follow-up BMD data of the previously selected cohort.
Methods: To estimate BMD dual-energy X-ray absorptiometry was used at baseline and 2 years later in 63 women with T1D and in 85 age-matched control subjects. HbA1C, IGF-1, IGF-binding protein-3, serum osteocalcin, and urine N-teleopeptide were also measured at follow-up.
Results: After adjusting for age, BMI and oral contraceptive use, BMD at year 2 persisted to be lower in women ≥20 years of age with T1D compared with control subjects at the total hip, femoral neck, and whole body. Lower BMD values were observed in cases <20 years of age compared with control subjects; however, the differences were not statistically significant. Lower BMD did not correlate with diabetes control, growth factors, or metabolic bone markers.
Conclusions: This study confirms lower BMD in young women with T1D compared to control subjects which appears to persist over time, particularly in women ≥20 years of age. Persistence of low BMD as well as failure to accrue bone density after age 20 years may contribute to the increased incidence of osteoporotic hip fractures documented in postmenopausal women with T1D.

Some studies have investigated the effects of diabetes-related metabolic and hormonal alterations on bone metabolism [17, 18]. However, very few studies have attempted to longitudinally characterize the natural history of BMD in patients with T1D. In this study, by performing a 2-year follow-up analysis, Mastrandrea et al. confirmed the lower BMD in the femoral neck and lateral spine in patients with T1D, especially in those older than 20 years. Furthermore, they documented that reduced values persisted during follow-up and that reduced BMD was associated with lower IGF1 levels in younger patients. Although this study has several limitations (the excessive number of women followed up compared to men, and the possible bias related to the selection of the patients enrolled) the persistently reduced BMD values during the follow-up clearly demonstrate that a complete and systematic characterization of bone mineral acquisition or turnover might be routinely adopted in all patients with T1D, especially during childhood and adolescence. Furthermore, better characterization of the exact mechanisms involved in the bone homeostasis in patients with T1D is needed. In fact, osteoporosis represent the most significant metabolic bone disease in patients with diabetes and is associated with an increased risk of the osteoporosis-related complications including hip fracture [19]. In particular, the characterization of markers of impaired bone homeostasis, able to identify patients at increased risk, are needed to use all the available preventive and therapeutic means in the daily care of patients with T1D.

A1C variability and the risk of microvascular complications in type 1 diabetes: data from the diabetes control and complications trial

Kilpatrick ES, Rigby AS, Atkin SL
Department of Clinical Biochemistry, Hull Royal Infirmary, Hull, UK
eric.kilpatrick@hey.nhs.uk
Diabetes Care 2008;31:2198–2202

Background: Debate remains as to whether short- or long-term glycemic instability confers an increased risk of microvascular complications in addition to that predicted by means of glycemia alone. In this study, Kilpatrick et al. analyzed data from the Diabetes Control and Complications Trial (DCCT) in order to assess whether HbA1c variability might influence the risk of retinopathy and nephropathy in patients with T1D.

Methods: During the DCCT HbA1c was collected quarterly in 1,441 individuals. The mean HbA1c and the SD of HbA1c variability after stabilization of glycemia (from 6 months onwards) were compared with the risk of retinopathy and nephropathy with adjustments for age, sex, disease duration, treatment group, and baseline HbA1c.

Results: By a multivariate Cox regression it was shown that the variability in HbA1c added to mean HbA1c in predicting the risk of development or progression of both retinopathy (hazard ratio 2.26 for every 1% increase in HbA1c SD [95% CI 1.63–3.14], p < 0.0001) and nephropathy (1.80 [1.37–2.42], p < 0.0001), in particular in conventionally treated patients.

Conclusions: This study documented that variability in HbA1c adds to the mean value in predicting microvascular complications in T1D. Thus, in contrast to analyses of DCCT data investigating the effect of short-term glucose instability on complication risk, longer-term fluctuations in glycemia seem to contribute to the development of retinopathy and nephropathy in patients with T1D.

In this study Kilpatrick et al. were able to confirm the role of HbA1c variability in the risk of diabetes complications. In fact, by using publicly accessible datasets collected by the DCCT (a 9-year randomized-controlled, follow-up study of 1,441 participants with T1D comparing the effect of intensive versus conventional insulin treatment on the risk of development of the microvascular complications) [20], they showed that the higher the HbA1c variability the greater the risk of developing both retinopathy and nephropathy. The risk was shown in the DCCT cohort overall and was also an individual feature of both treatment groups. In addition, the role of HbA1c variability was indirectly confirmed by the demonstration of a most pronounced effect among conventionally treated patients presumably due to the event rate or the range of variability or the spread of variability at any given mean HbA1c, which was larger than those for intensively treated patients. Overall, Kilpatrick et al. showed that the magnitude of the effect of HbA1c variability is marked, such that a 1% absolute increase in HbA1c-SD results in at least a doubling of retinopathy and an 80% increase in nephropathy risk. These findings are in contrast to those of a previous analysis of the DCCT data [21], which suggested that HbA1c variability had little effect on the risk of complications. However, in the previous study findings were probably distorted by the inclusion of all patient visits, even those visits before HbA1c stabilized at 6 months in intensively treated patients.

For clinicians involved in the care of patients with T1D it is essential to fully understand the relevant role of glycemic variability in the risk of developing micro- and macrovascular complications. In this perspective, recent technological and pharmacological advances have focused on reducing especially postprandial hyperglycemia which represents the main determinant of the increased glucose variability. Data from Kilpatrick et al. clearly show the importance of glucose variability and confirm data from the Pittsburgh Epidemiology Study which showed that HbA1c is an additional risk factor for the development of macrovascular complications [22]. In addition, although HbA1c is well known to represent the main predictor of diabetes-related complications, several studies have demonstrated a relevant role of postprandial and fasting hyperglycemia in metabolic control and diabetes complications. In fact, in patients with diabetes over quintiles of HbA1c both postprandial and fasting hyperglycemia are independent factors to be considered in order to reach the target of HbA1c and to reduce the risk of cardiovascular diseases [23, 24]. Thus, several postprandial events combine to make waves that may eventually wear down the endothelial mole. Similarly, instable metabolic control, as defined by HbA1c fluctuation, may act like a strong wind causing billows that strike the wall and may rapidly tear it down, amplifying the increased risk associated with impaired metabolic control. In order to reduce the risk of diabetes-related complications, patients and the diabetic team should cooperate to maintain not only HbA1c levels and glucose fluctuations as low as possible and but also to minimize HbA1c variability as little as possible.

Important for clinical practice

Institution of basal-bolus therapy at diagnosis for children with type 1 diabetes mellitus

Adhikari S, Adams-Huet B, Wang YC, Marks JF, White PC
Division of Pediatric Endocrinology, Department of Dietary Behavior, University of Texas Southwestern Medical Center, Dallas, Tex., USA
soumya.adhikari@childrens.com
Pediatrics 2009;123:e673–678

Background: Adhikari et al. evaluated whether the institution of basal-bolus therapy immediately after diagnosis improved glycemic control in the first year after diagnosis for children with newly diagnosed T1D.
Methods: The charts of 459 children ≥6 years of age who were diagnosed as having T1D between July 1, 2002, and June 30, 2006 (212 treated with basal-bolus therapy and 247 treated with a more-conventional neutral protamine Hagedorn regimen) were reviewed. Furthermore, Adhikari et al. analyzed data obtained at diagnosis and at quarterly clinic visits and compared groups by using repeated-measures, mixed-linear model analysis. The records of 198 children with preexisting T1D of >1-year duration who changed from the neutral protamine Hagedorn regimen to a basal-bolus regimen during the review period were also evaluated.
Results: Glargine-treated subjects with newly diagnosed diabetes had lower HbA1c levels 3, 6, 9, and 12 months after diagnosis than did neutral protamine Hagedorn-treated subjects (average HbA1c levels of 7.05% with glargine and 7.63% with neutral protamine Hagedorn, estimated across months 3, 6, 9, and 12, according to repeated-measures models adjusted for age at diagnosis and baseline HbA1c levels). Children with long-standing diabetes had no clinically important changes in their HbA1c levels in the first year after changing regimens.
Conclusions: Basal-bolus therapy with insulin glargine starting from the time of diagnosis of T1D was associated with improved glycemic control, in comparison with more-conventional neutral protamine Hagedorn regimens, during the first year after diagnosis.

This retrospective and large study reported by Adhikiri et al. adds relevant and additional findings to the complete definition of the safety and effectiveness, and especially on the ability to achieve better glycemic control reached by newer insulin analogs. In fact, by comparing data obtained in a total of 459 children older than 6 years of age and diagnosed as having T1DM, they showed a significant association on improved glycemic control obtained with a basal-bolus treatment (with glargine), used from the onset of diabetes. In particular, they reported that this treatment results in 0.58% lower HbA1c level compared to a scheme with neutral protamine Hagedorn. The effects on glycemic control were shown to be particularly relevant in older patients. In fact, after categorizing treatment responses according to age (dichotomized at 10.5 years), a greater treatment effect was observed for the oldest group (with a HbA1c difference of 0.86 vs. 0.37%). In contrast, Adhikiri et al. were not able to demonstrate similar effects in those patients (198 children with longstanding T1D diagnosed at >6 years of age) who changed from neutral protamine Hagedorn to glargine regimen.

Over the last decades the availability of newer insulin analogs has been shown to represent an important means aimed at improving metabolic control and quality of life [25]. Although several studies have demonstrated a significant improvement in glycemic control in children and adults by switching from neutral protamine Hagedorn to long-acting analogs [26], no data are available on the role of these new insulins used from the onset of T1D. In addition, these data introduce a relevant and already opened question. In fact improved glycemic control is well known to be associated with a greater duration of endogenous insulin secretory capacity [9, 13]. On the other hand preservation of β-cell mass determines better metabolic control resulting in a lower risk of diabetes-related complications [27, 28]. These effects are particularly relevant in adolescent patients in whom the pubertal-related effects negatively influence metabolic control. Although promising, there are relevant limitations, in particular the study design, in the data reported by Adhikiri et al. Therefore, prospective, randomized, controlled trials are needed with the aim of determining whether early institution of basal-bolus therapy with newer insulin analogs, started from the time of diagnosis of T1D, might positively affect β-cell mass.

Clinical trials, new treatments

GAD treatment and insulin secretion in recent-onset type 1 diabetes

Ludvigsson J, Faresjö M, Hjorth M, Axelsson S, Chéramy M, Pihl M, Vaarala O, Forsander G, Ivarsson S, Johansson C, Lindh A, Nilsson NO, Aman J, Ortqvist E, Zerhouni P, Casas R
Department of Clinical and Experimental Medicine, Faculty of Health Sciences, Linköping University, Linköping, Sweden
johnny.ludvigsson@lio.se
N Engl J Med 2008;359:1909–1920

Background: The 65-kD isoform of glutamic acid decarboxylase (GAD) is a major auto-antigen in patients with T1D. In this study the ability of alum-formulated GAD (GAD-alum) to reverse recent-onset T1D in patients 10 to 18 years of age was assessed.

Methods: Seventy young patients with T1D who had fasting C-peptide levels above 0.1 nmol/l (0.3 ng/ml) and GAD autoantibodies, recruited within 18 months after receiving the diagnosis of diabetes, were randomly assigned to receive subcutaneous injections of 20 μg of GAD-alum (35 patients) or placebo (alum alone, 35 patients) on study days 1 and 30. At day 1 and months 3, 9, 15, 21, and 30, a mixed-meal tolerance test was performed in all patients in order to stimulate residual insulin secretion (measured as the C-peptide level). The effect of GAD-alum on the immune system was also studied.

Results: Insulin secretion gradually decreased in both study groups. The study group had no significant effect on change in fasting C-peptide level after 15 months (the primary end point) compared to controls. Fasting C-peptide levels declined from baseline levels to significantly less over 30 months in the GAD-alum group than in the placebo group (–0.21 vs. –0.27 nmol/l [–0.62 vs. –0.81 ng/ml], p = 0.045), as did stimulated secretion measured as the area under the curve (–0.72 vs. –1.02 nmol/l/2 h [–2.20 vs. –3.08 ng/ml/2 h], p = 0.04). No protective effect was seen in patients treated 6 months or more after receiving the diagnosis. Adverse events appeared to be mild and similar in frequency between the 2 groups. The GAD-alum treatment induced a GAD-specific immune response.

Conclusions: GAD-alum may contribute to the preservation of residual insulin secretion in patients with recent-onset T1D, although insulin requirement is not modified 30 months after onset of clinical diabetes.

In this longitudinal, multicenter, placebo-controlled, randomized and relatively large study, Ludvigsson et al. were able to investigate whether subcutaneous administration of the 65-kD isoform of GAD, one of the major autoantigens in patients with T1D, would reduce or halt the loss of residual insulin secretion. Firstly, in this clinical trial two consecutive subcutaneous administrations of a recombinant human GAD in a standard vaccine formulation (a primary injection and a booster injection of 20 μg each) have been well tolerated. In fact, no relevant adverse events were documented during the entire study follow-up. In addition, a gradual loss of β-cell function was documented in both study groups as indicating by the progressive decrease from the baseline level in both fasting and stimulated C-peptide secretion. Furthermore, GAD-alum treatment was not associated with a change in fasting C-peptide level between baseline and month 15. At variance, in the GAD-alum group fasting as well as stimulated C-peptide levels showed a significantly smaller decline after 30 months, compared to the placebo group. However, an apparent protective effect of the GAD-alum treatment on C-peptide secretion was demonstrated only in patients treated for less than 6 months after diagnosis. In contrast, no effects on insulin requirement were document by GAD-alum treatment. Preservation of β-cell mass represents a relevant opportunity in patients with T1D [28]. In fact, it is well documented that even modest residual insulin secretion, with stimulated C-peptide levels of >0.2 nmol/l (0.6 ng/ml), has been reported to provide clinically meaningful benefits in terms of reducing long-term complications [27]. Previous studies and especially those with anti-CD3 monoclonal treatment [3] have shown minimal benefits which appear to be associated with relatively relevant adverse effects. The relatively safety and the similar duration and magnitude of the GAD-alum treatment encourage large-scale confirmatory studies with GAD-alum. In addition, further studies are needed to characterize the immunological mechanisms implicated in the GAD-alum-mediated modulation of autoimmunity. These results will provide further help to understand immune-mediated depletion of β cells in patients with T1D.

Effects of the selective serotonin reuptake inhibitor fluoxetine on counterregulatory responses to hypoglycemia in individuals with type 1 diabetes

Briscoe VJ, Ertl AC, Tate DB, Davis SN
Department of Medicine, Vanderbilt University, Nashville, Tenn., USA
steve.davis@vanderbilt.edu
Diabetes 2008;57:3315–3322

Background: Chronic administration of the serotonin reuptake inhibitor (SSRI) fluoxetine has been shown to augment counter-regulatory responses to hypoglycemia in healthy humans. However, virtually no information exists regarding the effects of fluoxetine on integrated physiological counter-regulatory responses during hypoglycemia in T1D. Thus, the specific aim of this study was to test whether in individuals with T1D 6-week use of the SSRI fluoxetine would amplify autonomic nervous system counter-regulatory responses to hypoglycemia.

Methods: 18 patients with T1D (14 men/4 women aged 19–48 years with BMI 25 ± 3 and HbA1C 7.0 ± 0.4%) participated in randomized, double-blind 2-hour hyperinsulinemic (9 pmol • kg^{-1} • min^{-1})-hypoglycemic clamp studies before and after 6 weeks of fluoxetine administration (n = 8) or identical placebo (n = 10). Glucose kinetics was determined by 3-tritiated glucose. Muscle sympathetic nerve activity was determined by microneurography.

Results: Hypoglycemia (2.8 ± 0.1 mmol/l) and insulinemia (646 ± 52 pmol/l) were similar during all clamp studies. Autonomic nervous system, neuroendocrine, and metabolic counter-regulatory responses remained unchanged in the placebo group. However, the key autonomic nervous system (epinephrine, norepinephrine, and muscle sympathetic nerve activity), metabolic (endogenous glucose production and lipolysis), and cardiovascular (systolic blood pressure) counter-regulatory responses during hypoglycemia were significantly increased by fluoxetine administration (p < 0.05).

Conclusions: Thus, 6-week administration of the SSRI fluoxetine can amplify the autonomic nervous system and metabolic counter-regulatory mechanisms during moderate hypoglycemia in patients with T1D. Consequently, the use of fluoxetine may be helpful in increasing epinephrine responses during hypoglycemia in clinical practice.

In this randomized, double-blind study Briscoe et al. were able to explore the effects on the autonomic nervous system, as well as the neuroendocrine and metabolic counter-regulatory mechanisms during hypoglycemia in patients with T1D before and after 6 weeks of fluoxetine (a selective serotonin reuptake inhibitor) compared to placebo administration. In particular, by using a 2-hour hyperinsulinemic-hypoglycemic clamp, they showed that a period of 6 weeks of high-dose fluoxetine significantly increases sympathetic nervous system, hypothalamic-pituitary-adrenal pathways, and metabolic (endogenous glucose production, lipolysis with increased glycerol and non-esterified fatty acids) counter-regulatory responses during hypoglycemia in patients with long-duration T1D. Interestingly, the most notable finding from the present study was the striking increase in epinephrine responses during hypoglycemia following fluoxetine. Despite equivalent insulin and glucose levels during the hypoglycemic clamps, fluoxetine resulted in a 90% increase in epinephrine levels. These findings are of great relevance in patients with T1D and a long diabetes duration. In fact, as the glucagon response to hypoglycemia is lost in patients with T1D with increasing disease duration

[29], epinephrine becomes the critical counter-regulatory hormone against acute hypoglycemia. Accompanying the amplified sympathetic nervous system responses were significant increases in blood pressure and heart rate during hypoglycemia following fluoxetine. Fluoxetine only amplified counter-regulatory responses during hypoglycemia and did not increase basal homeostatic mechanisms. Thus, there were no differences in baseline cardiovascular, metabolic, and neuroendocrine parameters following fluoxetine or placebo.

The reported effects of fluoxetine on physiological responses during hypoglycemia in a group of metabolically well-controlled young patients with T1D represents an important new perspective in the daily care of patients with diabetes. In fact, it is well know that hypoglycemia remains the major barrier to even near normalization of glucose in patients with T1D, especially in childhood [29]. Furthermore, patients with recurrent hypoglycemic episodes experience the dangerous 'hypoglycemia unawareness'. However, the dose of fluoxetine used in this study is higher than the average dose of the drug used in clinical practice [30] and therefore the similar effect of lower doses must be proven. In addition, the mechanisms of fluoxetine activity is not completely defined. Activation of a number of serotonergic receptors (5HT1A, 5HT1C, 5HT2, and 5HT3) has been demonstrated to increase autonomic nervous system outflow . Additionally, it is not defined whether the fluoxetine effect was being sensed at central (i.e., brain), peripheral (i.e., adrenal gland), or even both sites [31]. Therefore, it is important to perform further studies in order to thoroughly define the activity of selective serotonin reuptake inhibitors in improving counter-regulatory response to hypoglycemia in young patients with T1D.

New mechanisms

Selective death of autoreactive T cells in human diabetes by TNF or TNF receptor 2 agonism

Ban L, Zhang J, Wang L, Kuhtreiber W, Burger D, Faustman DL
Department of Immunobiology, Massachusetts General Hospital and Harvard Medical School, Boston, Mass., USA
faustuman@helix.mgh.harvard.edu
Proc Natl Acad Sci USA 2008;10:13644–13649

Background: As the immunosuppressive drugs are nonspecific, produce high levels of adverse effects, and are not based on mechanistic understanding of disease, their real application in human autoimmune diseases is limited. Destroying the rare autoreactive T lymphocytes causing autoimmune diseases would improve treatment. In animal models, TNF selectively kills autoreactive T cells, thereby hampering disease onset or progression. Here, Ban et al. attempted to determine, in fresh human blood, whether TNF or agonists of TNF selectively kill autoreactive T cells, while sparing normal T cells.

Methods: They isolated highly pure CD4 or CD8 T cells from patients with T1D (n = 675), other autoimmune diseases, and healthy controls (n = 512).

Results: By using a two cell death assays, they found that a subpopulation of CD8, but not CD4, T cells in patients' blood was vulnerable to TNF or TNF agonist-induced death. One agonist for the TNFR2 receptor exhibited a dose-response pattern of killing. In T1D, the subpopulation of T cells susceptible to TNF or TNFR2 agonist-induced death was traced specifically to autoreactive T cells to insulin, a known autoantigen. In addition, other activated and memory T-cell populations were resistant to TNF-triggered death.

Conclusions: Therefore, autoreactive T cells, although rare, can be selectively destroyed in isolated human blood. TNF and a TNFR2 agonist may offer highly targeted therapies, with the latter likely to be less systemically toxic.

In this in vitro study, the TNF's role as a selective killer of autoreactive CD8 T cells in humans was investigated. By exposing T cells (isolated from the blood specimens of patients with T1D as well other autoimmune diseases and normal control subjects) to TNF, and agonists that mimicked TNF's function (TNF-receptor-1 [TNFR1] or TNF-receptor-2 [TNF-R2]), they showed that TNF exposure kills a subset of human CD8 T cells from patients with T1D and other autoimmune diseases without any effect on CD4 T cells. In addition Ban et al. demonstrated that the death of this subpopulation of CD8 T cells was also triggered with a specific agonist for TNFR2 that mimics TNF's actions. In contrast, TNFR1 agonists did not trigger cell death of diabetic autoreactive T cells. Furthermore, these results showed that, in specimens from patients with T1D, a subpopulation of insulin autoreactive CD8 T cells specific for the HLA class I insulin-fragment died upon exposure to a TNFR2 agonist, confirming that the TNF pathway could be a target for new types of treatments. In contrast, activated CD8 T cells in diabetics to non-autoreactive peptides such as directed to CMV or EBV viral fragments, were resistant to TNF agonism, confirming the specificity of the TNF pathway as a targeted method of killing only autoreactive CD8 T cells. The capacity of a TNFR2 agonist to kill autoreactive diabetic CD8 T cells has relevant therapeutic implications for drug safety as potential therapeutic opportunity might be associated to minimal toxicity. Destruction of rare autoreactive T cells in autoimmune diseases represents an elusive therapeutic goal designed to produce marked benefit over current treatments that are nonspecific and plagued by adverse effects. A defective TNF signaling pathway, which leads to cell death, now provides, at least in vitro, a unique opportunity in human autoimmune diseases to kill only autoreactive T cells. The continuous progress in knowledge of the immunological mechanisms inducing the β-cell loss as well as the newer cytokines involved in immune system regulation, in addition to the newer formulation of highly selective drugs, will possibly offer new potential therapeutic opportunity in patients with T1D.

A microsphere-based vaccine prevents and reverses new-onset autoimmune diabetes

Phillips B, Nylander K, Harnaha J, Machen J, Lakomy R, Styche A, Gillis K, Brown L, Lafreniere D, Gallo M, Knox J, Hogeland K, Trucco M, Giannoukakis N
Diabetes Institute, Division of Immunogenetics, Department of Pediatrics, University of Pittsburgh School of Medicine, Pittsburgh, Penn., USA
ngiann1@pitt.edu

Diabetes 2008;57:1544–1555

Background: The aim of the study was to verify whether antisense oligonucleotide-formulated microspheres are efficacious to prevent T1D and to reverse new-onset disease.

Methods: Microspheres carrying antisense oligonucleotides to CD40, CD80, and CD86 were delivered into NOD mice. Glycemia was monitored to determine disease prevention and reversal. In recipients that remained and/or became diabetes free, spleen and lymph node T cells were enriched to determine the prevalence of Foxp3(+) putative regulatory T-cells (Treg cells). Splenocytes from diabetes-free microsphere-treated recipients were adoptively co-transferred with splenocytes from diabetic NOD mice into NOD-scid recipients. Live-animal in vivo imaging measured the microsphere accumulation pattern. To rule out nonspecific systemic immunosuppression, splenocytes from successfully treated recipients were pulsed with β-cell antigen or ovalbumin or co-cultured with allogenic splenocytes.

Results: T1D was prevented by microsphere adoption and, most importantly, the system exhibited a capacity to reverse clinical hyperglycemia, suggesting reversal of new-onset disease. The microspheres augmented Foxp3(+) Treg cells and induced hyporesponsiveness to NOD-derived pancreatic β-cell antigen, without compromising global immune responses to alloantigens and nominal antigens. T cells from successfully treated mice suppressed adoptive transfer of disease by diabetogenic splenocytes into secondary immunodeficient recipients. Finally, microspheres accumulated within the pancreas and the spleen after either intraperitoneal or subcutaneous injection. Dendritic cells from the spleens of microsphere-treated mice exhibit decreased cell surface CD40, CD80, and CD86.

Conclusions: This novel microsphere formulation represents the first diabetes-suppressive and reversing nucleic acid vaccine that confers an immunoregulatory phenotype to endogenous dendritic cells.

Starting from the possibility to confer functional immaturity (defined by the capacity to activate and maintain immunoregulatory, 'suppressive' cell networks) to the dendritic cells (using systemic and molecule-specific approaches) [32], Phillips et al. evaluated whether antisense oligonucleotide-formulated microspheres are able to prevent T1D and to reverse new-onset disease. In particular, by using a PROMAXX microsphere delivery system (which has been demonstrated to be neutral with respect to dendritic cell maturation state in vivo) they formulated a PROMAXX-microsphere-based vaccine characterized by a mixture of the CD40, CD80, and CD86 antisense oligonucleotides (AS-MSPs).

Francesco Chiarelli/Cosimo Giannini

Thereafter, the microspheres with AS-MSPs or with scrambled control sequences (SCR-MSP) were injected subcutaneously or intraperitoneally at a site anatomically proximal to the pancreatic lymph nodes, into 5- to 8-week-old NOD female mice. Thus they showed that one single injection of AS-MSP, at a site anatomically proximal to the pancreatic lymph nodes, significantly delayed onset of diabetes, and 8 consecutive injections were very efficacious in preventing the disease altogether. Similarly, they showed that injections performed soon after diabetes development were able to reverse diabetes. Furthermore, AS-MSP treatment was shown to increase the prevalence of Foxp3_ CD25_ putative regulatory T cells in vivo and to yield T cells hypo-responsive to NIT-1 cell lysate in vitro without inducing nonspecific immune suppression.

Given the repertoire of self-reactive, potentially pathogenic lymphocytes, therapeutic options to diminish autoimmune disease risk include deletion, reduced activation or increased regulation of self-reactive lymphocytes by means that mimic or promote physiological mechanisms of immunity [33]. Vaccination with self-antigen to promote self-antigen-specific tolerance, 'negative vaccination', may represent the most specific and potentially safest means of averting autoimmune disease. Although further studies are needed in order to deeply characterized the immune-mediated modulation achieved by this interesting technology, dendritic cell modulation represents an innovative and promising opportunity for diabetes treatment.

New genes

Meta-analysis of genome-wide association study data identifies additional type 1 diabetes risk loci

Cooper JD, Smyth DJ, Smiles AM, Plagnol V, Walker NM, Allen JE, Downes K, Barrett JC, Healy BC, Mychaleckyj JC, Warram JH, Todd JA
Juvenile Diabetes Research Foundation/Wellcome Trust Diabetes and Inflammation Laboratory, Department of Medical Genetics, Cambridge Institute for Medical Research, University of Cambridge, Addenbrooke's Hospital, Cambridge, UK
jason.cooper@cimr.cam.ac.uk
Nat Genet 2008;40:1399–1401

Methods: In this study a meta-analysis of data from 3 genome-wide association studies of T1D, testing 305,090 SNPs in 3,561 T1D cases and 4,646 controls of European ancestry was carried out by Cooper et al.

Results: The authors were able to demonstrate further support for 4q27 (IL2–IL21, $p = 1.9 \times 10^{-8}$) and, after genotyping an additional 6,225 cases, 6,946 controls and 2,828 families, obtained convincing evidence for 4 previously unknown and distinct risk loci in chromosome regions 6q15 (BACH2, $p = 4.7 \times 10^{-12}$), 10p15 (PRKCQ, $p = 3.7 \times 10^{-9}$), 15q24 (CTSH, $p = 3.2 \times 10^{-15}$) and 22q13 (C1QTNF6, $p = 2.0 \times 10^{-8}$).

Follow-up analysis of genome-wide association data identifies novel loci for type 1 diabetes

Grant SF, Qu HQ, Bradfield JP, Marchand L, Kim CE, Glessner JT, Grabs R, Taback SP, Frackelton EC, Eckert AW, Annaiah K, Lawson ML, Otieno FG, Santa E, Shaner JL, Smith RM, Skraban R, Imielinski M, Chiavacci RM, Grundmeier RW, Stanley CA, Kirsch SE, Waggott D, Paterson AD, Monos DS; DCCT/EDIC Research Group, Polychronakos C, Hakonarson H
Center for Applied Genomics, Abramson Research Center, The Children's Hospital of Philadelphia, Philadelphia, Penn., USA
hakonarson@chop.edu
Diabetes 2009;58:290–295

Background: Novel loci for T1D, a common multifactorial disease with a strong genetic component, have been shown in 2 recent genome-wide association studies. To fully utilize the genome-wide association data that Grant et al. had obtained by genotyping 563 T1D probands and 1,146 control subjects, as well as 483 case subject-parent trios, using the Illumina HumanHap550 BeadChip, authors designed a full stage 2 study to capture other possible association signals.

Methods: From the previously designed datasets, Grant et al. selected 982 markers with p < 0.05 in both genome-wide association cohorts. Genotyping these in an independent set of 636 nuclear families with 974 affected offspring revealed 75 markers that also had p < 0.05 in this third cohort. Among these, 6 single nucleotide polymorphisms in 5 novel loci also had p < 0.05 in the Wellcome Trust Case-Control Consortium dataset and were further tested in 1,303 T1D probands from the Diabetes Control and Complications Trial/Epidemiology of Diabetes Interventions and Complications (DCCT/EDIC) plus 1,673 control subjects.

Results: Two markers (rs9976767 and rs3757247) remained significant after adjusting for the number of tests in this last cohort; they reside in UBASH3A (OR 1.16; combined p = 2.33 × 10^{-8}) and BACH2 (1.13; combined p = 1.25 × 10^{-6}).

Conclusions: Additional loci associated with T1D have been revealed by evaluating a large number of statistical genome-wide association candidates in several independent cohorts. The two genes at these respective loci, UBASH3A and BACH2, are both biologically relevant to autoimmunity.

These 2 studies clearly show the ability of genome-wide analysis, especially if performed in a very large population-base database, to reveal new HLA or non-HLA risk loci for T1D. In particular, by forming a US case-control genome-wide association study from a smart meta-analysis of 3 genome-wide association studies, Cooper et al. were first able to provide further support for 4q27 (IL2–IL21) as an important T1D risk locus. More interestingly, they showed 4 previously unnoticed and different T1D risk loci (6q15, BACH2; 10p15, PRKCQ; 15q24, CTSH, and 22q13, C1QTNF6), increasing the total of T1D loci with convincing evidence from 10 [34] to 15 (including the HLA region). Similarly, by performing a full stage 2 study in which data from 4 independent studies were combined, Grant et al. were able to reveal 2 additional loci associated with T1D. In particular, they show 2 genes at these respective loci, UBASH3A (codifying for 2 proteins STS1 and STS2 which are critical regulators of the signaling pathways that control T-cell activation) and BACH2 (encoding for a group of proteins of the small Maf family that seem to function as regulators of the antibody response), which result both biologically relevant to autoimmunity.

In addition to the detection of these new T1D risk loci, both studies were able to demonstrate the effectiveness of combining evidence from GWA studies to find disease loci, showing that genome-wide analysis studies can be successfully performed using case and control data from different studies. Therefore, the rapid diffusion of new methods able to carry out whole-genome association studies using a large number of single nucleotide polymorphisms will offer not only the possibility to perform a large genetic analysis, but will also represent publicly available resource data to further improve the power and effectiveness of analysis directed to evidence new T1D loci risk. In the future these new gene-detecting tools will allow a complete characterization of genetic risk factors related to T1D and will possibly allow a population-based analysis of genetic risk for T1D.

Genome-wide association scan for diabetic nephropathy susceptibility genes in type 1 diabetes mellitus

Pezzolesi MG, Poznik GD, Mychaleckyj JC, Paterson AD, Barati MT, Klein JB, Ng DP, Placha G, Canani LH, Bochenski J, Waggott D, Merchant ML, Krolewski B, Mirea L, Wanic K, Katavetin P, Kure M, Wolkow P, Dunn JS, Smiles A, Walker WH, Boright AP, Bull SB; DCCT/EDIC Research Group, Doria A, Rogus JJ, Rich SS, Warram JH, Krolewski AS
Research Division, Joslin Diabetes Center, and Department of Medicine, Harvard Medical School, Boston, Mass., USA
andrzej.krolewski@joslin.harvard.edu
Diabetes 2009;58:1403–1410

Background: Despite extensive evidence for genetic susceptibility to diabetic nephropathy, limited success has been achieved in the identification of susceptibility genes and their variants. To search for diabetic nephropathy-related susceptibility genes, a genome-wide association scan was implemented on the Genetics of Kidneys in Diabetes collection.

Methods: Pezzolesi et al. genotyped approximately 360,000 single nucleotide polymorphisms (SNPs) in 820 cases (284 with proteinuria and 536 with end-stage renal disease) and 885 controls with T1D. Confirmation of implicated SNPs was sought in 1,304 participants of the DCCT/EDIC study, a long-term, prospective investigation of the development of diabetes-associated complications.

Results: A total of 13 SNPs located in 4 genomic loci were associated with diabetic nephropathy with p < 1 × 10^{-5}. The strongest association was at the FRMD3 (FERM domain containing 3) locus (OR = 1.45, p = 5.0 × 10^{-7}). A strong association was also identified at the CARS (cysteinyl-tRNA synthetase) locus (OR = 1.36, p = 3.1 × 10^{-6}). Associations between both loci and time to onset of diabetic nephropathy were supported in the DCCT/EDIC study (HR = 1.33, p = 0.02 and HR = 1.32, p = 0.01, respectively). The expression of both FRMD3 and CARS in the human kidney was demonstrated.
Conclusions: In this study Pezzolesi et al. were able to identify genetic associations for susceptibility to diabetic nephropathy at 2 novel candidate loci near the FRMD3 and CARS genes. Their identification implicates previously unsuspected pathways in the pathogenesis of this important late complication of T1D.

In this study Pezzolesi et al. attempt to identify loci associated with the risk of diabetic nephropathy in patients with T1D included in the Genetics of Kidneys in Diabetes (GoKinD) collection (made up of 935 patients with T1D and 944 control subjects) [35]. In particular by performing a genome-wide scan of the entire population they were able to detect some significant associations with variants located within 4 distinct chromosomal regions whose biology, interestingly, remains to be elucidated. In detail, the regions detected implicate: *FRMD3*, encoding 4.10 protein (a structural protein with unknown function) and a member of the 4.1 family of proteins (a cytoskeletal proteins); *CARS*, encoding cysteinyl-tRNA synthetase (a regulators of intracellular amino acid concentrations and protein biosynthesis in both the cytoplasm and mitochondria); *CHN2/CPVL*, a carboxypeptidase that is highly expressed in the kidney; and an intergenic region on chromosome 13q, as novel genes/genetic regions involved in the pathogenesis of diabetic nephropathy which might also involve two major genes closest to the associated SNPs, *MYO16* (myosin heavy-chain Myr 8) and *IRS2* (insulin receptor substrate 2). Although the limitations related to this study (such as the small sample size, the study design which is weighted with case subjects with end stage renal diseases and especially the need to elucidate the mechanism underlying the revealed associations) these findings contribute to the understanding of genetic susceptibility of diabetic nephropathy in T1D. In fact, although mounting clinical and epidemiological evidence has shown a main role of genetic factors in diabetic nephropathy, up to now no genes have been unequivocally demonstrated. However, these findings are not surprising as, similar to other complex genetic disorders, no single major gene contributing to an increased risk of disease has emerged [36]. A complete understanding of the genetic predisposing factors will be helpful in defining patients with diabetes at increased risk of developing micro- and macrovascular complications. Therefore, a multicenter-wide population-based study needs to be designed to further characterize the pathogenic role of these and other candidate genes identified as genetic determinant of the diabetes-related vascular complications.

Two new hormones

Plasma osteoprotegerin levels predict cardiovascular and all-cause mortality and deterioration of kidney function in type 1 diabetic patients with nephropathy

Jorsal A, Tarnow L, Flyvbjerg A, Parving HH, Rossing P, Rasmussen LM
Steno Diabetes Center, Gentofte, Denmark
ajrs@steno.dk
Diabetologia 2008;51:2100–2107

Background: Osteoprotegerin, a bone-related peptide, is produced by vascular cells and is involved in the process of vascular calcification. The aim of this study was to investigatethe predictive value of plasma levels of osteoprotegerin in relation to mortality, cardiovascular events and deterioration in kidney function in patients with T1D.
Methods: This prospective observational follow-up study included 397 patients with T1D and overt diabetic nephropathy (243 men; age [mean ± SD] 42.1 ± 10.6 years, duration of diabetes 28.3 ± 9.9 years, GFR 67 ± 28 ml min^{-1} 1.73 m^2) and a group of 176 patients with longstanding T1D and persistent normoalbuminuria (105 men; age 42.6 ± 9.7 years, duration of diabetes 27.6 ± 8.3 years).

Results: The median (range) follow-up period was 11.3 (0.0–12.9) years. Among patients with diabetic nephropathy, individuals with high osteoprotegerin levels (fourth quartile) had significantly higher all-cause mortality than patients with low levels (first quartile; covariate-adjusted hazard ratio [HR] 3.00 [1.24–7.27]). High osteoprotegerin levels also predicted cardiovascular mortality (covariate-adjusted HR 4.88 [1.57–15.14]). Furthermore, increased osteoprotegerin levels were associated with a significantly higher risk of progression to end-stage renal disease (covariate-adjusted HR 4.32 [1.45–12.87]) as well a higher rate of decline in GFR.
Conclusions: High levels of osteoprotegerin predict all-cause and cardiovascular mortality in patients with diabetic nephropathy. Furthermore, high levels of osteoprotegerin predict deterioration of kidney function towards end-stage renal disease.

In this long prospective observational study, Jorsal et al. were able to revealed a novel independent risk marker for all-cause and cardiovascular mortality in a relatively large population of patients with T1D and overt nephropathy. In fact, during a 11.3-year follow-up period they showed that the higher the osteoprotegerin quartile range, the higher , the risk of all-cause and cardiovascular mortality. They were also able to show that increased plasma osteoprotegerin concentrations predict deterioration of kidney function independent of potential influences of other well-known conventional cardiovascular and renal risk factors, including glomerular filtration rate. Although further larger and longer longitudinal studies are needed in order to confirm and validate these preliminary data, the identification of novel markers of cardiovascular diseases and deterioration of kidney function represents an important goal in patients with T1D. In fact, although microalbuminuria as well as HbA1c represent the best-available noninvasive and sensitive predictor of the risk of diabetic nephropathy as well as all-cause mortality and cardiovascular disease [37], some patients with microalbuminuria have advanced renal histopathological changes, and its full potential depends on longitudinal repeated measures [37]. Furthermore, although previous studies [20, 38] have demonstrated the importance of maintaining good glycemic control in the prevention of short- and long-term risk of complications, some patients develop chronic complications despite reasonable or even good metabolic control. Therefore, the identification of novel and highly sensitive and specific markers of risk of vascular complications in patients with T1D are needed.

Liraglutide, a long-acting human glucagon-like peptide 1 analog, improves glucose homeostasis in marginal mass islet transplantation in mice

Merani S, Truong W, Emamaullee JA, Toso C, Knudsen LB, Shapiro AM
Surgical Medical Research Institute, University of Alberta, Edmonton, Alta., Canada
shapiro@islet.ca
Endocrinology 2008;149:4322–4328

Background: The current scarcity of high-quality deceased pancreas donors represents a relevant factor able to minimize the widespread application of islet transplantation for treatment of labile T1D. Opportunities for the improvement of current techniques include optimization of islet isolation and purification, use of culture with pharmacological insulinotropic agents, strategies to reduce graft rejection and inflammation, and the search for alternative insulin-producing tissue.
Methods: In this study Merani et al. reported findings on the efficacy of the long-acting human glucagon-like peptide 1 analog, liraglutide, in a mouse model of marginal mass islet transplantation. In streptozotocin-induced diabetic BALB/c mice liraglutide was administered (200 µg/kg s.c. twice daily) after a marginal mass syngeneic islet transplant.
Results: In liraglutide-treated animals the time-to-normoglycemia was significantly shorter (median 1 vs. 7 days; p = 0.0003), even in recipients receiving sirolimus (median 1 vs. 72.5 days; p < 0.0001). Furthermore, improved glucose tolerance, as assessed by an intraperitoneal glucose tolerance test, was shown in liraglutide-treated animals. Liraglutide discontinuation on postoperative day 90 resulted in diminished glucose tolerance during the intraperitoneal glucose tolerance test, whereas a late-start liraglutide therapy 90 days after transplant resulted in no improvement. These findings suggest that liraglutide therapy mediates early and late insulinotropic effects. In accordance with this hypothesis, insulin/terminal deoxynucleotidyl transferase-mediated deoxyuridine 5-triphosphate nick end-labeling fluorescence microscopy showed reduced transplanted β-cell apoptosis in liraglutide-treated recipients 48 h after transplant. In addition, liraglutide resulted in improved glucose-dependent insulin secretion.

                                          Francesco Chiarelli/Cosimo Giannini

Conclusions: In conclusion, this study showed that liraglutide has a beneficial impact on the engraftment and function of syngeneic islet transplants in mice, when administered continuously starting on the day of transplant.

In this study Merani et al. attempted to evaluate whether liraglutide, a glucagon-like peptide 1 (GLP-1) analog, might represent a new clinically applicable therapeutic opportunity able to prolong and improved transplanted islet in patients with T1D. In particular, after transplanting diabetic BALB/c animals with a marginal mass of 250 syngeneic islets, animals were randomized to 4 treatment groups: vehicle; liraglutide; sirolimus (an immunosuppressive drug); or sirolimus plus liraglutide. Thus, they showed that liraglutide administration reduced the time required to achieve normoglycemia (time to engraftment) in transplanted animals as well as provided better long-term glycemic control and improved glucose homeostasis in the marginal mass islet transplant model without the need for exogenous insulin. Furthermore, they also demonstrated that these characteristics of liraglutide are present even when sirolimus is administered concurrently. In addition Merani et al. have offered relevant information on the time of liraglutide administration as well on the mechanism of liraglutide action. In fact, they clarified that liraglutide must be administered both immediately after islet transplantation and continuously thereafter to maximize its beneficial effects. In addition, they also showed that liraglutide administration results in both reduced β-cell apoptosis and improved glucose-dependent insulin secretion. Although further investigation on liraglutide in the field of islet transplantation are needed, the effect of liraglutide on β-cell activity is promising. In fact, although islet transplantation is an emerging therapeutic option for the treatment of select labile T1D, several barriers prevent its broad application, even within a selected group of patients [39]. In particular, the frequently documented insulin requirement even after islet transplantation and the insurgence of islet allograft rejection minimize its application [39]. Because of the liraglutide effects on reduced apoptosis in transplanted β cells and on improved glucose metabolism, it might be speculated that a complete characterization of the GLP-1 analog-related actions would offer relevant help by delaying islet allo-rejection and by inducing a complete insulin independency.

Review

Clinical review 2: The 'metabolic memory': is more than just tight glucose control necessary to prevent diabetic complications?

Ceriello A, Ihnat MA, Thorpe JE
Warwick Medical School, University of Warwick, Coventry, UK
antonio.ceriello@warwick.ac.uk
J Clin Endocrinol Metab 2009;94:410–415

Background: The concept of a 'metabolic memory', that is of diabetic vascular stresses persisting after glucose normalization, has been supported both in the laboratory and in the clinic and in T1D as well as in T2D.

Methods: Using PubMed sources, Ceriello et al. searched for publications on diabetic micro- and macro-vascular complications using terms such as persistence, prolongation, sustained, and 'memory', and focused on the mechanistic basis behind this metabolic memory.

Results: They found that as early as the mid-1980s this memory phenomenon was described in diabetic animals and isolated cells exposed to high glucose followed by normalized glucose and then, beginning around 2002, in results from large clinical trials such as the DCCT-EDIC and the United Kingdom Prospective Diabetes Study. Furthermore, mechanisms for propagating this memory appear focused on the non-enzymatic glycation of cellular proteins and lipids and on an excess of cellular reactive oxygen and nitrogen species, in particular originating at the level of glycated mitochondrial proteins and perhaps acting in concert with one another to maintain stress signaling independent of glucose levels.

Conclusions: The relevant role of this metabolic memory suggests either the need for early aggressive treatment aiming to 'normalize' metabolic control or the addition of agents which reduce cellular reactive species and glycation in order to minimize long-term diabetic complications.

During the last 50 years several in vitro and in vivo (both in animals and humans), studies have clearly demonstrated that hyperglycemia represents the major determinant of the development and progression of diabetes related micro- and macrovascular complications [21, 38]. Further studies have unequivocally demonstrated that the effects of hyperglycemia exposure persist even after a complete metabolic normalization introducing the concept of the 'metabolic memory'. By reviewing published data using the PubMed source, Ceriello et al. attempt to give a complete view of the in vitro and in vivo evidence of the existing 'metabolic memory' in patients with diabetes. In particular, by unifying different evidence, they clearly showed that hyperglycemia has long-lasting deleterious effects both in T1D and T2D and that glycemic control, if not started at a very early stage of the disease, is not sufficient to completely reduce the risk of vascular complications. In addition, Cerriello et al. described the main mechanisms implicated in 'metabolic memory'. This evidence raises many questions regarding the therapeutic management of diabetes. In particular, the existence of the metabolic memory suggests that very early aggressive treatment of hyperglycemia is mandatory. As it is documented that despite the awareness of the importance of maintaining good glycemic control, treatment of diabetes is inadequate, especially in childhood [40]. Therefore, Cerriello et al. prospect a future strategy consisting not only in an early aggressive treatment of hyperglycemia, but with the simultaneous use of compounds active on advanced glycated end-product formation, together with compounds capable of specifically targeting mitochondrial reactive species which have been shown to play the main role in the instauration of a metabolic memory. This strategy might have the potential to reduce the deleterious effects of metabolic memory and hyperglycemia on diabetic complications.

Shared and distinct genetic variants in type 1 diabetes and celiac disease

Smyth DJ, Plagnol V, Walker NM, Cooper JD, Downes K, Yang JH, Howson JM, Stevens H, McManus R, Wijmenga C, Heap GA, Dubois PC, Clayton DG, Hunt KA, van Heel DA, Todd JA
Juvenile Diabetes Research Foundation-Wellcome Trust Diabetes and Inflammation Laboratory, Department of Medical Genetics, Cambridge Institute for Medical Research, University of Cambridge, Addenbrooke's Hospital, Cambridge, UK
john.todd@cimr.cam.ac.uk
N Engl J Med 2008;359:2767–2777

Background: Two inflammatory disorders, T1D and celiac disease, are frequently associated in populations, suggesting a common genetic origin. Since the HLA class II genes on chromosome 6p21 are associated in both diseases , Smyth et al. tested whether non-HLA loci are shared.
Methods: They evaluated the association between T1D and 8 loci related to the risk of celiac disease by genotyping and statistical analyses of DNA samples from 8,064 patients with T1D, 9,339 control subjects, and 2,828 families providing 3,064 parent–child trios (consisting of an affected child and both biologic parents). They also investigated 18 loci associated with T1D in 2,560 patients with celiac disease and 9,339 control subjects.
Results: Three celiac disease loci – RGS1 on chromosome 1q31, IL18RAP on chromosome 2q12, and TAGAP on chromosome 6q25 – were associated with T1D ($p < 1.00 \times 10^{-4}$). The 32-bp insertion-deletion variant on chromosome 3p21 was newly identified as a T1D locus ($p = 1.81 \times 10^{-8}$) and was also associated with celiac disease, along with PTPN2 on chromosome 18p11 and CTLA4 on chromosome 2q33, bringing the total number of loci with evidence of a shared association to 7, including SH2B3 on chromosome 12q24. The effects of the IL18RAP and TAGAP alleles confer protection in T1D and susceptibility in celiac disease. INS on chromosome 11p15, IL2RA on chromosome 10p15, and PTPN22 on chromosome 1p13 in T1D, and IL12A on 3q25 and LPP on 3q28 in celiac disease were shown to be loci with distinct effects in the two diseases.
Conclusions: A genetic susceptibility to both T1D and celiac disease shares common alleles. Therefore, common biologic mechanisms, such as autoimmunity-related tissue damage and intolerance to dietary antigens, may be etiologic features of both diseases.

     Francesco Chiarelli/Cosimo Giannini

By genotyping and statistically analyzing data from a large population, Smyth et al. explored the existence of non HLA-related loci associated with T1D and celiac disease and shared by the 2 diseases. In particular, according to the results obtained by previously published genome-wide association studies, they genotyped single-nucleotide polymorphisms (SNPs) from 8 celiac disease loci and from 15 T1D loci as well as from 3 other major genes (IL7R, CD226, and the 32-bp insertion–deletion variant in CCR5).

According to previous studies, Smyth et al. provided further evidence that 21 non-HLA loci are associated with T1D and 11 non-HLA loci are associated with celiac disease. In addition, in patients with T1D statistical analysis showed that 3 of the non-HLA regions associated with celiac diseases (in particular RGS1 on chromosome 1q31, IL18RAP on chromosome 2q12, and TAGAP on chromosome 6q25) proved to be strong evidence for the association with diabetes. On the other hand, in patients with celiac disease, Smyth et al. demonstrated in a logistic regression analysis that 7 T1D loci (RGS1, TAGAP, IL18RAP, CTLA4 on chromosome 2q33, CCR5 on chromosome 3p21, SH2B3 on chromosome 12q24, and PTPN2 on chromosome 18p119) are convincing evidence of an association with the disease. In addition, RGS1, CTLA4, SH2B3, and PTPN2 showed the same direction of association in the 2 diseases, constituting evidence for shared causal variants. In contrast, the minor alleles of the SNPs rs917997 (IL18RAP) and rs1738074 (TAGAP) were negatively associated with T1D, whereas these minor alleles were positively associated with celiac disease.

In conclusion, 7 chromosome regions, 3 celiac disease loci, associated with T1D (RGS1, IL18RAP, and TAGAP), and 2 T1D loci, associated with celiac disease (CCR5 and PTPN2), are shared between the 2 diseases, giving clear evidence of a common genetic susceptibility pattern. As these loci are directly involved in different cellular or immunological functions, the complete characterization of the genetic-dependent determinant shared by both diseases will help to offer further pieces of the complex puzzle describing these multifaceted diseases. In addition, full investigation of any possible association between the different genetic risk determinants and the natural history of diabetes or celiac onset in both these autoimmune diseases will offer further help for evaluating new approaches to preventing or retarding their onset.

Iodine and tri-iodo-thyronine reduce the incidence of type 1 diabetes mellitus in the autoimmune prone BB rats

Hartoft-Nielsen ML, Rasmussen AK, Bock T, Feldt-Rasmussen U, Kaas A, Buschard K
Department of Endocrinology, Rigshospitalet, University Hospital of Copenhagen, Copenhagen, Denmark
ma-lars@dadlnet.dk
Autoimmunity 2009;42:131–138

Background: Thyroid hormones modulate the immune system and metabolism, influence insulin secretion, and cause decreased glucose tolerance. Although it has been described that thyroid hormones are able to change the incidence of spontaneous autoimmune thyroiditis in Bio-Breeding/Worcester (BB) rats, whether these hormones do or do not affect the development of T1D is still unknown. The aim of this study was to investigate the influence of changes in thyroid function during postnatal development on the prevalence of T1D in BB rats and the influence of T3 on the β-cell mass in non-diabetic Wistar rats.

Methods: BB rats were treated with sodium iodine (NaI) or thyroid-stimulating hormone (TSH) neonatally, or with tri-iodo-thyronine (T$_3$) during adolescence. The incidence of T1D and the degree of insulitis were evaluated at the age of 19 weeks. By unbiased stereological methods, the influence of T$_3$ treatment on the β-cell mass was evaluated in Wistar rats.

Results: The incidence of T1D in control BB rats was 68% at the age of 19 weeks. NaI and T$_3$ reduced the incidence, whereas TSH had no effect. In Wistar rats T$_3$ treatment increased the β-cell mass per body-weight.

Conclusions: The modulation of thyroid function during postnatal development may affect the precipitation of T1D in genetically susceptible individuals.

In this study Hartoft-Nielsen et al. were able, for the first time, to investigate the influence of thyroid hormones on the incidence of T1D in rats. In particular, by performing analysis in the BB rat (a well-established animal model with a spontaneous incidence of about 50% for T1D and autoimmune thyroiditis), they showed that treatment with thyroid hormone and iodine significantly reduces the incidence of T1D in BB rats. In fact, in male rats, iodine given immediately postpartum and thereafter daily for the first 6 days reduced the incidence of T1D; in contrast, no effects on the T1D development were documented after TSH administration (given immediately postpartum and daily for the first 3 days during the first 3 weeks). Similar to iodine treatment, the authors reported that T_3 given during adolescence reduced the incidence of T1D but only significantly in female rats, with a protective effect of iodine which seems to be stronger than the protective effect of T_3. Although these results appear quite interesting, the mechanisms of action for the reduced incidence of T1D after the iodine and T_3 treatment are not known and several hypothesis might be postulated. In fact, for both treatments the effect could be a direct influence on the β cells or a more indirect effect on the immune system. For example, treatment could act by influencing the functional state of β cells and therefore the important balance between apoptosis, replication and neogenesis. This might be caused by a reduced endogenous insulin secretion and reduced amount of antigens on the β-cell surface [41]. Furthermore, resting β cells are less vulnerable to a destructive effect of proinflammatory cytokines. In addition, as the treatment is given earlier, different mechanisms might be moved on for iodine treatment. In particular, as documented in β cells treated neonatally with stimulatory drugs, iodine might cause an early maturation of the β cells, resulting in a stronger recognition of the β cells as 'self' by the immune system. However, up to now no exact mechanisms have been defined. Finally, because of the influence of T_3 on glucose metabolism, and of the influence of iodine and T_3 on metabolism in general [42], the complete characterization of the underling mechanisms represents an important tool to be defined in order to offer new prospective views involved in the development of T1D and autoimmune thyroiditis.

References

1. Shoda LK, Young DL, Ramanujan S, Whiting CC, Atkinson MA, Bluestone JA, et al: A comprehensive review of interventions in the NOD mouse and implications for translation. Immunity 2005;23:115–126.
2. Lee DD, Grossman E, Chong AS: Cellular therapies for type 1 diabetes. Horm Metab Res 2008;40:147–154.
3. Keymeulen B, Vandemeulebroucke E, Ziegler AG, Mathieu C, Kaufman L, Hale G, et al: Insulin needs after CD3-antibody therapy in new-onset type 1 diabetes. N Engl J Med 2005;352:2598–2608.
4. Hochedlinger K, Jaenisch R: Nuclear reprogramming and pluripotency. Nature 2006;441:1061–1067.
5. Orkin SH, Zon LI: Hematopoiesis: an evolving paradigm for stem cell biology. Cell 2008;132:631–644.
6. Pearl EJ, Horb ME: Promoting ectopic pancreatic fates: pancreas development and future diabetes therapies. Clin Genet 2008;74:316–324.
7. Skyler JS, Krischer JP, Wolfsdorf J, Cowie C, Palmer JP, Greenbaum C, et al: Effects of oral insulin in relatives of patients with type 1 diabetes: the Diabetes Prevention Trial – Type 1. Diabetes Care 2005;28:1068–1076.
8. Diabetes Prevention Trial–Type 1 Diabetes Study Group: Effects of insulin in relatives of patients with type 1 diabetes mellitus. N Engl J Med 2002;346:1685–1691.
9. Kobayashi T, Maruyama T, Shimada A, Kasuga A, Kanatsuka A, Takei I, et al: Insulin intervention to preserve beta cells in slowly progressive insulin-dependent (type 1) diabetes mellitus. Ann NY Acad Sci 2002;958:117–130.
10. Toma A, Laika T, Haddouk S, Luce S, Briand JP, Camoin L, et al: Recognition of human proinsulin leader sequence by class I-restricted T-cells in HLA-A*0201 transgenic mice and in human type 1 diabetes. Diabetes 2009;58:394–402.
11. Keller RJ, Eisenbarth GS, Jackson RA: Insulin prophylaxis in individuals at high risk of type I diabetes. Lancet 1993;341:927–928.
12. Montanya E, Fernandez-Castaner M, Soler J: Improved metabolic control preserved beta-cell function two years after diagnosis of insulin-dependent diabetes mellitus. Diabetes Metab 1997;23:314–319.
13. Effect of intensive therapy on residual beta-cell function in patients with type 1 diabetes in the diabetes control and complications trial. A randomized, controlled trial. The Diabetes Control and Complications Trial Research Group. Ann Intern Med 1998;128:517–523.
14. Vang T, Miletic AV, Arimura Y, Tautz L, Rickert RC, Mustelin T: Protein tyrosine phosphatases in autoimmunity. Annu Rev Immunol 2008;26:29–55.
15. Magro F, Costa C: Long-standing remission of Crohn's disease under imatinib therapy in a patient with Crohn's disease. Inflamm Bowel Dis 2006;12:1087–1089.
16. Hagerkvist R, Sandler S, Mokhtari D, Welsh N: Amelioration of diabetes by imatinib mesylate (Gleevec): role of beta-cell NF-kappaB activation and anti-apoptotic preconditioning. FASEB J 2007;21:618–628.
17. Liu EY, Wactawski-Wende J, Donahue RP, Dmochowski J, Hovey KM, Quattrin T: Does low bone mineral density start in post-teenage years in women with type 1 diabetes? Diabetes Care 2003;26:2365–2369.
18. Rakel A, Sheehy O, Rahme E, LeLorier J: Osteoporosis among patients with type 1 and type 2 diabetes. Diabetes Metab 2008;34:193–205.
19. Forsen L, Meyer HE, Midthjell K, Edna TH: Diabetes mellitus and the incidence of hip fracture: results from the Nord-Trondelag Health Survey. Diabetologia 1999;42:920–925.
20. The effect of intensive treatment of diabetes on the development and progression of long-term complications in insulin-dependent diabetes mellitus. The Diabetes Control and Complications Trial Research Group. N Engl J Med 1993;329:977–986.
21. The relationship of glycemic exposure (HbA1c) to the risk of development and progression of retinopathy in the diabetes control and complications trial. Diabetes 1995;44:968–983.
22. Prince CT, Becker DJ, Costacou T, Miller RG, Orchard TJ: Changes in glycaemic control and risk of coronary artery disease in type 1 diabetes mellitus: findings from the Pittsburgh Epidemiology of Diabetes Complications Study (EDC). Diabetologia 2007;50:2280–2288.

23. Monnier L, Lapinski H, Colette C: Contributions of fasting and postprandial plasma glucose increments to the overall diurnal hyperglycemia of type 2 diabetic patients: variations with increasing levels of HbA(1c). Diabetes Care 2003;26:881–885.
24. Coutinho M, Gerstein HC, Wang Y, Yusuf S: The relationship between glucose and incident cardiovascular events. A metaregression analysis of published data from 20 studies of 95,783 individuals followed for 12.4 years. Diabetes Care 1999;22:233–240.
25. Roach P: New insulin analogues and routes of delivery: pharmacodynamic and clinical considerations. Clin Pharmacokinet 2008;47:595–610.
26. Gough SC: A review of human and analogue insulin trials. Diabetes Res Clin Pract 2007;77:1–15.
27. Steffes MW, Sibley S, Jackson M, Thomas W: Beta-cell function and the development of diabetes-related complications in the diabetes control and complications trial. Diabetes Care 2003;26:832–836.
28. Nakanishi K, Watanabe C: Rate of beta-cell destruction in type 1 diabetes influences the development of diabetic retinopathy: protective effect of residual beta-cell function for more than 10 years. J Clin Endocrinol Metab 2008;93:4759–4766.
29. Cryer PE: Hypoglycemia unawareness in IDDM. Diabetes Care 1993;16(suppl 3):40–47.
30. Schleis T: Realities of the fluoxetine-to-sertraline switch. Am J Health Syst Pharm 1995;52:423; author reply 4, 8.
31. Carvalho F, Barros D, Silva J, Rezende E, Soares M, Fregoneze J, et al: Hyperglycemia induced by acute central fluoxetine administration: role of the central CRH system and 5-HT3 receptors. Neuropeptides 2004;38:98–105.
32. McCurry KR, Colvin BL, Zahorchak AF, Thomson AW: Regulatory dendritic cell therapy in organ transplantation. Transpl Int 2006;19:525–538.
33. Harrison LC: Vaccination against self to prevent autoimmune disease: the type 1 diabetes model. Immunol Cell Biol 2008;86:139–145.
34. Hakonarson H, Qu HQ, Bradfield JP, Marchand L, Kim CE, Glessner JT, et al: A novel susceptibility locus for type 1 diabetes on Chr12q13 identified by a genome-wide association study. Diabetes 2008;57:1143–1146.
35. Mueller PW, Rogus JJ, Cleary PA, Zhao Y, Smiles AM, Steffes MW, et al: Genetics of Kidneys in Diabetes (GoKinD) study: a genetics collection available for identifying genetic susceptibility factors for diabetic nephropathy in type 1 diabetes. J Am Soc Nephrol 2006;17:1782–1790.
36. Scott LJ, Mohlke KL, Bonnycastle LL, Willer CJ, Li Y, Duren WL, et al: A genome-wide association study of type 2 diabetes in Finns detects multiple susceptibility variants. Science 2007;316:1341–1345.
37. Mogensen CE, Poulsen PL: Microalbuminuria, glycemic control, and blood pressure predicting outcome in diabetes type 1 and type 2. Kidney Int Suppl 2004;92:S40–S41.
38. Effect of intensive therapy on the microvascular complications of type 1 diabetes mellitus. JAMA 2002;287:2563–2569.
39. Leitão CB, Cure P, Tharavanij T, Baidal DA, Alejandro R: Current challenges in islet transplantation. Curr Diab Rep 2008;8:324–331.
40. Danne T, Mortensen HB, Hougaard P, Lynggaard H, Aanstoot HJ, Chiarelli F, et al: Persistent differences among centers over 3 years in glycemic control and hypoglycemia in a study of 3,805 children and adolescents with type 1 diabetes from the Hvidore Study Group. Diabetes Care 2001;24:1342–1347.
41. Atkinson MA, Maclaren NK, Luchetta R: Insulitis and diabetes in NOD mice reduced by prophylactic insulin therapy. Diabetes 1990;39:933–937.
42. Chidakel A, Mentuccia D, Celi FS: Peripheral metabolism of thyroid hormone and glucose homeostasis. Thyroid 2005;15:899–903.

Obesity and Weight Regulation

Martin Wabitsch, Sina Horenburg, Christian Denzer, Julia von Schnurbein, Michaela Keuper, Daniel Tews, Anja Moss, Carsten Posovszky and Pamela Fischer-Posovszky

Division of Pediatric Endocrinology and Diabetes, Obesity Unit, Department of Pediatrics, University of Ulm, Ulm, Germany

Once more, the recent literature on obesity and weight regulation demonstrates the activity and interest of this field of science. For the Yearbook selection this year, only articles published in journals with a high impact factor were considered, assuming that relevant findings were published in these journals.

The highlights are papers about the further functional characterization of the fat mass- and obesity-associated (FTO) gene, about strong evidence of a continuous turnover of adipocytes in white adipose tissue, about brown adipose tissue in man as a target for the regulation of homeostasis, and about factors influencing weight maintenance after weight loss therapy. Furthermore, evidence-based recommendations on prevention and treatment of obesity in children and adolescents are now available.

New insights into the function of fat mass-and obesity-associated (FTO) gene

Fat mass-and obesity-associated (FTO) gene variant is associated with obesity: longitudinal analyses in two cohort studies and functional test

Qi L, Kang K, Zhang C, van Dam RM, Kraft P, Hunter D, Lee CH, Hu FB
Department of Nutrition, Harvard School of Public Health, Boston, Mass., USA
nhlqi@channing.harvard.edu
Diabetes 2008;57:3145–3151

Background: A huge number of polymorphisms influencing weight and BMI have been identified. The best reproducible association exists for variants in the FTO gene. So far however, little is known about the function of FTO, its influence on metabolism and time-related changes in the influence on BMI.

Methods: 2,287 men and 3,520 women from two prospective cohorts (Nurses` Health Study and Health Professional Follow-Up Study) were genotyped for the common variant rs9939609. Plasma adiponectin and leptin were measured in a subset of diabetic men (n=854) and women (n=987). Expression of FTO was tested in adipocytes from mice lacking the leptin-receptor (db/db mice) and in wild-type mouse macrophages.

Results: Rs9939609 was associated with increased BMI and risk for overweight/obesity in men and women both in young adulthood and later in life. The association between this polymorphism and obesity risk showed a tendency to decline with increasing age in men.

Heterozygosity and homozygosity for the risk allele were associated with type 2 diabetes in both men and women and with lower adiponectin and higher leptin levels in women. However, these associations became non-significant when adjusted for BMI.

FTO was expressed in several metabolically active tissues in humans and wild-type C56BL/6 mice. In db/db mice FTO expression in white adipocytes was reduced by 50%.

Conclusion: The study confirms an association between a common FTO variant and BMI over a wide age-range. Observed connections between this variant and diabetes-risk or changes in adipocytokine levels were mediated via BMI. Db/db mice showed a decreased expression in FTO.

Increasing heritability of BMI and stronger associations with the FTO gene over childhood

Haworth CM, Carnell S, Meaburn EL, Davis OS, Plomin R, Wardle J
Social, Genetic and Developmental Psychiatry Centre, Institute of Psychiatry, King's College London, London, UK
Claire.Haworth@iop.kcl.ac.uk
Obesity (Silver Spring) 2008;16:2663–2668

Background: Twin research has been pivotal in identifying the substantial genetic impact on individual differences in BMI. A huge number of polymorphisms influencing weight and BMI have been identified; with the best reproducible association for variants in the FTO gene. However, the magnitude of genetic influence on BMI seems to change with age. Up to date very few longitudinal twin analysis have been performed to asses this age-dependency.

Methods: Repeated BMI assessments at 4, 7, 10 and 11 years of age were performed in a longitudinal sample of >7000 children from the Twins Early Development Study in the United Kingdom. Analyses for the FTO polymorphism rs9939609 were conducted in one member of each pair, for which DNA material was available (around 2800 children).

Results: The differences between monozygotic and dicygotic twins in twin-correlation for BMI increased from age 4 to age 11 whereas shared environmental influence decreased. The association between the FTO variant and BMI rose in parallel to the gain in heritability, going from $R^2 < 0.001$ at age 4 to $R^2 = 0.01$ at age 11.

Conclusion: The findings suggest that either expression of FTO becomes stronger throughout childhood or that children increasingly select an environment suiting their genetic propensities.

Both articles address the important issue of the mechanisms underlying the influence of genes on BMI. Variants in the FTO gene are well established among the potential factors [1–3], different population studies yield wildly differing results concerning the magnitude of this influence. At least in part this might be attributable to different age ranges in the groups examined. Although longitudinal studies avoid some of the confounding factors identified in cross-sectional studies, few studies longitudinal studies on the influence of gene variants on BMI exist. In the first article long-term changes in two large general populations are examined. In the second the more specific aspects of longitudinal twin studies are used. The twin study shows a clear age-dependency with an increased influence of age. According to the population study this influence might vane in later years, however, these changes were non-significant. These articles highlight the complexity of gene/environment interactions and add yet another puzzle piece to our understanding.

Inactivation of the FTO gene protects from obesity

Fischer J, Koch L, Emmerling C, Vierkotten J, Peters T, Brüning JC, Rüther U
Institute for Animal Developmental and Molecular Biology, Heinrich Heine University, Düsseldorf, Germany
Nature 2009;458(7240):894–898

Background: Recently, a strong correlation between polymorphisms in the human FTO gene and body mass index was identified by several independent genome-wide association studies. Common risk variants in the first intron of this gene define a risk allele predisposing to obesity. Homozygous carriers of the risk allele were in average ~3 kg heavier and had a 1.67-fold increased risk of obesity then control persons. However, the functional impact of FTO in energy homeostasis remains elusive.

Methods: $Fto^{-/-}$ mice were generated by replacement of exons 2 and 3 of the *Fto* gene by a neomycin resistance cassette. The deletion success was verified by western blot and qRT-PCR analysis in different tissues. Given the suggested function of FTO in energy metabolism, $Fto^{-/-}$ mice and controls were analysed concerning their body composition, energy homeostasis and physical activity.

Results: The deletion of Fto in mice leads to a growth retardation 2 days after birth onwards and a reduction in lean and fat mass, despite decreased physical activity and relative hyperphagia. This leanless develops as a consequence of increased energy expenditure and systemic sympathetic activation.

Conclusion: This study provides data that Fto is a functional mediator of energy homeostasis by the control of energy expenditure.

This study provides functional data about the role of *Fto* (fat mass and obesity associated) in energy metabolism of mice. This is important since its functional relevance in metabolism is unclear. Common gene variants in the first intron of this gene have recently been found by genome wide analyses to be associated with traits of obesity. Fischer et al. generated mice lacking this gene and compared them with wildtype and heterozygous (*Fto*^{+/−}) mice. *Fto*^{−/−} mice did not differ in body weight during embryonic development, but growth retardation became apparent at postnatal day 2 and remains stable throughout the entire lifespan of these mice. After six weeks, the body weight between homozygous and wt mice differed by approximately 30–40%, whereas heterozygous mice did not show any significant weight reduction. This reduction in weight was associated with a significant loss of white adipose tissue, with nearly complete loss after 15 months. Interestingly, this reduction in weight and fat was not due to a lower food intake of the mutants. In fact, these mice ate more in proportion to their body weight compared to wildtype animals. Moreover, both groups of mutant mice gained less weight on a high fat diet. Instead, *Fto*^{−/−} mice show an increased energy expenditure, while their physical activity was decreased. The authors conclude that the increase in energy expenditure was due to a higher activity of the sympathetic system, shown by enhanced levels of adrenaline and noradrenaline. The authors suggest that *FTO* risk alleles might lead to an altered expression of FTO resulting in a higher individual susceptibility to obesity. It would be interesting to identify the molecular pathways by which FTO influences the sympathetic system. Additionally, tissue-specific knock-outs in areas which are relevant to energy homeostasis and metabolism are needed. The sympathetic system might turn out as as a substantial mediator for the action of FTO.

Adipose tissue revisited
Strong evidence for fat cell turnover in white adipose tissue: target for pharmaceutical intervention?

Dynamics of fat cell turnover in humans

Spalding KL, Arner E, Westermark PO, Bernard S, Buchholz BA, Bergmann O, Blomqvist L, Hoffstedt J, Naslund E, Britton T, Concha H, Hassan M, Ryden M, Frisen J, Arner P
Department of Cell and Molecular Biology, Karolinska Institutet, Stockholm, Sweden
kirsty.spalding@ki.se
Nature 2008;453:783–787

Background: Obesity together with its enhanced risk of cardiovascular diseases and metabolic disorders like type 2 diabetes is increasing in an epidemic manner. The size of the adipose tissue mass is determined by the number of fat cells as well as their volume. The increased lipid storage in already existing adipocytes is thought to be the most important mechanism by which the fat mass expands during obesity.

Methods: The authors combined previously observed data concerning the number of adipocytes in children and adolescents with data about the number of adipocytes from lean and obese adults before and after a major weight loss. Additionally, they measured the adipocyte turnover rate in lean and obese adults by analyzing the integration of atmospheric ^{14}C derived from nuclear bomb tests during the cold war into the genomic DNA of fat cells via accelerator mass spectrometry.

Results: The major results of this paper are that the number of adipocytes is set during childhood and shows only slight variations during adulthood. Even after a significant weight loss the authors could only detect a decreased adipocyte volume but no changes in the number of adipocytes. They observed, however, a remarkable turnover rate of the adipocytes. Approximately 10% of fat cells were renewed annually at all adult ages and levels of body fat index. Neither death rate nor the generation of new adipocytes was altered in early onset obesity, suggesting a tight regulation of fat cell number in this condition during adulthood.

Conclusion: The high adipocyte turnover offers a new target towards pharmacological therapy of obesity and it will be important to identify the molecular feedback mechanisms controlling adipocyte turnover.

To date the knowledge about adipocyte cell turnover in humans is very restricted. In animal experiments incorporation of labelled nucleotides can be used to study cell turnover but due to its potential toxicity it is not possible to perform this method in humans. In this study, the authors came up with a clever solution by utilizing the rapid increase in atmospheric ^{14}C levels which resulted from nuclear bomb tests during 1955–1963. In 1963 the ban of these nuclear tests resulted in a drop in atmospheric ^{14}C to the levels before the cold war. Once the ^{14}C is integrated into the genomic DNA of an adipocyte, it remains until the cell dies and degrades its DNA. Monitoring ^{14}C incorporation, the authors were able to date the generation of the adipocytes in adipose tissue of humans who grew up during the time of decreasing atmospheric ^{14}C levels.

It was previously shown that obesity is associated with an increased infiltration of macrophages into the adipose tissue which indicates an elevated death rate of adipocytes [7]. In contrast, Spalding et al. could not observe differences between cell death rates in lean and obese patients. One explanation may be the small sample size of 13 lean and 14 obese subjects. However, there is a trend toward increased death rate and decreased age of the adipocytes in obese subjects. The finding that there is a pool of early committed white adipocyte precursors in the mural cell compartment of the adipose vasculature [8] supports the idea of a constant turnover of adipocytes during lifespan and supplies a putative source for the new adipocytes. Thus, unlike previous contention, new fat cells are continually being born to replace their dead predecessors. The average age of a fat cell seems to be about 10 years in both lean and obese individuals, and the number of fat cells as a proportion of all cells remains constant in each weight group. But the total number of new fat cells was higher in obese subjects, suggesting that they are replenishing an existing larger pool. In summary, this paper offers a new possible pharmacological target for treating obesity, therefore emphasizing the high impact of research on the molecular mechanisms underlying this adipocyte turnover.

White fat progenitor cells reside in the adipose vasculature

Tang W, Zeve D, Suh JM, Bosnakovski D, Kyba M, Hammer RE, Tallquist MD, Graff JM
Department of Developmental Biology, University of Texas Southwestern Medical Center, Dallas, Tex., USA
Science 2008;322:583–586

Background: Adipocytes form throughout life, with the most marked expansion of the lineage occurring during the postnatal period. Endogenous adipocyte progenitors probably reside in the adipose stromal-vascular fraction (SVF), a heterogeneous mixture of cells. Peroxisome proliferator-activated receptor γ(PPARγ), a central regulator of fat formation, is necessary and sufficient for adipogenesis. Thus, marking PPARγ-expressing cells in vivo might provide insight into adipose lineage specification.
Methods: The authors generated PPARγ-reporter strains to isolate proliferating and renewing adipogenic progenitors. PPARγ-GFP-positive cells were localized to the vasculature, and their adipogenic potential was observed.
Results: The SV compartment of adipose depots contained PPARγ-expressing cells which behaved as an amplifying population and contributed to the adipocyte lineage. These progenitors were already committed, either prenatally or early in postnatal life and resided in the mural cell compartment of the adipose vasculature, but not in the vasculature of other tissues. They were phenotypically distinct from adipocytes and other SV cells and had a unique molecular signature. The precursors were adipogenic and also expressed mural cell markers.
Conclusion: A population of early committed white adipocyte precursors appears to be mural cells that reside in the vasculature of adipose tissue. Thus, the adipose vasculature might function as a progenitor niche providing signals for adipocyte development.

Although adipocytes are postmitotic, white adipose tissue mass retains the ability to expand throughout adult life by an increase in adipocyte number [9]. Recent studies suggest that approximately 10% of the body's fat cells are regenerated each year [10]. Nevertheless, there is only limited knowledge on the identity and localization of adipocyte precursors in vivo. In the present publication, Tang et al. identified an adipogenic cell population expressing both PPARγ and mural markers. These proliferating progenitors were committed either prenatally or early in life and resided in the mural cell compartment of adipose vasculature. The authors conclude that the adipose vasculature appears to function as a progenitor niche and may provide signals for adipocyte development. Their data support the previous finding of preadipocytes existing in the adipose vasculature [11] and contradict the classical idea that adipocyte formation occurs later during development.

Identification and importance of brown adipose tissue in adult humans

Cypess AM, Lehman S, Williams G, Tal I, Rodman D, Goldfine AB, Kuo FC, Palmer EL, Tseng YH, Doria A, Kolodny GM, Kahn CR
Research Division, Joslin Diabetes Center, Boston, Mass., USA
N Engl J Med 2009;360:1509–1517

Background: While brown adipose tissue (BAT) is known to regulate energy expenditure in rodents, it was regarded to have no physiologic relevance in adult humans.
Methods: 1,972 patients were analyzed by ^{18}F-fluorodeoxyglucose (^{18}F-FDG) positron-emission tomographic and computed tomographic (PET-CT) scans in order to identify BAT. PET-CT data were related to clinical data. UCP-1 immunohistochemistry was performed on biopsy specimens from putative BAT depots.
Results: By PET-CT, remarkable depots of BATe depots were identified in regions from the neck to the thorax. Females had a 2-fold higher mass of BAT and higher ^{18}F-FDG uptake activity. BAT was inversely correlated to body mass index.
Conclusion: Substantial amounts of BAT were identified in adult humans. An inverse correlation of the amount of BAT with BMI suggests a potential role of BAT in human metabolism.

Functional brown adipose tissue in healthy adults

Virtanen KA, Lidell ME, Orava J, Heglind M, Westergren R, Niemi T, Taittonen M, Laine J, Savisto NJ, Enerback S, Nuutila P
Turku PET Center, University of Turku, Turku, Finland
N Engl J Med 2009;360:1518–1525

Background: While BAT helps maintain normal body temperature in newborn infants, it was considered to have no physiologic relevance in adults.
Methods: 5 healthy subjects underwent ^{18}F-fluorodeoxyglucose (^{18}F-FDG) positron-emission tomographic and computed tomographic (PET-CT) scans during cold exposure or during warm temperature. BAT tissue samples were subjected to immunohistochemistry and quantitative RT-PCR using primers specific for BAT marker genes.
Results: Cold-induced glucose uptake was increased by a factor of 15 in supraclavicular BAT in all 5 patients compared to an increase by a factor of 4 in white adipose tissue. Expression of BAT markers such as UCP-1 and DIO2 (deiodonase, iodothyronine, type 2) was demonstrated in BAT specimens.
Conclusion: BAT is present in adult humans.

Cold-activated brown adipose tissue in healthy men

van Marken Lichtenbelt WD, Vanhommerig JW, Smulders NM, Drossaerts JM, Kemerink GJ, Bouvy ND, Schrauwen P, Teule GJ
Department of Human Biology, Nutrition and Toxicology Research Institute Maastricht, The Netherlands
markenlichtenbelt@hb.unimaas.nl
N Engl J Med 2009;360:1500–1508

Background: Studies in animals indicate that BAT is important for the regulation of body weight.
Methods: 24 healthy men (10 lean, BMI <25,and 14 overweight, BMI >25) were studied under thermoneutral conditions (22°C) or during mild cold exposure (16°C). BAT was determined by ^{18}F-fluorodeoxyglucose (^{18}F-FDG) positron-emission tomographic and computed tomographic (PET-CT) scan. Body composition and energy expenditure were measured by dual-energy X-ray absorptiometry and indirect calorimetry.
Results: During cold exposure, BAT activity was found in 23 subjects. The activity was lower in overweight compared to lean subjects. The percent of body fat and BMI were negatively correlated with BAT, while the resting metabolic rate had a positive correlation.
Conclusion: BAT is present in adult humans. Its activity is reduced with overweight or obesity.

¹⁸F-FDG PET-CT measures uptake of ^{18}F-labelled deoxyglucose into metabolically active tissues and is usually used in the diagnosis of neoplasms and their metastases. PET-CT radiologists knew of a bizarre dark knots and stripes along the neck and paraspinally that occur more frequently when their patients were exposed to excessive air-conditioning, but we only now understand that these represent BAT. The 3 above-mentioned studies used this method to identify metabolically highly active BAT depots.

The common message from these studies is that BAT is present and active in adult humans, and its presence and activity are inversely associated with obesity and indexes of the metabolic syndrome.

The major shortcoming of these studies is the lack of a direct correlation between cold-stimulated changes in energy expenditure and BAT activity. This could be secondary to the inability of the PET-CT technique to measure the activity of small nests of BAT.

However, these studies point to a potential 'natural' intervention to trigger energy expenditure by turning down the heat and burning calories.

This conclusion is certainly an oversimplification. Nonetheless, BAT provides a target for pharmacologic and environmental interventions, aimed at modulating energy expenditure.

A new weapon in the fight against obesity and diabetes: SIRT1 activation

Specific SIRT1 activation mimics low energy levels and protects against diet-induced metabolic disorders by enhancing fat oxidation

Feige JN, Lagouge M, Canto C, Strehle A, Houten SM, Milne JC, Lambert PD, Mataki C, Elliott PJ, Auwerx J
Institut de Génétique et de Biologie Moléculaire et Cellulaire, CNRS/INSERM/Université Louis Pasteur, Illkirch, France
admin.auwerx@epfl.ch
Cell Metab 2008;8:347–358

Background: The NAD⁺-dependent deacetylase SIRT1 controls metabolic processes in response to low nutrient availability. New, selective activators of Sirt1 such as SRT1720 are currently tested for suitability as therapeutic agents for the treatment of metabolic disorders.
Methods: Male 7-week-old C57BL/6J mice were fed a standard or HF diet supplemented or not with SRT1720. Animals were phenotyped in terms of body weight, food intake, muscle, liver and adipose tissue function.
Results: SRT1720 administration robustly enhances endurance running performance and strongly protects from diet-induced obesity and insulin resistance by enhancing oxidative metabolism in skeletal muscle, liver, and brown adipose tissue. These metabolic effects of SRT1720 are mediated by the induction of a genetic network controlling fatty acid oxidation through a multifaceted mechanism that involves direct deacetylation of PGC-1α, FOXO1, and p53 and the indirect stimulation of AMPK signaling through a global metabolic adaptation mimicking low energy levels.
Conclusion: This study further validates SIRT1 as a target for the treatment of metabolic disorders and characterizes the mechanisms underlying the therapeutic potential of SIRT1 activation.

Calorie restriction has been shown to delay age-related diseases and to extend lifespan in numerous species including mammals. It has long been assumed that the extension of life span by calorie restriction is mediated in a passive way by lowering oxidative stress, DNA damage and apoptosis. Ongoing studies now show that the response to calorie restriction is a highly regulated process and SIRT1 has been identified as the key molecular player. One natural activator of Sirt1, the polyphenolic substance resveratrol, is found in grapes and red wine. Resveratrol came to our attention because it was linked to the so-called French paradox, which describes the fact that French people have a lower risk of developing cardiovascular disease compared to other Europeans. This finding was linked to the moderate consumption of red wine and to the substance resveratrol. Resveratrol has since been shown to limit diet-induced obesity, to increase energy efficiency and to prevent diabetes in mice.

Since resveratrol exerts versatile functions by activating several intracellular pathways, researchers have now developed small molecule drugs which are much more potent than resveratrol and specifically target Sirt1.

 Martin Wabitsch et al.

Preclinical studies with SIRT1 activators have demonstrated potential importance in multiple disease areas, including type 2 diabetes and related complications, mitochondrial disorders, cardiovascular disease, inflammation, neurodegenerative diseases, and cancer. Early clinical studies have demonstrated promising results in type 2 diabetes.

Weight loss maintenance – an everlasting challenge

Lifestyle intervention in obese children with variations in the melanocortin 4 receptor gene

Reinehr T, Hebebrand J, Friedel S, Toschke AM, Brumm H, Biebermann H, Hinney A
Department of Pediatric Nutrition Medicine, Vestische Hospital for Children and Adolescents Datteln, University of Witten/Herdecke, Datteln, Germany
T.Reinehr@kinderklinik-datteln.de
Obesity (Silver Spring) 2009;17:382–389

Background: The melanocortin 4 receptor (MC4R) is a critical regulator of energy homeostasis in men and mutations in the MC4R gene leading to reduced receptor function are assumed to have a major effect on body weight. Although functionally relevant mutations in the MC4R gene are reported to have a considerable prevalence in obese children and adolescents, little is known about the impact of these mutations on the effect of a lifestyle intervention program.

Methods: A cohort of 514 overweight children aged 5–16 years participating in a 1-year multidisciplinary lifestyle intervention program was screened for mutations in the MC4R gene. Children carrying a MC4R mutation leading to reduced receptor function (group A) were each matched with 5 subjects without MC4R mutations (group B). All study participants underwent comprehensive metabolic phenotyping.

Results: 16 children (3.1%) were identified with nonsynonymous mutations leading to reduced receptor function and 17 children (2.7%) with MC4R variations not leading to reduced receptor function. Nine of the total of 16 children of group A (56%) and 46 of the 80 children of group B (58%) started the intervention. Furthermore, 1 subject in group A and 5 subjects in group B dropped out of the intervention program. BMI z-score was reduced in both groups to a similar degree at the end of the 1-year intervention. In contrast, only children without MC4R mutations (group B) maintained the weight loss over a 1-year post-intervention follow-up period, whereas BMI z-score in carriers of MC4R mutations (group A) did not differ significantly from baseline after follow-up (intention to treat analysis). Children in groups A and B did not differ with regard to anthropometrical markers, hormone profile, or cardiovascular risk factors.

Conclusion: The study demonstrates that children affected by MC4R mutations can lose weight by multidisciplinary lifestyle intervention but seem to have difficulties in maintaining weight loss over short-term follow-up.

Since the cloning of the fourth member of the melanocortin receptor family [12] and the first descriptions of the clinical phenotype of severe obesity associated with mutations in its gene [13, 14], MC4R mutations have become one of the best investigated genetic causes of obesity. Reported prevalence rates of up to 5.8% for MC4R deficiency make these mutations potentially the most common form of monogenic obesity in humans. Even the existence of a 'MC4R syndrome' characterized amongst others by early onset obesity, increased linear growth, hyperphagia, and pronounced hyperinsulinemia has been proposed [15]. In their present study, Reinehr et al. add to the field of MC4R research important information on the impact of reduced MC4R function on the chances of success of an outpatient weight management program for affected individuals. En passant four novel MC4R mutations were identified and functionally characterized. The present study demonstrates that carriers of MC4R mutations can achieve significant weight loss under the conditions of an intensive outpatient lifestyle intervention program, but only 1 year after the end of intervention there was no detectable change of BMI z-score in the MC4R group compared to baseline, while non-mutated children sustained their degree of weight loss. Furthermore, Reinehr et al. were unable to identify clinical or laboratory markers pointing to MC4R mutations, therefore questioning – as do other authors – the idea of a 'MC4R syndrome'. In summary, the present study provides further data on the impact of MC4R mutations on weight status, and advocates MC4R mutation screening at least in obese children and adolescents with a strong family history of obesity, obese siblings or rapid weight gain after obesity interventions. Nonetheless, the key question of how to treat patients with a strong genetic predisposition for obesity remains unanswered.

Leptin reverses weight loss-induced changes in regional neural activity responses to visual food stimuli

Rosenbaum M, Sy M, Pavlovich K, Leibel RL, Hirsch J
Department of Pediatrics, Division of Molecular Genetics, Naomi Berrie Diabetes Center, Columbia University Medical Center/New York Presbyterian Medical Center, New York, NY, USA
mr475@columbia.edu
J Clin Invest 2008;118:2583–2591

Backround: Increased hunger and food intake during diet are critical problems in the clinical management of obesity. Therefore, physiological changes in neuronal activity regulating energy intake and expenditure during starvation/diet are of special interest.
Methods: Brain-region specific neural activity was examined by functional MRI in 6 obese subjects. Responses to food-related visual cues were assessed during states of normal weight and after stabilization at a 10% reduced body weight, while the patients received either injections of leptin or placebo.
Results: Weight loss-elicited changes in neural activity were partly reversible by leptin treatment. Specifically, weight loss-induced increases in neural activity-response in the brainstem, culmen, parahippocampal gyrus, inferior and middle frontal gyri, middle temporal gyrus and lingual gyrus were reversed by leptin, as were decreases in activity in the hypothalamus, cingulated gyrus and middle frontal gyrus.
Conclusion: Weight loss elicits changes in neuronal activity in areas known to be involved in the regulatory, emotional, and cognitive control of food intake. These changes were partly reversible by leptin, indicating that leptin levels might play an important role in increased feelings of hunger during diet.

The discovery of the anorectic hormone leptin [16] provoked an enthusiastic response worldwide in the hope of finally having found a medical treatment for obesity. The subsequent realization that obesity as such represents a state of leptin resistance and that leptin treatment seems to be effective only in rare states of leptin deficiency [17] was disillusioning. During diet, leptin levels are decreased and Rosenbaum et al. have shown before that restoration of leptin levels to pre-weight loss levels reverses several metabolic and behavioral changes induced by diet [18]. In this article they now show elegantly that this reversal in behavioral changes has a correlation with changes in neuronal activity, thereby highlighting the importance of specific brain areas in regulating energy homeostasis mediated by leptin. These findings overlap at least in part with changes seen by Farooqi et al. [19] in leptin-deficient children before and after treatment with leptin.

Intestinal gluconeogenesis is a key factor for early metabolic changes after gastric bypass but not after gastric lap-band in mice

Troy S, Soty M, Ribeiro L, Laval L, Migrenne S, Fioramonti X, Pillot B, Fauveau V, Aubert R, Viollet B, Foretz M, Leclerc J, Duchampt A, Zitoun C, Thorens B, Magnan C, Mithieux G, Andreelli F
Institut National de la Santé et de la Recherche Médicale, U695, Faculté de Médecine Xavier Bichat, Université Paris 7, Paris, France
Cell Metab 2008;8:201–211

Background: Gastric bypass surgery also has immediate metabolic benefits that precede any substantial weight loss. The aim of the present study was to compare early metabolic changes after gastric bypass versus gastric lap-band (GLB) in mice.

Martin Wabitsch et al.

Methods: Energy and glucose metabolism following two experimental bariatric surgical procedures were compared to sham-operated high-fat diet-induced obese C57Bl6 and RIPGLUT1 × GLUT2$^{-/-}$ mice. In the first procedure a restrictive GLB was positioned around the upper stomach to create a small proximal and large distal gastric pouch. Alternatively, the pyloric sphincter was ligatured, followed by an enterogastric anastomosis (EGA) allowing a bypass of the duodenum and proximal jejunum as a surrogate for Roux-en-Y gastric bypass (RYGB). Food intake, body weight and composition as well as metabolic effects of bariatric surgery in mice were assessed.

Results: Food intake was significantly decreased in EGA mice, while the body fat loss was similar compared to sham-control and GLB mice. In addition, insulin sensitivity and intestinal gluconeogenesis increased after the EGA procedure independent of the GLP-1 action, but not after gastric banding (GLB). All EGA effects could be blocked in GLUT-2 knockout mice and in mice with portal vein denervation.

Conclusion: This study provides evidence that the beneficial effects of the EGA procedure on food intake and glucose homeostasis involve intestinal gluconeogenesis and its detection via a GLUT-2 and hepato-portal sensor pathway.

Bariatric bypass surgery is an increasingly popular treatment option for obese patients, and adolescents are being operated more frequently than ever before. It has traditionally been assumed that bariatric operations cause weight loss through gastric restriction, intestinal malabsorption, or both. Long-term total mortality especially from diabetes, heart disease and cancer was significantly reduced after gastric bypass surgery. Unexpectedly, the typical RYGB procedure seems to have the potential to also reduce type 2 diabetes mellitus even in patients without obesity. Although there is growing interest in using RYGB, the mechanisms mediating the metabolic effects of this procedure remain poorly understood. Potential mechanisms underlying the direct anti-diabetes effects of RYGB include enhanced nutrient stimulation of lower intestinal hormones (e.g. glucagon-like peptide-1), altered physiology from excluding ingested nutrients from the upper intestine, compromised ghrelin secretion, modulation of intestinal nutrient sensing and regulation of insulin sensitivity. The mechanistic model by Troy et al. using a gastric bypass model in mice proposes that glucose produced by defined intestinal segments is secreted directly into the portal vein where changes in blood glucose are detected by sensory fibers presumably projecting to central nervous system circuits controlling food intake, insulin secretion and nutrient partitioning. Elucidating the physiologic mechanisms underlying these surgical procedures should be an important research priority and might lead to new pharmaceuticals that would obviate the need for surgery.

Food for thought

Adenotonsillectomy and the development of overweight

Wijga AH, Scholtens S, Wieringa MH, Kerkhof M, Gerritsen J, Brunekreef B, Smit HA
National Institute for Public Health and the Environment, Centre for Prevention and Health Services Research, Bilthoven, The Netherlands
alet.wijga@rivm.nl
Pediatrics 2009;123:1095–1101

Background: Although some studies have shown that after adenotonsillectomy in childhood weight gain was accelerated, this finding has not been considered as a risk factor for overweight and obesity in children yet. The aim of this study was to investigate the association between adenotonsillectomy and the subsequent development of overweight in the general population.

Methods: The study sample included 3,963 children enrolled in the Dutch Prevention and Incidence of Asthma and Mite Allergy birth cohort. Annual questionnaires completed by the parents provided data on weight and height as well as on covariate factors known to influence weight development. Weight and height at 8 years of age has been measured.

Results: Undergoing adenotonsillectomy from birth to age 7 was significantly associated with overweight and obesity at 8 years of age. Being overweight at 2 years of age did not predict an increased risk of adenotonsillectomy at older ages.

Conclusion: These longitudinal data on weight and height in the years before and after surgery suggest that adenotonsillectomy form a turning point between a period of growth faltering and a period of catch-up growth, which might explain the increased risk of developing overweight after the operation.

Limitations of this study include loss to follow-up for the medical examination where weight and height were measured and that most data were parentally reported.
The cumulative incidence of adenotonsillectomy up to age 8 years was 12%, for adenotonsillectomy it was 15%. These numbers are rather high compared to the incidences in other countries.
Children who underwent the operation had a higher prevalence of low maternal education, maternal overweight, smoking, and no breastfeeding. After controlling for these factors, the authors concluded that operations were independently associated with the risk for overweight and obesity at age 8 years.

Growth and growth biomarker changes after adenotonsillectomy: systematic review and meta-analysis

Bonuck KA, Freeman K, Henderson J
Department of Family and Social Medicine, Albert Einstein College of Medicine, Mazer, Bronx, N.Y., USA
bonuck@montefiore.org

Arch Dis Child 2009;94:83–91

Background: It is well established that sleep disordered breathing in children secondary to adenotonsillar hypertrophy is a risk factor for growth failure. Adenotonsillectomy itself is associated with increases in height, IGF-1 and/or IGFBP-3 and interestingly also in weight. So far only small cohorts including less than 100 children were not able to strengthen the hypothesis of a causal relationship.
Methods: This is a systematic review and meta-analysis including studies from 1980 to 2007 for anthropometrics, the meta-analysis included studies presenting z scores or percentiles.
Results: Twenty of 211 studies met the review criteria. The meta-analysis found significant increases in weight and height z-scores, and IGF-1 and IGFBP-3 serum levels after adenotonsillectomy.
Conclusion: The findings suggest that primary care providers and specialists should consider sleep disordered breathing secondary to adenotonsillar hypertrophy when screening, treating and referring children with growth failure. Adenotonsillectomy might be followed by excessive weight gain and the development of overweight.

It is established that sleep disordered breathing which is characterized by snoring, mouth breathing and obstructive sleep apnea, is a risk factor for growth failure. Adenotonsillar hypertrophy is the primary factor associated with sleep disordered breathing in children.
Several possible mechanisms might explain a relationship between sleep disordered breathing and growth failure. Sleep disordered breathing interrupts slow-wave sleep, when growth hormone is preferentially secreted. Impaired growth hormone secretion results in decreased IGF-1 and/or IGFBP-3 levels. Sleep disordered breathing can also lead to growth failure by the associated increases energy expenditure during sleep and the reduced appetite induced by pharyngeal dysphagia associated with adenotonsillar hypertrophy. Sleep disordered breathing is also associated with increased motor activity during the day which might lead to an increased total energy expenditure.
After adenotonsillectomy these alterations are normalized. The meta-analysis for differences in before and after weight, which was based on 11 studies enrolling a total of 390 children, showed that the operation favored weight increases in addition to resulting in an increased height velocity and increases in IGF-1 and IGFBP-3 serum concentrations.
This review focused on longitudinal growth and growth biomarker changes after adenotonsillectomy. However, it also evaluated the changes in weight.
These results of clinical studies open an interesting field of research involving sleep disordered breathing and the regulation of longitudinal growth, appetite, and energy homeostasis.

Clinical review: treatment of pediatric obesity: a systematic review and meta-analysis of randomized trials

McGovern L, Johnson JN, Paulo R, Hettinger A, Singhal V, Kamath C, Erwin PJ, Montori VM
Department of Pediatrics, Mayo Clinic, Rochester, Minn., USA
J Clin Endocrinol Metab 2008;93:4600–4605

Background: The Endocrine Society decided to formulate clinical practice guidelines for the management of pediatric obesity. In doing so, it formed a task force to develop these recommendations.
Methods: In a first step a systematic review of the literature on the treatment of pediatric obesity was conducted. Literature was searched until February 2006. Eligible studies were randomized trials of overweight children and adolescents assessing the effect of nonsurgical interventions on obesity outcomes.
Results: Short-term medications were effective as demonstrated for sibutramine and orlistat. In addition studies focusing on an increase in physical activity also showed moderate effects on the reduction of percent body fat only. Combined lifestyle interventions led to small changes in BMI.
Conclusions: This report briefly summarizes the findings of a systematic review and a meta-analysis of randomized trials. It can be concluded that medications and combined lifestyle interventions show short-term efficacy with small changes in overweight. The long-term efficacy and safety of such treatment programs is unclear.

Clinical review: behavioral interventions to prevent childhood obesity: a systematic review and metaanalyses of randomized trials

Kamath CC, Vickers KS, Ehrlich A, McGovern L, Johnson J, Singhal V, Paulo R, Hettinger A, Erwin PJ, Montori VM
Knowledge and Encounter Research Unit, Mayo Clinic, Rochester, Minn., USA
J Clin Endocrinol Metab 2008;93:4606–4615

Background: Experts have implicated both physical activity and dietary behavior in the causal path of obesity. Consequently targeting these lifestyle behaviors have been the aims of studies to prevent childhood obesity. However, the efficacy of such programs to prevent pediatric obesity remain unclear so far.
Methods: A literature search was performed until February 2006. Eligible studies were randomized trials assessing the impact of interventions on both lifestyle behaviors and body mass index (BMI).
Results: The available randomized controlled trials to prevent pediatric obesity showed that small changes in their respective target behavior can be achieved. However, this is not associated with significant changes in BMI compared with controls. Further exploration through hypothesis-generating subgroup analysis found: (1) there was no sex-treatment interaction; (2) trials in children found larger reductions in sedentary activity than trials in adolescents; (3) trials of treatments for >6 months found larger reductions in sedentary activity and BMI than shorter trials, and (4) no significant interaction was found between interventional components and their effect on target behaviors or BMI compared with controls.
Conclusion: Obesity prevention programs may cause small changes in target behaviors but no significant effect on BMI compared with controls.

Prevention and treatment of pediatric obesity: an endocrine society clinical practice guideline based on expert opinion

August GP, Caprio S, Fennoy I, Freemark M, Kaufman FR, Lustig RH, Silverstein JH, Speiser PW, Styne DM, Montori VM
George Washington University School of Medicine, Washington, D.C., USA
J Clin Endocrinol Metab 2008;93:4576–4599

Background: The Clinical Guideline Subcommittee of the Endocrine Society identified pediatric obesity as a priority area requiring practice guidelines and appointed a task force to formulate evidence-based recommendations.

Methods: The task force uses systematic reviews of available evidence to give key recommendations. The Grading of Recommendations Assessment, Development, and Evaluation (GRADE) method was applied.

Results: Each recommendation given is followed by a description of the evidence, the values that panelists considered in making the recommendation, and in some instances remarks with technical comments or caveats.

Conclusion: These recommendations are very helpful for practitioners treating obese children and for people of the public health system involved in prevention programs for pediatric obesity.

Interventions for treating obesity in children (review)

Oude Luttikhuis H, Baur L, Jansen H, Shrewsbury VA, O'Malley C, Stolk RP, Summerbell CD
Beatrix Children'S Hospital and Department of Epidemiology; University Medical Center Groningen, The Netherlands
h.oudeluttikhuis@bkk.umcg.nl

Cochrane Database Syst Rev 2009;1:CD001872. DOI: 10.1002/14651858.CD001872.pub2

Background: More information is needed about the best way to treat obesity in children and adolescents.

Methods: A literature research was performed (1985 to May 2008). Defined selection criteria were applied.

Results: 64 studies were included (54 studies on lifestyle treatments and 10 studies on drug treatments). No surgical treatment studies were suitable to include in this review. The analysis of study data showed that lifestyle programs can slightly reduce the level of overweight 6 and 12 months after the beginning of the program. There is an additional effect of orlistat and sibutramine, although a range of adverse effects was also noted. There are not sufficient data on the long-term outcome of such treatment programs.

Conclusion: Combined behavioral lifestyle intervention compared to standard care or self help can produce significant and clinical meaningful reduction in overweight in children and adolescents during the first months.

Huge efforts have been made to review and analyze the available results from studies investigating the effect of treatment programs and prevention programs on childhood overweight and obesity. It is a valuable result of all the above-mentioned reviews that these data have been put together and the main outcomes are now easily available for practitioners and scientists in the field.

However, it has to be concluded that so far all efforts comprising intensive multi-professional long-term (up to 12 months) care result only in modest reductions in overweight. In addition the effective programs are only available for a minority of the children and the large majority of obese children and adolescents is not able to enter in such programs due to lack of motivation and social, familial, or financial support.

Therefore new ways have to be found to tackle the problem of childhood obesity probably with an emphasis on public health measures aiming at changing the living environment of these children.

References

1. Frayling TM, Timpson NJ, Weedon MN, Zeggini E, Freathy RM, Lindgren CM, Perry JR, Elliott KS, Lango H, Rayner NW, Shields B, Harries LW, Barrett JC, Ellard S, Groves CJ, Knight B, Patch AM, Ness AR, Ebrahim S, Lawlor DA, Ring SM, Ben-Shlomo Y, Jarvelin MR, Sovio U, Bennett AJ, Melzer D, Ferrucci L, Loos RJ, Barroso I, Wareham NJ, Karpe F, Owen KR, Cardon LR, Walker M, Hitman GA, Palmer CN, Doney AS, Morris AD, Smith GD, Hattersley AT, McCarthy MI: A common variant in the FTO gene is associated with body mass index and predisposes to childhood and adult obesity. Science 2007;316:889–894.

2. Renstrom F, Payne F, Nordstrom A, Brito EC, Rolandsson O, Hallmans G, Barroso I, Nordstrom P, Franks PW: Replication and extension of genome-wide association study results for obesity in 4923 adults from northern Sweden. Hum Mol Genet 2009;18:1489–1496.

3. Thorleifsson G, Walters GB, Gudbjartsson DF, Steinthorsdottir V, Sulem P, Helgadottir A, Styrkarsdottir U, Gretarsdottir S, Thorlacius S, Jonsdottir I, Jonsdottir T, Olafsdottir EJ, Olafsdottir GH, Jonsson T, Jonsson F, Borch-Johnsen K, Hansen T, Andersen G, Jorgensen T, Lauritzen T, Aben KK, Verbeek AL, Roeleveld N, Kampman E, Yanek LR, Becker LC, Tryggvadottir L, Rafnar T, Becker DM, Gulcher J, Kiemeney LA, Pedersen O, Kong A, Thorsteinsdottir U, Stefansson K: Genome-wide association yields new sequence variants at seven loci that associate with measures of obesity. Nat Genet 2009;41:18–24.

4. van Hoek M, Dehghan A, Witteman JC, van Duijn CM, Uitterlinden AG, Oostra BA, Hofman A, Sijbrands EJ, Janssens AC: Predicting type 2 diabetes based on polymorphisms from genome-wide association studies: a population-based study. Diabetes 2008;57:3122–3128.

5. Ng MC, Park KS, Oh B, Tam CH, Cho YM, Shin HD, Lam VK, Ma RC, So WY, Cho YS, Kim HL, Lee HK, Chan JC, Cho NH: Implication of genetic variants near TCF7L2, SLC30A8, HHEX, CDKAL1, CDKN2A/B, IGF2BP2, and FTO in type 2 diabetes and obesity in 6,719 Asians. Diabetes 2008;57:2226–2233.

6. Stratigopoulos G, Padilla SL, LeDuc CA, Watson E, Hattersley AT, McCarthy MI, Zeltser LM, Chung WK, Leibel RL: Regulation of Fto/Ftm gene expression in mice and humans. Am J Physiol Regul Integr Comp Physiol 2008;294:R1185–R1196.

7. Weisberg SP, McCann D, Desai M, Rosenbaum M, Leibel RL, Ferrante AW Jr: Obesity is associated with macrophage accumulation in adipose tissue. J Clin Invest 2003;112:1796–1808.

8. Tang W, Zeve D, Suh JM, Bosnakovski D, Kyba M, Hammer RE, Tallquist MD, Graff JM: White fat progenitor cells reside in the adipose vasculature. Science 2008;322:583–586.

9. Prins JB, O'Rahilly S: Regulation of adipose cell number in man. Clin Sci (Lond) 1997;92:3–11.

10. Spalding KL, Arner E, Westermark PO, Bernard S, Buchholz BA, Bergmann O, Blomqvist L, Hoffstedt J, Näslund E, Britton T, Concha H, Hassan M, Rydén M, Frisén J, Arner P: Dynamics of fat cell turnover in humans. Nature 2008;453:783–787.

11. Sengenès C, Lolmède K, Zakaroff-Girard A, Busse R, Bouloumié A: Preadipocytes in the human subcutaneous adipose tissue display distinct features from the adult mesenchymal and hematopoietic stem cells. J Cell Physiol 2005;205:114–122.

12. Gantz I, Miwa H, Konda Y, Shimoto Y, Tashiro T, Watson SJ, DelValle J, Yamada T: Molecular cloning, expression, and gene localization of a fourth melanocortin receptor. J Biol Chem 1993;268:15174–15179.

13. Vaisse C, Clement K, Guy-Grand B, Froguel P: A frameshift mutation in human MC4R is associated with a dominant form of obesity. Nat Genet 1998;20:113–114.

14. Yeo GS, Farooqi IS, Aminian S, Halsall DJ, Stanhope RG, O'Rahilly S: A frameshift mutation in MC4R associated with dominantly inherited human obesity. Nat Genet 1998;20:111–112.

15. Farooqi IS, Keogh JM, Yeo GS, Lank EJ, Cheetham T, O'Rahilly S: Clinical spectrum of obesity and mutations in the melanocortin 4 receptor gene. N Engl J Med 2003;348:1085–1095.

16. Zhang Y, Proenca R, Maffei M, Barone M, Leopold L, Friedman JM: Positional cloning of the mouse obese gene and its human homologue. Nature 1994;372:425–432.

17. Heymsfield SB, Greenberg AS, Fujioka K, Dixon RM, Kushner R, Hunt T, Lubina JA, Patane J, Self B, Hunt P, McCamish M: Recombinant leptin for weight loss in obese and lean adults: a randomized, controlled, dose-escalation trial. JAMA 1999;282:1568–1575.

18. Rosenbaum M, Goldsmith R, Bloomfield D, Magnano A, Weimer L, Heymsfield S, Gallagher D, Mayer L, Murphy E, Leibel RL: Low-dose leptin reverses skeletal muscle, autonomic, and neuroendocrine adaptations to maintenance of reduced weight. J Clin Invest 2005;115:3579–3586.

19. Farooqi IS, Bullmore E, Keogh J, Gillard J, O'Rahilly S, Fletcher PC: Leptin regulates striatal regions and human eating behavior. Science 2007;317:1355.

Type 2 Diabetes, Metabolic Syndrome, Lipid Metabolism

Orit Pinhas-Hamiel

Pediatric Endocrine and Diabetes Unit, Safra Children's Hospital, Sheba Medical Center Ramat-Gan, and Juvenile Diabetes Center Maccabi Health Care Services, Tel-Aviv University Sackler School of Medicine, Tel-Aviv, Israel

The occurrence of type 2 diabetes (T2DM) in youth has been established and numerous reports about prevalence, incidence, and clinical characteristics of these adolescents are continuously documented from all over the world [1]. The highlights of this year's section include: population genetics studies shedding light on both susceptibility to develop T2DM and on novel disease mechanisms; new data on complications of T2DM in youth, and the outcome of a new treatment modality – bariatric surgery in adolescents with T2DM.

Several works have aimed to identify children and adolescents who are at increased risk of developing T2DM. The impact of intrauterine exposure to both maternal obesity and maternal diabetes and the impact of medications such as atypical antipsychotic drugs and valproic acid, on impaired glucose metabolism, the metabolic syndrome and T2DM are reviewed. In parallel the reliability of our diagnostic methods for impaired glucose metabolism in obese children is highlighted as well. In addition, evidence for the efficacy and side effects of various pharmacologic medications in obese children and in adolescents with polycystic ovary syndromes (PCOS) is reviewed. The last section reviews clinical practice recommendations for children with diabetes and dyslipidemia for children with elevated LDL cholesterol and with hypertriglyceridemia.

New mechanism: insights in the pathogenesis of impaired fasting glucose and T2DM

A variant near MTNR1B is associated with increased fasting plasma glucose levels and type 2 diabetes risk

Bouatia-Naji N, Bonnefond A, Cavalcanti-Proenca C, Sparsø T, Holmkvist J, Marchand M, Delplanque J, Lobbens S, Rocheleau G, Durand E, De Graeve F, Chevre JC, Borch-Johnsen K, Hartikainen AL, Ruokonen A, Tichet J, Marre M, Weill J, Heude B, Tauber M, Lemaire K, Schuit F, Elliott P, Jorgensen T, Charpentier G, Hadjadj S, Cauchi S, Vaxillaire M, Sladek R, Visvikis-Siest S, Balkau B, Levy-Marchal C, Pattou F, Meyre D, Blakemore AI, Jarvelin MR, Walley AJ, Hansen T, Dina C, Pedersen O, Froguel P
CNRS-UMR-8090, Institute of Biology and Lille 2 University, Pasteur Institute, Lille, France
Nat Genet 2009;41:89–94

Background: Genetic variation involved in glucose homeostasis may explain susceptibility to insulin resistance and T2DM.

Methods: A genome-wide association for fasting plasma glucose was done in 2,151 nondiabetic French subjects. The contribution of a single nucleotide polymorphism (SNP) to pancreatic β-cell function and diabetes was further studied in 16,094 Europeans.

Results: A SNP, rs1387153, on chromosome 11 was identified as a modulator of fasting plasma glucose. This SNP is located near to MTNR1B which encodes the melatonin receptor. In European populations (n = 16,094), the rs1387153 T allele was associated with increased fasting plasma glucose, T2DM and risk of developing hyperglycemia or diabetes over a 9-year period. RT-PCR analyses confirm the presence of MT2 transcripts in neural tissues and show MT2 expression in human pancreatic islets and β cells.

Conclusions: Data suggest a possible link between circadian rhythm regulation and glucose homeostasis through the melatonin signaling pathway.

G-allele of intronic rs10830963 in MTNR1B confers increased risk of impaired fasting glycemia and type 2 diabetes through an impaired glucose-stimulated insulin release: studies involving 19,605 Europeans

Sparsø T, Bonnefond A, Andersson E, Bouatia-Naji N, Holmkvist J, Wegner L, Grarup N, Gjesing AP, Banasik K, Cavalcanti-Proenca C, Marchand M, Vaxillaire M, Charpentier G, Jarvelin MR, Tichet J, Balkau B, Marre M, Levy-Marchal C, Faerch K, Borch-Johnsen K, Jorgensen T, Madsbad S, Poulsen P, Vaag A, Dina C, Hansen T, Pedersen O, Froguel P
Steno Diabetes Center, Gentofte, Denmark
tspr@steno.dk
Diabetes 2009;58:1450–1456

Background: rs10830963, a SNP, is an intronic variant in MTNR1B that showed the strongest signal to fasting plasma glucose using in silico studies.

Methods: Direct genotyping of rs10830963 was done in a large European descent population. The associations of this SNP were studied with isolated impaired fasting glycemia (i-IFG), isolated impaired glucose tolerance (i-IGT), T2DM and measures of insulin release and peripheral and hepatic insulin sensitivity.

Results: The MTNR1B intronic variant, rs10830963, carried most of the effect on FPG and showed the strongest association with FPG and T2D. Further analyses revealed that the rs10830963-G allele increased the risk of i-IFG but not i-IGT. It was associated with a decreased insulin release after oral and intravenous glucose challenges but not after injection of tolbutamide. In elderly twins it was associated to hepatic insulin resistance.

Conclusions: The G-allele of MTNR1B rs10830963 increases risk of T2DM through a state of i-IFG and not through i-IGT. The same allele associates with estimates of β-cell dysfunction and hepatic insulin resistance.

These two fascinating studies lighten the association between melatonin and impaired glucose metabolism.

Melatonin is a neurohormone that regulates the circadian rhythm by translating photoperiodic information from the eyes to the brain. Melatonin functions via two receptors: MT1 and MT2, encoded by MTNR1A and MTNR1B, respectively.

Bouatia-Naji and his colleagues confirmed the expression of MTNR1B in the retina, in the circadian rhythm control center in the brain and in pancreatic tissue, suggesting a role of melatonin in the regulation of insulin secretion. Indeed in healthy individuals, melatonin secretion peaks in the middle of the night, and gradually falls during the day in an opposite manner to insulin levels. Both melatonin secretion and circadian rhythm are impaired in T2DM.

In genome-wide association studies a SNP, rs1387153, was found to be in association with fasting plasma glucose among lean and obese adults and children, and was associated with an increased risk of T2DM. This SNP maps within a 62.1-kb linkage disequilibrium block on chromosome 11 and is located in the 5′ region of the gene encoding the melatonin receptor 1B. In the study by Sparsø et al., another SNP, rs10830963, located in the only intron of MTNR1B, was studied as the source of the association signal on fasting plasma glucose and T2DM in more than 11,300 individuals. The G-allele of rs10830963 was associated with increased risk of isolated IFG with the combined IFG and IGT phenotype as well as with overt T2DM but not with isolated IGT, suggesting that this SNP predisposes to T2DM via a state of impaired fasting but not through postprandial glucose levels. Decreased serum insulin levels post-OGTT and post-IVGTT suggest that carriers of the diabetogenic risk allele in MTNR1B may have pancreatic β-cell dysfunction.

Among both adults and children, sleep restriction increases the risk for obesity. Moreover, among adults, sleep duration significantly correlates with the metabolic syndrome and is an independent risk factor for T2DM [2].

Several biological mechanisms through which sleep duration may lead to diabetes have been suggested including elevated evening cortisol level, increase in sympathetic tone which has an inhibitory effect on pancreatic function, reduction in leptin. Now we learn about the role of melatonin in the regulation of glucose homeostasis. Stay tuned, this may open new therapeutic opportunities for T2DM.

     Orit Pinhas-Hamiel

Single nucleotide transcription factor 7-like 2 (TCF7L2) gene polymorphisms in anti-islet autoantibody-negative patients at onset of diabetes

Yu J, Steck AK, Babu S, Yu L, Miao D, McFann K, Hutton J, Eisenbarth GS, Klingensmith G
University of Colorado Health Sciences Center, Aurora, Colo., USA
jeesuk_yu@yahoo.com
J Clin Endocrinol Metab 2009;94:504–510

Background: Genetic variants within the transcription factor 7-like 2 (TCF7L2) gene were associated with the development of T2DM in adults from various ethnic groups. The aim of this study was to evaluate whether single nucleotide polymorphisms (SNPs) of transcription TCF7L2 gene are associated with the development of islet autoantibody-negative diabetes vs. islet autoantibody-positive diabetes in young patients and whether these SNPs are associated with specific clinical phenotypes.
Methods: Two noncoding variants in the TCF7L2 gene, rs12255372 and rs7903146, were genotyped in 893 subjects less than age 25 at the onset of diabetes and normal controls.
Results: A total of 140 patients (15.7%) were negative for all islet autoantibodies. The allele and genotype frequencies of two SNPs showed that these are associated (odds ratio up to 4) with the development of diabetes in the autoantibody-negative diabetic cohort, but not in the autoantibody-positive diabetic cohort.
Conclusions: TCF7L2 T2DM susceptibility alleles are associated with islet autoantibody-negative but not autoantibody-positive new onset diabetes in young patients.

TCF7L2 belongs to a subfamily of TCF7-like high-mobility group box-containing transcription factors and maps to chromosome 10q25. The TCF7L2 gene product is part of the Wnt signaling pathway. Emerging new evidence, recently reviewed [3], reveals that Wnt signaling influences endocrine pancreas development and modulates mature β-cell functions including insulin secretion, survival and proliferation. TCF7L2 also modulates adipogenesis and regulates GLP-1 production. Among adults, TCF7L2 genes are associated with the development of T2DM diabetes.

With the increasing incidence of childhood obesity it would be helpful to know who those at high risk of developing T2DM are. Moreover, in a child with new onset diabetes and overlapping diabetes phenotype, additional tools to define the type of diabetes are often needed. To date, diagnosis of T2DM has been by exclusion, mainly those with negative antibodies for type 1 diabetes mellitus (T1DM) are diagnosed with T2DM. The key finding of this study was that TCF7L2 CT/TT genotypes can help distinguish between young subjects autoantibody-positive and autoantibody-negative diabetes patients.

Important for clinical practice: at-risk groups for prediabetes and type 2 diabetes mellitus

Association of intrauterine exposure to maternal diabetes and obesity with type 2 diabetes in youth: the SEARCH case-control study

Dabelea D, Mayer-Davis EJ, Lamichhane AP, D'Agostino RB, Jr., Liese AD, Vehik KS, Narayan KM, Zeitler P, Hamman RF
Department of Preventive Medicine and Biometrics, University of Colorado Denver, Denver, Colo., USA
dana.dabelea@uchsc.edu
Diabetes Care 2008;31:1422–1426

Background: The association between in utero exposure to maternal diabetes and obesity and T2DM in diverse youths was studied.
Methods: In the SEARCH case-control study, 79 youths with T2DM and 190 nondiabetic control youths aged 10–22 years were studied. In utero exposures to maternal diabetes and obesity were recalled by biological mothers.

Results: Youths with T2DM were more likely to have been exposed to maternal diabetes or obesity in utero than were nondiabetic control youths (p < 0.0001 for each). Exposure to maternal diabetes led to a 5.7-fold increase and exposure to maternal obesity to a 2.8-fold increased risk to T2DM in the offspring after adjusting for offspring age, sex, and race/ethnicity. Adjustment for other perinatal and socioeconomic factors did not alter these associations. When offspring BMI was added, the OR for the association between in utero exposure to obesity and T2DM was attenuated toward the null (OR 1.1 [0.5–2.4]). Overall, of T2DM in youths could be attributed to intrauterine exposure to maternal diabetes and obesity.

Conclusions: Intrauterine exposures to maternal diabetes and obesity are strongly associated with T2DM in youth. Prevention efforts may need to target, in addition to childhood obesity, the increasing number of pregnancies complicated by obesity and diabetes

Association between maternal diabetes in utero and age at offspring's diagnosis of type 2 diabetes

Pettitt DJ, Lawrence JM, Beyer J, Hillier TA, Liese AD, Mayer-Davis B, Loots B, Imperatore G, Liu L, Dolan LM, Linder B, Dabelea D

Sansum Diabetes Research Institute, Santa Barbara, Calif., USA

dpettitt@sansum.org

Diabetes Care 2008;31:2126–2130

Background: The age of diabetes diagnosis in youths who have a parent with diabetes by diabetes type and timing of diagnosis of the parent's diabetes in relation to the youth's birth were studied.

Methods: The cohort comprised SEARCH for Diabetes in Youth Study participants with a diabetic parent.

Results: Youths with T2DM were more likely to have a parent with either type 1 or T2DM (mother 39.3%, father 21.2%) than youths with type 1 diabetes (5.3 and 6.7%, respectively, p < 0.001 for each). T2DM was diagnosed 1.68 years earlier among those exposed to diabetes in utero than among those whose mothers' diabetes was diagnosed later (p = 0.018, controlled for maternal diagnosis age, paternal diabetes, sex, and race/ethnicity). Age at diagnosis of type 1 diabetes for youths with and without in utero exposure did not differ significantly. Paternal age at diagnosis of diabetes and its relation to child's birth were not associated with age at diagnosis of offspring.

Conclusions: T2DM was diagnosed at younger ages among those exposed to hyperglycemia in utero. Among youths with type 1 diabetes, the effect of the intrauterine exposure was not significant when controlled for the mother's age of diagnosis.

It has been said before that 'The fathers have eaten sour grapes, and the children's teeth are set on edge' [Jeremiah Chapter 31(28)]. Increased maternal pre-pregnancy weight [4] and increased gestational weight gain are associated with increased risk of offspring obesity [5]. Maternal weight loss by bariatric surgery prevents transmission of obesity to children [6]. Using data from the SEARCH study, a multicenter survey of youths with diabetes diagnosed before age 20 years, we now learn that exposure to maternal obesity was also associated with a 2.8-fold risk for T2DM in adolescents and that exposure to maternal diabetes in utero was associated with a 5.7-fold risk for T2DM in adolescents. Moreover, in a study limited to diabetic youths, T2DM was diagnosed in younger ages in those exposed to diabetic intrauterine environment, whereas no difference was observed in subjects with type 1 diabetes.

These studied are specifically interesting in light of emerging data on epigenetics and obesity. Epigenetics refers to changes in gene expression that are not caused by changes in the underlying DNA sequence, but rather in other mechanisms. Yet these changes may remain through cell divisions and therefore are trans-generational. DNA methylation is one of the mechanisms that enables to either switched 'on or off' gene expression. During differentiation of the early embryo there are potential 'critical windows' when environment could affect methylation. Nutrition during early life can affect DNA methylation.

The Agouti viable yellow (A^{vy}) mouse is a model of genetic obesity. The A^{vy} mice are hyperphagic, obese with a yellow coat because the agouti protein impairs both the satiety mechanism at the melanocortin 4 receptor and pigmentation in hair follicles. In this mice model, it has been recently demonstrated that maternal obesity causes trans-generational amplification of body weight [7]. This trans-generational amplification of body weight can be prevented by a methyl-supplemented diet that induces DNA hypermethylation during pregnancy, suggesting epigenetic mechanisms involved in this process. Taken together, these data imply that assisting pregnant women to meet the recommended weight gain during pregnancy may be an important strategy for preventing pediatric obesity and T2DM.

Pre-teen insulin resistance predicts weight gain, impaired fasting glucose, and type 2 diabetes at age 18–19 years: a 10-year prospective study of black and white girls

Morrison JA, Glueck CJ, Horn PS, Schreiber GB, Wang P
Division of Cardiology, Cincinnati Children's Hospital Medical Center, Cincinnati, Ohio, USA
john.morrison@cchmc.org

Am J Clin Nutr 2008;88:778–788

Background: The roles of pre-teen insulin resistance and insulin in weight gain and the development of IFG and T2DM were assessed.

Methods: In a prospective cohort study, body habitus and fasting insulin and glucose were measured in girls aged 9–10 and 18–19 years. Multiple 3-D diet records were collected.

Results: At age 18–19 years there were 5 incident cases of T2DM, 37 cases of IFG, and 597 non-cases. Baseline insulin, HOMA-IR, IFG, the change in HOMA-IR during follow-up, and baseline insulin × total caloric intake interaction predicted IFG and T2DM at age 18–19 years. In multivariate analyses, the 10-year change in homeostatic model assessment of insulin resistance (HOMA-IR) and the age 9–10 years HOMA-IR × percentage of calories from fat interaction were positive predictors of 10-year changes in BMI.

Conclusions: Pre-teen IFG, insulin resistance (and insulin), and rapidly increasing insulin resistance during adolescence identifies girls who are at greater risk of future IFG and T2DM. In addition, insulin resistance, interacting with high-fat diets, identifies girls who are at risk of greater weight gain. These findings could open avenues to primary prevention of obesity, IFG, and T2DM in children.

The interactions of hyperinsulinemia and obesity are complex. Many scientists believe that this is a case of the 'chicken or the egg' – hyperinsulinemia contributes to obesity, but obesity in turn worsens insulin resistance, leading to IFG and T2DM.

In this 10-year tracking study, factors that may predict obesity, central obesity, IFG and T2DM were studied. Elevated insulin levels at age 9–10 years and HOMA-IR were found to have a central role in predicting future obesity and impaired glucose metabolism. Moreover, the interaction of poor dietary intake, i.e. increased intake of fat calories with hyperinsulinemia, further increases the ability to identify those children who are at risk.

The ability to predict upcoming health problems and to take preventive steps is a key point in health care. The findings of this study may help clinicians to identify young children with poor eating habits and hyperinsulinemia and treat them intensively to prevent future morbidity.

Parental diabetes, pubertal stage, and extreme obesity are the main risk factors for prediabetes in children and adolescents: a simple risk score to identify children at risk for prediabetes

Reinehr T, Wabitsch M, Kleber M, de Sousa G, Denzer C, Toschke AM
Department of Pediatric Nutrition Medicine, Vestische Hospital for Children and Adolescents, University of Witten/Herdecke, Datteln, Germany

Pediatr Diabetes 2008; Epub ahead of print

Background: Prediabetes is defined as impaired fasting glucose (IFG) or impaired glucose tolerance, and its prevalence parallels the increase of obesity. However, it is unclear who the children that should be screened for prediabetes are.

Methods: The authors studied 437 overweight children and adolescents to identify risk factors for prediabetes. A risk score for prediabetes was calculated and examined in a second, independent cohort of 567 overweight youths. History of T2DM in parents and grandparents, degree of overweight, age, pubertal stage, birth weight, hypertension, dyslipidemia, acanthosis nigricans, and abdominal obesity were considered as potential risk factors.

Results: The frequency of prediabetes was 6% in the first cohort and 17% in the second one. The strongest association was observed for history of parental diabetes with a 6.3- to 9.5-fold risk, followed by pubertal stage with a 5.5- to 6.2-fold risk and by extreme obesity with a 3.3- to 5.0-fold increased risk.

Conclusions: The main risk factors for prediabetes were parental diabetes, pubertal stage, and extreme obesity. Screening for prediabetes seems meaningful in subjects with either a parental history of T2DM or a combination of extreme obesity and pubertal stage and detected nearly 90% of the overweight children and adolescents with prediabetes.

According to recent data in 2003–2006 [8], 16.3% of children and adolescents aged 2–19 years were at or above the 95th percentile, and 31.9% were at or above the 85th percentile. In light of the increasing rates of obesity it is clear that strict criteria for those who need to be screened are necessary to separate the wheat from the chaff. The authors aimed to identify risk factor for prediabetes in overweight children and adolescents. In this study, overweight was defined as BMI above the 90th percentile, obesity as BMI above the 97th percentile and extreme obesity as BMI above the 99.5 percentile. Interestingly, potential predictors such as diabetes in grandparents, gender, birth weight, hypertension, dyslipidemia, acanthosis nigricans, and abdominal obesity were not significantly associated to prediabetes. The authors developed a risk score for OGTT of at least 2 points where parental diabetes scores 2 points, positive puberty scores 1 point, and extreme obesity score 1 point. This risk score had a sensitivity of 90%. These findings need to be studied in other ethnic populations, but it seems reasonable to screen only those with extreme obesity rather than those with overweight and to exclude history in grandparents. Another particularly high-risk population to target for screening recently described is overweight siblings of children diagnosed with T2DM. Siblings had 4 times greater odds of having abnormal glucose tolerance compared with other overweight children [9].

New concerns: reliability of our screening tools

Reproducibility of the oral glucose tolerance test in overweight children

Libman IM, Barinas-Mitchell E, Bartucci A, Robertson R, Arslanian S
Children's Hospital of Pittsburgh, and Department of Epidemiology, Graduate School of Public Health, Center for Exercise and Health-Fitness Research, University of Pittsburgh, Pittsburgh, Pa., USA
ingrid.libman@chp.edu
J Clin Endocrinol Metab 2008;93:4231–4237

Background: The oral glucose tolerance test (OGTT) is used to test for diabetes, insulin resistance and the metabolic syndrome. The reproducibility of the test in overweight children was evaluated.

Methods: 60 overweight youths aged 8–17 years completed 2 OGTTs with an interval time between tests of 1–25 days. Insulin sensitivity was assessed by additional surrogate measures.

Results: Of the 10 subjects with impaired glucose tolerance (IGT) during the first test, only 3 (30%) had abnormal results during the second test. The percent positive agreement between the first and second OGTT was low for both impaired fasting glucose and IGT (22.2 and 27.3%, respectively). Fasting blood glucose had higher reproducibility compared with the 2-hour glucose. Obese youths with discordant OGTT results are more insulin-resistant.

Conclusions: These data show poor reproducibility of the OGTT in obese youths, in particular for the 2-hour plasma glucose.

Treating obesity is often futile, and in adolescents may carry the risk of developing eating disorders. Therefore, pediatricians need to select those patients who are at high risk for secondary morbidity of obesity. The metabolic syndrome is a cluster of physiologic markers including obesity, insulin resistance, dyslipidemia, and hypertension. The importance of the diagnosis of the metabolic syndrome is that it helps to identify those individuals at risk of developing diabetes and cardiovascular disease.

The definition established by the World Health Organization (WHO) diabetes group includes insulin resistance or its surrogates, IGT or diabetes as essential component. Similarly, the ADA recommends a fasting blood glucose method be used in obese children for screening. It is therefore essential to know the reliability of these tests. It is important to note that fasting indices represent different aspects of glucose homeostasis compared with indices derived from oral glucose stimulation. Fasting serum glucose levels reflect hepatic gluconeogenesis and basal pancreatic insulin release, while glucose levels after oral glucose stimulation reflect several different mechanisms including glucose absorption, gastrointestinal hormones, neural stimulation and pancreatic β-cell response. Among adults, longitudinal outcome studies of diabetes show worse outcomes in terms of cardiovascular morbidity and mortality in those diagnosed on the basis of the 2-hour plasma glucose result, as part of the OGTT. There is no clear-cut consensus on the role of OGTT in both clinical practice and research in children.

Reading this work we learn that the correlation and reproducibility of the 2-hour OGTT is worse than fasting glucose. Based on both OGTTs, 6 of 60 (10%) had IFG in the first test and 3 of 60 (5%) in the second test. Only 1 child had IFG in both tests. Based on both OGTTs, 10 of 60 (17%) had IGT in the first test and 12 of 60 (20%) in the second test. Only 3 children had IGT in both tests. This observation raises doubts about making a reliable diagnosis of glucose metabolism abnormalities outside diabetes. The OGTT is clearly less convenient, costs more and now we learn it is less reproducible, therefore fasting plasma glucose measurements should be preferred as a routine clinical test in children.

New concerns: complications in youths with T2DM

Macroalbuminuria and renal pathology in First Nation youth with type 2 diabetes

Sellers EA, Blydt-Hansen TD, Dean HJ, Gibson IW, Birk PE, Ogborn M
Department of Pediatrics and Child Health, University of Manitoba, Winnipeg, B.C., Canada
esellers@exchange.hsc.mb.ca
Diabetes Care 2009;32:786–790

Background: The prevalence of macroalbuminuria, clinical characteristics and renal pathological changes associated with macroalbuminuria were studied in a population of Canadian First Nation children and adolescents with T2DM.

Methods: In a retrospective chart review data on microalbuminuria (≥3 mg/mmol creatinine [26.5 mg/g]) and macroalbuminuria (≥28 mg/mmol creatinine [247.5 mg/g]), estimated glomerular filtration rate, renal pathology, and aggravating risk factors such as poor glycemic control, obesity, hypertension, glomerular hyperfiltration, hypercholesterolemia, smoking, and exposure to diabetes in utero were studied.

Results: Among 90 children and adolescents with T2DM, 53% had at least one random urine albumin-to-creatinine ratio consisting of the diagnosis of microalbuminuria at or within 8 years of diagnosis of diabetes. A total of 10 subjects had renal biopsies performed. None had classic diabetic nephropathy in biopsy. Nine of 10 exhibited immune complex disease or glomerulosclerosis.

Conclusions: This study suggests that the diagnosis of renal disease in children with T2DM cannot be reliably determined by clinical and laboratory findings and renal biopsy is necessary for accurate diagnosis.

There are only limited data regarding the microvascular complications of adolescents with T2DM. Initial reports from Pima Indians and Maori (New Zealand) with T2DM diagnosed during childhood demonstrate that microalbuminuria was present in up to one-fifth of the patients at diagnosis. After 10 years of follow-up, above 50% of the patients had microalbuminuria and 16% had macroalbuminuria. Studies comparing the prevalence of microalbuminuria in patients with childhood-onset T2DM and T1DM also suggest that adolescents with T2DM have more rapid progression of nephropathy.

This study by Seller and her colleagues teaches us that things are much more complicated than they look at first glance. They follow the Canadian First Nation children in whom the prevalence of T2DM in children aged 4–19 years is 1%.

Interestingly, Canadian First Nation children without diabetes have an increased rate of both congenital and acquired primary renal disease, mainly glomerulosclerosis. 90 youths with T2DM were studied. Their mean age was 15.2 years and mean duration of diabetes was 2.5 years (range 0.4–5). About one-third of them had microalbuminuria at diagnosis and more than half had at least one pathological test during follow-up. 10 subjects (9%) with persistent macroalbuminuria had renal biopsy. The biopsy results demonstrate that no one had sufficient histological changes to make a definitive diagnosis of diabetic nephropathy. Immune complex disease and glomerulosclerosis were the most common etiology of macroalbuminuria in this young population. These results are indeed surprising as nephropathy was intuitively thought to be secondary to poor control diabetes and obesity. Most interestingly, the population of the Canadian First Nation children has a private polymorphism in the hepatic nuclear factor (HNF)-1α gene. This is a transcription factor expressed in many tissues including the liver, intestine, pancreatic β cells, and kidney. It appears that the HNF-1α gene is associated with early-onset diabetes in this population and also is involved in the differentiation of the nephron and thus the authors speculated that this polymorphism may play a role in the development of the renal pathology found in this population. The effect of obesity on renal function and the impact of exposure to diabetes in utero are discussed. Most importantly, the authors conclude that diagnosis of renal disease cannot rely on laboratory findings and biopsy is necessary for accurate diagnosis.

Adolescents with type 2 diabetes: early indications of focal retinal neuropathy, retinal thinning, and venular dilation

Bronson-Castain KW, Bearse MA, Jr., Neuville J, Jonasdottir S, King-Hooper B, Barez S, Schneck ME, Adams AJ
Graduate Program in Vision Science, School of Optometry, University of California, Berkeley, Calif., USA
kbc@berkeley.edu
Retina 2009;29:618–626

Background: The eye provides a unique window into the neural and vascular health of a patient with diabetes. The present study is the first of its kind to examine the neural retinal function, structure and retinal vascular health in adolescents with T2DM.

Methods: Focal neural responses were tested using multifocal electroretinography. Optical coherence tomography was utilized to measure retinal thickness. Digital fundus photographs were examined for the presence of retinopathy and to measure vascular caliber using retinal vessel analysis. 15 adolescents diagnosed with T2DM, aged 13–21 years with a mean diabetes duration of 2.1 ± 1.3 years, were tested and compared with 26 age-matched control subjects were also tested.

Results: Multifocal electroretinograms of the T2DM group were significantly delayed by 0.49 ms. The diabetic group also showed significant retinal thinning (10.3 µm) and significant venular dilation (16.2 µm).

Conclusions: The present study shows early indications of focal retinal neuropathy, retinal thinning, and venular dilation in adolescents with T2DM.

The present study is the first to examine structural and neural measures in eyes of adolescents with T2DM. Among adults with T2DM, vascular and neural changes in the eye occur before any documented vision change. Three different methods were performed: (1) Multifocal electroretinogram (mfERG), a noninvasive clinical tool which enables the recording of electrical potentials from multiple, small areas of the central retina and thus assesses retinal neuropathy. (2) Optical coherence tomography (OCT), a noninvasive, noncontact, transpupillary imaging technology which can image retinal structures and enables measurement of retinal thickness. (3) Digital fundus photographs for measuring vascular caliber. Abnormalities in the three parameters studied were demonstrated in adolescents with T2DM. Firstly, 40% of the subjects in the diabetes group presented with abnormal mfERG compared with 8% of the control subjects, and are thus considered to have functionally abnormal retinas. Secondly, retinal thickness of the diabetic group was thinner than that of the control group. Among adults with T2DM, changes in retinal thickness and nerve fiber are thought to be due to neural tissue loss. Finally, venular caliber of adolescents with T2DM was significantly larger than that of our control group. In adults, venular dilation has been associated with carotid artery disease, cerebrovascular disease, measures of atherosclerosis and diabetic nephropathy. The retinal changes in adolescent with T2DM were unexpected given the relatively short duration of diabetes. These data strengthen the recommendation of the ADA to study all adolescents with T2DM at diagnosis.

Structural and functional cardiac abnormalities in adolescent girls with poorly controlled type 2 diabetes

Whalley GA, Gusso S, Hofman P, Cutfield W, Poppe KK, Doughty RN, Baldi JC
Department of Medicine, Faculty of Medicine and Health Sciences, The University of Auckland, Auckland, New Zealand
g.whalley@auckland.ac.nz
Diabetes Care 2009;32:883–888

Background: The main cause of death in adults with T2DM is cardiovascular disease. The cardiovascular status of adolescent-onset T2DM was studied.
Methods: Echocardiography and Doppler measurements were performed in 8 adolescents with T2DM, 11 with T1DM and 20 nondiabetic control subjects of whom 9 were lean and 11 overweight.
Results: Subjects with T2DM had larger left ventricular dimensions and left ventricular mass, which persisted when indexed to height. Diastolic filling was impaired in both diabetic groups, and systolic longitudinal function was lower in the T2DM group. Half of the group with T2DM met the published criteria for left ventricular hypertrophy and left ventricular dilatation, 25% had evidence of elevated left ventricular filling pressure in association with structural abnormalities.
Conclusions: This study has demonstrated preclinical abnormalities of cardiac structure and function in adolescent girls with T2DM, despite the short duration of diabetes and highlights the potential high cardiovascular risk occurring in adolescent T2DM.

This is the first study aimed to determine whether cardiac structural and functional abnormalities occur in adolescents with T2DM. Eight girls with T2DM, mean age of 14.9 ± 1.1 years, mean duration of diabetes 20 months and mean BMI 38.3 ± 7.4 kg/m², were studied and compared to age-matched T1DM, to lean and overweight control subjects. Studying cardiac structure, adolescents with T2DM had the largest heart reflected by left ventricular diameter, mass and left atrial area. This was significantly different from both lean and T1DM groups, but similar to the overweight group. Studying cardiac function, the T2DM subjects had lower diastolic and systolic longitudinal myocardial motion and higher left ventricular filling pressure. Only 1 of 8 patients with T2DM had no abnormalities compared to 10 of 11 subjects with type 1 diabetes. Based on these data, the authors hypothesized that these abnormal findings are related to obesity rather than diabetes per se and that diabetes further augmented cardiac abnormalities. The authors state that although the prognostic implications of the abnormalities detected are not known, they may progress toward clinical syndrome of heart failure. Recently, a 17-year-old male, whose weight was 140 kg, BMI 48 kg/m², who presented with a crushing pain radiating to the left shoulder and arm was reported [10]. He had elevated cardiac enzymes and was diagnosed with inferior myocardial infarction. No other risk factors for coronary artery disease were detected. The day is not far away when adolescents will leave the pediatrician's office with aspirin, antihypertensive medications and sublingual vasodilators. Adolescents with severe obesity, specifically those with T2DM, need routine cardiac evaluation. Intervention studies to prevent further progress of cardiac abnormalities are needed.

Clinical trials, new treatments: for prediabetes and for T2DM in adolescents

Short-term metabolic and cardiovascular effects of metformin in markedly obese adolescents with normal glucose tolerance

Burgert TS, Duran EJ, Goldberg-Gell R, Dziura J, Yeckel CW, Katz S, Tamborlane WV, Caprio S
Department of Pediatrics, Yale University School of Medicine, New Haven, Conn., USA
tania.burgert@yale.edu
Pediatr Diabetes 2008;9:567–576

Background: Metformin is an insulin sensitizer currently used as an adjunct to the treatment of some of the complications of childhood obesity besides T2DM. The metabolic and clinical effects of metformin in obese children with normal glucose tolerance were studied.

Methods: In a 4-month double-blind clinical trial in 28 obese adolescents with a mean BMI of 40.3 ± 5.7 kg/m², subjects were randomized to metformin (n = 15, dose 1,500 mg daily) or placebo (n = 13).

Results: The treatment with metformin was well tolerated and associated with a significant decreased BMI as well as with a reduction in subcutaneous fat, particularly the deep subcutaneous fat as assessed by magnetic resonance imaging. After intervention, the metformin group had a 35% improvement in insulin sensitivity compared with the placebo group. However, when adjusted for differences in baseline insulin sensitivity, significance was lost. While there was no change in inflammatory cytokines or lipid parameters, cardiovascular function as assessed by heart rate recovery after exercise improved with metformin and worsened in placebo.

Conclusions: Short-term use of metformin is well tolerated by obese children with normal glucose tolerance and has a beneficial effect on BMI and autonomic control of the heart as well as a trend toward improved insulin sensitivity. Thus, long-term treatment with MET may provide a means to ameliorate the cardiometabolic consequences of adolescent obesity.

This study is an additional contribution to several earlier works about the impact of metformin on weight loss and metabolic parameters in obese adolescents. As insulin resistance is a major player in comorbidities of obesity such as T2DM, hypertension and dyslipidemia, it seems logical to try to suppress elevated insulin levels to improve metabolic abnormalities. Moreover, studies among adults show a positive effect on weight loss. In this double-blind placebo-controlled intervention, the effects of metformin on metabolic parameters and fat partitioning were studied in obese children. In addition, an attempt to assess the effect of metformin on physiological measures of cardiovascular risk was taken. Heart rate recovery after exercise was studied after a self-paced exercise step test. During exercise there is a sympathetic dominance associated with increased heart rate. In the recovery period after exercise there is reactivation of parasympathetic tone with a drop in heart rate. A large drop in heart rate after exercise indicates an intact parasympathetic response whereas poor recovery rate has been associated insulin resistance and higher risk of developing T2DM. After 4 months those who were treated with metformin had: (1) a significantly lower BMI than the placebo group; (2) a reduction in deep subcutaneous fat; (3) an increase in heart rate recovery that paralleled the change in BMI, and (4) there was no change in lipid profile and CRP. Metformin treatment had short-term beneficial effects in obese children.

The impact of metformin, oral contraceptives, and lifestyle modification on polycystic ovary syndrome in obese adolescent women in two randomized, placebo-controlled clinical trials

Hoeger K, Davidson K, Kochman L, Cherry T, Kopin L, Guzick DS
Department of Obstetrics and Gynecology, University of Rochester Medical Center, Rochester, New York, N.Y., USA
Kathy_hoeger@urmc.rochester.edu

J Clin Endocrinol Metab 2008;93:4299–4306

Background: The effects of metformin, oral contraceptives (OCs), and/or lifestyle modification in obese adolescents with PCOS were studied.

Methods: A total of 79 obese adolescent women with PCOS were randomized to metformin, placebo, a lifestyle modification program, or OC. In the combined treatment trial, all subjects received lifestyle modification and OC and were randomized to metformin or placebo. Serum concentrations of androgens and lipids were measured.

Results: Lifestyle modification alone resulted in a 59% reduction in free androgen index with a 122% increase in SHBG. OC resulted in a significant decrease in total testosterone (44%) and free androgen index (86%) but also resulted in an increase in C-reactive protein (39.7%) and cholesterol (14%). The combination of lifestyle modification, OC, and metformin resulted in a 55% decrease in total testosterone, as compared to 33% with combined treatment and placebo, a 4% reduction in waist circumference, and a significant increase in HDL (46%).

Conclusions: In these preliminary trials, both lifestyle modification and OCs significantly reduce androgens and increase SHBG in obese adolescents with PCOS. Metformin, in combination with lifestyle modification and OC, reduces central adiposity, reduces total testosterone, and increases HDL, but does not enhance overall weight reduction.

This is a two-stage study on different treatment modalities of obese adolescent girls with PCOS. In a 'single treatment trial', 43 obese adolescent girls with PCOS were randomized to one of four arms: metformin, OC, lifestyle modification or placebo. Nine subjects did not complete the trial. In girls treated with OC there was a significant reduction in weight, in androgen levels, and in plasminogen activator inhibitor, however these positive changes were accompanied by an increase in CRP and LDL cholesterol. Lifestyle modification resulted in a significant reduction in androgens, in diastolic blood pressure and plasminogen activator inhibitor levels, however these were associated with compliance problems. Metformin treatment resulted in reduction in triglyceride levels with no change in BMI, fasting insulin or menstrual cycles. As OC and lifestyle modification resulted in improvement, the second stage study built was the 'combined treatment trial'. All 36 participants received lifestyle modification and OC, and were randomized to either metformin or placebo. While metformin did not induce weight loss it was associated with reduction in central obesity, albeit with significant increase in CRP levels. The importance of this study is that it increases the uncertainty of the benefits of different treatments. It seems that we fix one thing but break another. The bottom line as usual is that we need larger studies for a longer time.

Reversal of type 2 diabetes mellitus and improvements in cardiovascular risk factors after surgical weight loss in adolescents

Inge TH, Miyano G, Bean J, Helmrath M, Courcoulas A, Harmon CM, Chen MK, Wilson K, Daniels SR, Garcia VF, Brandt ML, Dolan LM

Division of Pediatric Surgery, Cincinnati Children's Hospital Medical Center, Cincinnati, Ohio, USA
thomas.inge@cchmc.org
Pediatrics 2009;123:214–222

Background: T2DM is associated with obesity, dyslipidemia, and hypertension, all well-known risk factors for cardiovascular disease. Surgical weight loss has resulted in a marked reduction of these risk factors in adults. The impact of gastric bypass on metabolic dysfunction and cardiovascular risk in adolescents with T2DM was studied.
Methods: Eleven adolescents who underwent Roux-en-Y gastric bypass at 5 centers were studied. Anthropometric, hemodynamic, and biochemical measures and surgical complications were analyzed. Data were compared with 67 adolescents with T2DM who were treated medically.
Results: Adolescents who underwent Roux-en-Y gastric bypass were extremely obese with a mean BMI of 50 ± 5.9 kg/m^2 with numerous cardiovascular risk factors. After surgery there was evidence of remission of T2DM in all but 1 patient. Significant improvements in BMI (–34%), fasting blood glucose (–41%), fasting insulin concentrations (–81%), hemoglobin A_{1c} levels (7.3–5.6%), and insulin sensitivity were also seen. There were significant improvements in serum lipid levels and blood pressure. In comparison, adolescents with T2DM who were followed during 1 year of medical treatment demonstrated stable body weight and no significant change in blood pressure or in diabetic medication use. Medically managed patients had significantly improved hemoglobin A_{1c} levels over 1 year (baseline: 7.85 ± 2.3%; 1 year: 7.1 ± 2%).
Conclusions: Extremely obese diabetic adolescents experience significant weight loss and remission of T2DM after Roux-en-Y gastric bypass. Improvements in insulin resistance, β-cell function, and cardiovascular risk factors support Roux-en-Y gastric bypass as an intervention that improves the health of these adolescents. Although the long-term efficacy of Roux-en-Y gastric bypass is not known, these findings suggest that Roux-en-Y gastric bypass is an effective option for the treatment of extremely obese adolescents with T2DM.

According to the recently published guidelines of the Endocrine Society, bariatric surgery was suggested for adolescents who have reached their adult height with BMI ≥50 kg/m^2 or BMI ≥40 kg/m^2 with severe comorbidities in whom lifestyle modifications and/or pharmacotherapy have failed [11]. The Roux-en-Y anastomosis is named after César Roux, the surgeon who first described the method and the stick-figure representation. An estimated 2,700 adolescent bariatric surgeries were performed between 1996 and 2003 [12]. While there was only little variation in the annual case volume in adolescent bariatric surgeries between 1996 and 2000, the number more than tripled from 2000 to 2003. In 2007 the NIH launched a prospective study called Teen-LABS (Longitudinal Assessment of Bariatric Surgery) to help determine if bariatric surgery is appropriate for adolescents. The study is planned for 5 years and we are waiting for data about obesity-related medical problems, other health risk factors, and quality of life before and after surgery. Meanwhile, we learn about the outcome of morbid obese adolescents with T2DM who underwent Roux-en-Y gastric bypass. The authors report that in addition to improved glycemic control, diabetic adolescents undergoing Roux-en-Y gastric bypass had significant improvements in measures of fatty liver disease, blood pressure, serum triglycerides, and total cholesterol. Among adults, T2DM was resolved in 77% of the patients and improved in 86% after bariatric procedures. Several antidiabetic properties are suggested [13], including decreased secretion of ghrelin, an exaggerated postprandial PYY response, contributing to appetite loss, and also increased glucagon-like peptide 1 (GLP-1) levels. One final point, based on 1 operated patient who did not experience resolution of diabetes even though at 3 years after surgery his BMI was reduced to 23 kg/m^2, the authors suggest that over time, there may be β-cell dysfunction that may not be recoverable even after bariatric surgery. Therefore, a greater benefit may be derived by reducing insulin resistance earlier in the course of T2DM to prevent β-cell fatigue, perhaps before the requirement of insulin therapy.

Food for thought: Medications increasing the risk for impaired glucose metabolism and T2DM

Metabolic and cardiovascular adverse events associated with antipsychotic treatment in children and adolescents

McIntyre RS, Jerrell JM
Department of Psychiatry and Pharmacology, Mood Disorders Psychopharmacology Unit, University Health Network, Toronto, Ont., Canada
roger.mcintyre@uhn.on.ca

Arch Pediatr Adolesc Med 2008;162:929–935

Background: The metabolic disturbances and cardiovascular events in children and adolescents treated with antipsychotics were studied.
Methods: In a retrospective cohort design, a treatment cohort of 4,140 children and adolescents prescribed 1 of 5 atypical or 2 conventional antipsychotics, and a random sample of 4,500 children not treated with psychotropic medications were compared.
Results: Compared with the control sample, the treated cohort had a higher prevalence of obesity (odds ratio [OR] 2.13), T2DM (OR 3.23), cardiovascular conditions (OR 2.70), and orthostatic hypotension (OR 1.64). Patients exposed to multiple antipsychotics were at significantly higher risk for incident obesity/weight gain (OR 2.28), T2DM (OR 2.36), and dyslipidemia (OR 5.26). Cardiovascular events were more likely to occur in those treated with conventional (OR 4.34) or multiple (OR 1.57) antipsychotics and mood stabilizers (OR 1.31).
Conclusions: Antipsychotics are associated with several metabolic and cardiovascular-related adverse events in pediatric populations, especially when multiple antipsychotics or classes of psychotropic medications are co-prescribed, controlling for individual risk factors.

In the United States, prescriptions for atypical antipsychotic drugs for youths increased 500% from approximately 201,000 in 1993 to 1,224,000 in 2002. The majority of prescriptions of an antipsychotic were for nonpsychotic conditions including disruptive behavior disorders (37.8%), mood disorders (31.8%), pervasive developmental disorders or mental retardation (17.3%). Only 14.2% were given to schizophrenia and bipolar disorder [14]. According to IMS Health, a private firm that tracks drug trends, the overall sales of atypical antipsychotics drugs past all other classes, reaching USD 14.6 billion in 2008. Therefore the public health implications of wide off-label use of this class are so important.

In this study we learn that the odds of developing obesity, T2DM, or dyslipidemia were higher for girls, adolescents 13 years and older and those exposed to multiple antipsychotics. It took 2–3 years between initiation of antipsychotic therapy and the incident of comorbidity. Importantly, patients with preexisting obesity and hypertension had a 4.5-fold increased risk of developing T2DM.

Cardiovascular events, defined as myocardial infarction, ischemic pulmonary heart disease, cardiomyopathy and arrhythmias, were higher in those treated with conventional antipsychotics or exposed to multiple antipsychotics. Overall, 25% of the children and adolescents treated with antipsychotic treatment had 1–3 comorbid chronic medical conditions in addition to their psychiatric disorder. The authors should be commended for this important study. The current emerging evidence provides support that the benefits and risks of antipsychotic treatment should be weighted considering the possible toxic effects.

Effect of valproic acid treatment on body composition, leptin and the soluble leptin receptor in epileptic children

Rauchenzauner M, Haberlandt E, Scholl-Burgi S, Karall D, Schoenherr E, Tatarczyk T, Engl J, Laimer M, Luef G, Ebenbichler CF
Department of Pediatrics IV, Division of Neuropediatrics, Medical University Innsbruck, Innsbruck, Austria
Markus_Rauchenzauner@hotmail.com

Epilepsy Res 2008;80:142–149

Background: The aim of the study was to determine the influence of valproic acid treatment on leptin, the soluble leptin receptor (sOB-R), the sOB-R/leptin ratio, body composition and insulin resistance in epileptic children.

Methods: Body composition, glucose homeostasis, leptin levels, sOB-R and the sOB-R/leptin ratio were determined in a cross-sectional cohort study of children >6 years with idiopathic epilepsy treated with antiepileptic drugs for at least 6 months.

Results: 87 children were on treatment with VPA, and 55 on other antiepileptic drugs. VPA-treated children had significantly higher BMI standard deviation scores, body fat, serum insulin concentrations and homeostasis model assessment (HOMA) index. Leptin concentrations were significantly higher and the sOB-R/leptin ratio was significantly lower when compared to the non-VPA group. Overweight VPA-treated children showed lower sOB-R concentrations and a lower sOB-R/leptin ratio (each p < 0.001) as well as higher body fat and leptin levels (each p < 0.001) compared to lean VPA-treated children.

Conclusion: VPA monotherapy was associated with higher body weight, body fat and serum leptin concentrations as well as impaired glucose homeostasis. Low sOB-R concentrations and a low sOB-R/leptin ratio in overweight VPA-treated patients might contribute to disturbances in glucose homeostasis and to the development of the metabolic syndrome in these children later in life.

This is yet another group of children that needs special attention because of the increased risk to significant metabolic complications secondary to treatment. Epilepsy is one of the most common neurological diseases, and VPA is one of the most widely prescribed antiepileptic drugs. One of the most common side effects of VPA is weight gain. In addition, hyperinsulinemia and increased prevalence of polycystic ovary syndromes (PCOS) in women with epilepsy and different features of the metabolic syndrome were reported. In this study the authors aimed to characterize the influence of VPA treatment on the adipocytokine axis. In the current study, higher fat mass was not only demonstrated in overweight VPA-treated children but also in lean VPA-treated children compared to lean controls. Similarly, hyperleptinemia in VPA-treated children was independent of body weight. Thus, VPA modifies leptin levels through the increase of body weight. In addition, overweight VPA-treated children had higher leptin levels, a lower sOB-R and lower sOB-R/leptin ratio compared to lean VPA-treated patients, possibly contributing to disturbances in glucose homeostasis and the development of the metabolic syndrome.

Among adults, insulin resistance caused by antipsychotic agents and valproic acid was corrected with insulin sensitizers without compromising their psychotropic effect [15]. Studies aimed at assessing the efficacy of metformin in preventing VPA-induced weight gain and hyperinsulinemia in children are needed.

Dyslipidemia in youth with diabetes: to treat or not to treat?

Maahs DM, Wadwa RP, Bishop F, Daniels SR, Rewers M, Klingensmith GJ
Barbara Davis Center for Childhood Diabetes, University of Colorado Health Sciences Center, Aurora, Colo., USA
David.Maahs@uchsc.edu
J Pediatr 2008;153:458–465

Background: Both T1D and T2D are increasing in youth and manifesting at younger ages, implying a longer burden of disease and earlier onset of vascular complications. Given that dyslipidemia is an important and potentially modifiable CVD risk factor, data for clinical decision-making regarding screening criteria and treatment of dyslipidemia in this high-risk population are of significant public health importance.
Methods: Recent data and current recommendations on dyslipidemia in youths with DM were reviewed.
Results: The authors emphasize that because no prospective data exist on safety, cost, or outcomes on dyslipidemia medications in adolescents with DM, it is uncertain how aggressively CVD risk factors should be treated in this population. Arguments against aggressive treatment include lack of data on safety, efficacy, and outcome, and even on surrogate marker data; intraindividual and interindividual variability; medication cost; potential life-long treatment, and data suggesting that early vascular lesions can regress with treatment in adulthood. Conversely, arguments for aggressive treatment include safety in adults with DM and in youth with familial hypercholesterolemia; data from landmark studies on the presence of early atherosclerosis in youth; increased risk of coronary heart disease in young adults with DM compared with nondiabetics; a preponderance of data indicating a reduced risk of coronary heart disease with statin treatment in adults; tracking of lipids from youth to adulthood.
Conclusions: Clinicians still need to adjust existing guidelines to individual patients and carefully weigh the possible benefits of treating cholesterol problems in children with diabetes against the safety, cost, and other concerns.

Recent studies have shown that cholesterol problems are widespread among children with diabetes. In the SEARCH for Diabetes in Youth Study, the prevalence of abnormal lipids was higher in T2DM than in T1DM: 33 vs. 19% had total cholesterol concentration >200 mg/dl; 24 vs. 15% had LDL-C concentration >130 mg/dl; 29 vs. 10% had triglyceride concentration >150 mg/dl, and 44 vs. 12% had HDL cholesterol concentration <40 mg/dl [16]. Only 1% of those with T1DM and 5% of T2DM were receiving pharmacologic therapy for dyslipidemia.

As demonstrated in this review, the juries are still out on the intensity needed to treat children with diabetes and dyslipidemia. Two important concepts should be mentioned. The first one is lipotoxicity, i.e. the exposure of the β-cell to excessive levels of lipids may be a cause of worsening β-cell function. In this view, failure to correct hyperlipidemia dooms the β-cell to a continual assault that perpetuates the downward spiral to β-cell dysfunction and β-cell death [17]. In vitro, prolonged exposure of insulin-secreting cells to elevated levels of fatty acids is associated with poor insulin secretion, impairment of insulin gene expression, and apoptosis of the β cell. The second intriguing concept raised in this review is the possible negative 'vasculometabolic memory' analogous to that of 'metabolic memory' in diabetes. The idea of 'metabolic memory' is that early abnormal environment may be remembered in the target organ and may have persistent effects. In diabetes, good metabolic control, achieved early in the course of diabetes, substantially reduces development of microvascular complications. It is tempting to extrapolate this concept to abnormal lipids level as well. If so, it is possible that early treatment of dyslipidemia is necessary to prevent lifelong atherosclerosis.

Lipid screening and cardiovascular health in childhood

Daniels SR, Greer FR, et al: Committee on Nutrition
Pediatrics 2008;122:198–208

Background: Given the current epidemic of childhood obesity with the subsequent increasing risk of T2DM, hypertension, and cardiovascular disease in older children and adults, there was a need of new guidelines.
Methods: A literature search designed to identify appropriate observational studies, clinical trials, reviews, meta-analyses and systematic reviews.
Results: The approach to screening children and adolescents with a fasting lipid profile remains a targeted approach. Overweight children belong to a special risk category of children and are in need of cholesterol screening regardless of family history or other risk factors.
Conclusions: For patients 8 years and older with an LDL concentration of ≥190 mg/dl, or ≥160 mg/dl with a family history of early heart disease or with two additional risk factors, pharmacologic intervention should be considered.

There was a big commotion after the publication of the new policy statement including editorials in leading medical journals [18, 19], daily newspapers, news and internet postings. The current guidelines still support targeted screening, i.e. children and adolescents with a positive family history of dyslipidemia or premature CVD (≤55 years of age for men and ≤65 years of age for women), children with unknown family history or those with other CVD risk factors, such as hypertension, cigarette smoking, or diabetes mellitus and the new inclusion of overweight and obesity. This targeted screening should take place after 2 years of age but no later than 10 years of age. The most controversial recommendations were pharmacologic intervention beginning at age 8 years and the inclusion of statins as first-line of pharmacological therapy. Repeated concerns were the paucity of long term efficacy and the poor long-term safety data in children and adolescents available to date. The response to concerns regarding the lack of strong evidence in terms of primary prevention of adult-onset CVD was that it is unlikely that such evidence will be available as these studies last for several decades.

Guidelines are recommendations for therapy, but they do not restrict therapeutic freedom.

The science of medicine should be supported by the 'art of care'. Each physician will need to decide for each child if and when pharmacological therapy is needed.

One final point, although no professional organization recommends universal screening, in a recent review by Kwiterovich [20] it was suggested that 'each child and adolescent should ideally have an assessment of their plasma lipids and lipoproteins'.

Spectrum and management of hypertriglyceridemia among children in clinical practice

Manlhiot C, Larsson P, Gurofsky RC, Smith RW, Fillingham C, Clarizia NA, Chahal N, Clarke JT, McCrindle BW
Division of Cardiology, Labatt Family Heart Centre, Hospital for Sick Children, University of Toronto, Toronto, Ont., Canada
Pediatrics 2009;123:458–465

Background: The prevalence of hypertriglyceridemia in youths will likely increase as a consequence of childhood obesity and increased screening for dyslipidemias. Factors associated with increased triglyceride (TG) levels and treatment options were studied.
Methods: Clinical review of data for 76 patients who had at least one elevated TG level (>4 mmol/l [>350 mg/dl]) was performed.
Results: Hypertriglyceridemia was secondary to lifestyle factors in 17% of the patients. The rest had primary hypertriglyceridemia, with 43% having familial combined hypertriglyceridemia and hypercholesterolemia (type II), 33% having primary hypertriglyceridemia (type IV), 5% having familial lipase deficiency (type I), and 2% having hyperlipoproteinemia E2/E2 phenotype (type III). TG levels were highest in type I and III hypertriglyceridemia (>10 mmol/l [>900 mg/dl]). A total of 45% received drug therapy as part of TG level management (bile acid-binding resins, fibrates, statins). TG levels were found to decrease over time with the use of fibrates, to increase with the use of bile acid-binding resins, and not to change with the use of statins.

Conclusions: Lifestyle modifications remain the primary therapeutic avenue for the management of pediatric hypertriglyceridemia. An algorithm for the management of this heterogeneous population to guide clinicians in their treatment decisions is proposed.

This is a clinical experience of a single pediatric lipid disorder clinic over 33 years. During this time period, 76 children at a median age of 11.6 years (range 5.1–20.3) with hypertriglyceridemia were followed. Most patients were asymptomatic and were referred because of family history or by a routine examination. During their entire follow-up periods, almost half of the patients were given lipid-lowering medications. The authors report that the use of fibrates was associated with the most significant decrease in TG levels and that the use of statins did not affect TG level. TG levels increased with the use of bile acid-binding resins. According to a proposed algorithm the decision of treatment was based on TG levels. With TG levels between 150 and 450 mg/dl, lifestyle changes should be prioritized and ω–3 can be supplementary. With TG levels between 450 and 900 mg/dl, decision on treatment is dependent on a complete lipid profile. For isolated TG levels, fibrates should be considered whereas if LDL-C is elevated as well, statins should be considered. About one-fifth of overweight children have elevated TG levels so it appears that we will need to study the long-term impact of ω–3, diet and medication on TG levels.

Food for Thought

Mirthful laughter, as adjunct therapy in diabetic care, increases HDL cholesterol and attenuates inflammatory cytokines and HS-CRP and possible CVD risk

Berk L, Tan S
Loma Linda University, Loma Linda, CA Oak Crest Health Research Institute, Loma Linda, Calif., USA
122nd Annual Meeting of the American Physiological Society, April 18–22, 2009, New Orleans, La., USA

Background: Psychosocial status has a role in maintaining health and preventing disease. The effect of 'mirthful laughter' on individuals with diabetes was studied.

Methods: A group of 20 high-risk diabetic patients with hypertension and hyperlipidemia were divided into two groups: laughter group and control group. Both groups were started on standard medications for diabetes, hypertension and hyperlipidemia. Subjects were followed for 12 months and levels of stress hormones epinephrine and norepinephrine, HDL cholesterol, inflammatory cytokines TNF, IFN, IL-6 and C-reactive proteins were measured. The laughter group viewed self-selected humor for 30 min in addition to the standard therapies described above.

Results: Patients in the laughter group had lower epinephrine and norepinephrine levels by the second month, suggesting lower stress levels. The laughter group also had lower levels of TNF, IFN, IL-6 and C-reactive protein levels, indicating lower levels of inflammation and increased HDL cholesterol. At the end of 1 year, the research team saw significant improvement in the laughter group: HDL cholesterol had risen by 26% compared with and only 3% in control group. Harmful C-reactive proteins decreased 66% in the laughter group vs. 26% for the control group.

Conclusion: The study suggests that the addition of an adjunct therapeutic mirthful laughter Rx (a potential modulator of positive mood state) to standard diabetes care may lower stress and inflammatory response and increase good cholesterol levels.

The first and last abstract of this chapter speak for themselves. Finally positive messages: sleep more and have a mirthful laughter –your weight and cardiovascular risk factors will improve.

References
1. Mayer-Davis EJ, Bell RA, Dabelea D, et al: The many faces of diabetes in American youth: type 1 and type 2 diabetes in five race and ethnic populations: the SEARCH for Diabetes in Youth Study. Diabetes Care 2009;32(suppl 2):S99–S101.
2. Gottlieb DJ, Punjabi NM, Newman AB, et al: Association of sleep time with diabetes mellitus and impaired glucose tolerance. Arch Intern Med 2005;165:863–867.

3. Welters HJ, Kulkarni RN: Wnt signaling: relevance to β-cell biology and diabetes. Trends Endocrinol Metab 2008;19:349–355.
4. Tequeanes AL, Gigante DP, Assuncao MC, et al: Maternal anthropometry is associated with the body mass index and waist:height ratio of offspring at 23 years of age. J Nutr 2009;139:750–754.
5. Oken E, Rifas-Shiman SL, Field AE, et al: Maternal gestational weight gain and offspring weight in adolescence. Obstet Gynecol 2008;112:999–1006.
6. Kral JG, Biron S, Simard S, et al: Large maternal weight loss from obesity surgery prevents transmission of obesity to children who were followed for 2 to 18 years. Pediatrics 2006;118:e1644–e1649.
7. Waterland RA, Travisano M, Tahiliani KG, et al: Methyl donor supplementation prevents transgenerational amplification of obesity. Int J Obes (Lond) 2008;32:1373–1379.
8. Ogden CL, Carroll MD, Flegal KM: High body mass index for age among US children and adolescents, 2003–2006. JAMA 2008;299:2401–2405.
9. Magge SN, Stettler N, Jawad AF, et al: Increased prevalence of abnormal glucose tolerance among obese siblings of children with type 2 diabetes. J Pediatr 2009;154:562–566.
10. El-Menyar AA, Gomaa MM, Arafa SE: Obesity: a risk factor for acute myocardial infarction with angiographically patent epicardial coronary vessels in an adolescent. Med Princ Pract 2006;15:449–452.
11. August GP, Caprio S, Fennoy I, et al: Prevention and treatment of pediatric obesity: an endocrine society clinical practice guideline based on expert opinion. J Clin Endocrinol Metab 2008;93:4576–4599.
12. Tsai WS, Inge TH, Burd RS: Bariatric surgery in adolescents: recent national trends in use and in-hospital outcome. Arch Pediatr Adolesc Med 2007;161:217–221.
13. Spanakis E, Gragnoli C: Bariatric surgery, safety and type 2 diabetes. Obes Surg 2009;19:363–368.
14. Olfson M, Blanco C, Liu L, et al: National trends in the outpatient treatment of children and adolescents with antipsychotic drugs. Arch Gen Psychiatry 2006;63:679–685.
15. Bahtiyar G, Weiss K, Sacerdote AS: Novel endocrine disrupter effects of classic and atypical antipsychotic agents and divalproex: induction of adrenal hyperandrogenism, reversible with metformin or rosiglitazone. Endocr Pract 2007;13:601–608.
16. Kershnar AK, Daniels SR, Imperatore G, et al: Lipid abnormalities are prevalent in youth with type 1 and type 2 diabetes: the SEARCH for Diabetes in Youth Study. J Pediatr 2006;149:314–319.
17. Poitout V, Robertson RP: Glucolipotoxicity: fuel excess and β-cell dysfunction. Endocr Rev 2008;29:351–366.
18. De Ferranti S, Ludwig DS: Storm over statins – the controversy surrounding pharmacologic treatment of children. N Engl J Med 2008;359:1309–1312.
19. Tanne JH: US paediatricians and cardiologists are criticised for recommending statins for children. BMJ 2008;337:a813.
20. Kwiterovich PO Jr: Recognition and management of dyslipidemia in children and adolescents. J Clin Endocrinol Metab 2008;93:4200–4209.

Population Genetics and Pharmacogenetics

Ken K. Ong[a,b]
[a]Medical Research Council Epidemiology Unit, Cambridge, UK
[b]Department of Paediatrics, University of Cambridge, UK

A clear indication of the increasing prominence of population genetics in pediatric endocrinology is that these papers are becoming a regular feature across the other chapters of the Yearbook. For example, in other chapters this year look out for the summaries of major genetic association studies of type 1 diabetes [1–3], blood glucose levels [4, 5] and bone mineral density [6], and also for an example of the emerging role of pharmacogenetics in a study of a vitamin D receptor genotype [7]. In the last year, genome-wide association (GWA) studies have continued to lead on new discoveries of single nucleotide polymorphisms (SNPs) in genes or chromosomal positions (loci) that had previously not been suspected of acting in the various disease or physiological pathways. Indeed, the pace of discovery has increased with the pooling of existing data into large international consortia for meta-analyses; type 1 diabetes [1], obesity [see Willer et al. below], and blood pressure [8] are examples of such highly fruitful collaborations.

So what uses do these genetic discoveries have? There is widespread acceptance that the effect sizes of individual SNPs are much lower than were previously thought. For example, an odds ratio of >1.3 is now considered to be a large genetic effect, and nearly all of the 18 new SNPs for type 1 diabetes have odds ratios of <1.2 [1]. This means that such variants do not have, and possibly may never have, sufficient power to predict future disease risks in individuals [see Lyssenko et al. and Meigs et al. below]. New studies looking at using copy number variation or low-frequency polymorphisms may identify loci with larger effect sizes and greater ability to predict disease risks. The current discoveries have started to inform new animal models of disease, such as the Fto knockout mouse [9] [see chapter on Obesity and Weight Regulation], but it is far too early to expect any impact on drug discovery.

For the time being, recognition of new loci for common traits (e.g. age at menarche) will hopefully inform the identification of rare mutations or chromosomal microdeletions that cause severe clinical conditions (e.g. precocious puberty or hypogonadotrophic hypogonadism). In combination with international clinical collaborations, this could inform genetic counseling for affected families [see Firth et al. below]. Secondly, by Mendelian randomization principles the use of these robust variants as 'instrumental variables' to demonstrate causal effects between exposures and disease outcomes is a very powerful new epidemiological tool [see comments on Sulem et al., Perry et al., Liu et al. and Eriksson et al. below].

Mechanism of the year: high throughput sequencing

Rare variants of IFIH1, a gene implicated in antiviral responses, protect against type 1 diabetes

Nejentsev S, Walker N, Riches D, Egholm M, Todd JA
Juvenile Diabetes Research Foundation/Wellcome Trust Diabetes and Inflammation Laboratory, Cambridge Institute for Medical Research, University of Cambridge, Cambridge, UK
Science 2009;324:387–389

Background: Genome-wide association (GWA) studies have identified genomic regions contributing to common human diseases, but they often do not identify the precise causative genes and sequence variants.
Methods: In order to identify specific causative variants for type 1 diabetes (T1D), the authors resequenced exons and splice sites of 10 candidate genes in pools of DNA from 480 patients and 480 controls and tested their association with T1D in over 30,000 participants.

Results: Four rare variants were identified which were associated with lower T1D risk independent of each other (odds ratio 0.51–0.74; p = 1.3 × 10^{-3} to 2.1 × 10^{-16}) in IFIH1 (interferon-induced with helicase C domain 1), a gene located in a region previously associated with T1D in GWA studies. These variants are predicted to alter the expression and structure of IFIH1.

Conclusions: These findings firmly establish the role in T1D of IFIH1 in melanoma differentiation-associated protein 5, a cytoplasmic helicase that mediates induction of interferon response to viral RNA. Furthermore, this study demonstrates that resequencing studies can pinpoint disease-causing genes in genomic regions initially identified by GWA studies.

In Yearbook 2008 we highlighted the new generation of very high-throughput DNA sequencing technologies that was used to report James Watson's DNA sequence [10]. The current paper now describes the first application of this technology in the study of complex disease. GWA studies have benefited greatly from the presence of linkage disequilibrium. This means that in many regions of our genome, numerous individual genetic variants tend to be inherited together. This means that we need to genotype 'only' a few hundred thousand variants in order to effectively 'capture' the effects of almost all the millions of common variants that exist. However the major downside is that once an association is identified, it is often not at all clear which variant or even which gene is primarily, or causally, responsible. One solution is to use large-scale gene sequencing to identify rare variants that have much larger disease associations. In contrast to the 'common' variants (with allele frequencies of >5%) that are typically analyzed in GWA studies, the 4 'rare' variants associated with type 1 diabetes mellitus (T1DM) in this study had allele frequencies of around 0.5–2%. However, their relatively large odds ratios for association with T1DM helped to pinpoint the IFIH1 gene as responsible for the association signal on chromosome 2q24 from the authors' previous GWA study. In essence this study now causally links IFIH1 to T1DM risk. IFIH1 is a cytoplasmic protein that recognizes RNA of picornaviruses, including enteroviruses. Enteroviral infection is more common among prediabetic and newly diagnosed T1D patients and has been suggested to trigger the appearance of autoantibodies. Upon infection, IFIH1 senses the presence of viral RNA, triggers activation of NF-κB and interferon regulatory factor pathways, and induces an antiviral interferon-β response. Variants, which are predicted to reduce function of the IFIH1 protein, would reduce the antiviral response and decrease the risk of T1D.

New paradigms: a catalog of rare events

DECIPHER: Database of Chromosomal Imbalance and Phenotype in Humans using Ensembl Resources

Firth HV, Richards SM, Bevan AP, Clayton S, Corpas M, Rajan D, Van Vooren S, Moreau Y, Pettett RM, Carter NP
Cambridge University Department of Medical Genetics, Addenbrooke's Hospital, Cambridge, UK
Am J Hum Genet 2009;84:524–533

Background: Many patients with developmental disorders have submicroscopic chromosomal deletions or duplications that, by affecting the copy number of dosage-sensitive genes or by disrupting normal gene expression, lead to disease. However, the extremely rare nature of many aberrations makes genotype-phenotype correlations uncertain and therefore limits clinical interpretation. Identification of patients who share the same genomic rearrangements and similar phenotypic features enables new syndromes to be defined.

Methods: The authors have developed an interactive web-based database called DECIPHER (Database of Chromosomal Imbalance and Phenotype in Humans Using Ensembl Resources) which incorporates a suite of tools designed to aid the interpretation of submicroscopic chromosomal imbalance, inversions, and translocations.

Results: DECIPHER enhances genetic counseling by retrieving relevant information from a variety of bioinformatics resources. Known and predicted genes within a chromosomal aberration are listed in the DECIPHER patient report, and genes of recognized clinical importance are highlighted and prioritized. DECIPHER enables clinical scientists worldwide to maintain records of phenotype and chromosome

Ken K. Ong

rearrangement for their patients and, with informed consent, share this information with the wider research community through the genome browser Ensembl.

Conclusions: By sharing cases worldwide, groups of rare cases with similar phenotypes and genomic structural rearrangements can be identified. Such cooperation will facilitate the delineation of new syndromes and also further our understanding of gene function.

We often see patients with growth and developmental disorders who we think are surely 'syndromic'. However, even when our genetic analyses identify chromosomal microdeletions or other aberrations, in many cases these genomic alterations occur in chromosomal regions of unknown significance, and we are therefore no clearer to providing the family with prognostic information about their growth or future health risks. This paper reports on an international network of academic centers of clinical genetics which has developed an online tool to increase medical knowledge about microdeletions and duplications and thereby improve the medical care and genetic advice for individuals/families with these conditions (see website: https://decipher.sanger.ac.uk/). This network will also inform scientific research by providing greater certainty in the pathogenic nature of genomic rearrangements and therefore the study of genes which affect human development and health. This will be of increasing importance as high throughput sequencing techniques pick up greater numbers of potentially disruptive mutations in individual genomes.

New genetic associations: a large harvest of new genes for BMI and obesity

Six new loci associated with body mass index highlight a neuronal influence on body weight regulation

Willer CJ, Speliotes EK, Loos RJ, Li S, Lindgren CM, Heid IM, Berndt SI, Elliott AL, Jackson AU, Lamina C, Lettre G, Lim N, Lyon HN, McCarroll SA, Papadakis K, Qi L, Randall JC, Roccasecca RM, Sanna S, Scheet P, Weedon MN, Wheeler E, Zhao JH, Jacobs LC, Prokopenko I, Soranzo N, Tanaka T, Timpson NJ, Almgren P, Bennett A, Bergman RN, Bingham SA, Bonnycastle LL, Brown M, Burtt NP, Chines P, Coin L, Collins FS, Connell JM, Cooper C, Smith GD, Dennison EM, Deodhar P, Elliott P, Erdos MR, Estrada K, Evans DM, Gianniny L, Gieger C, Gillson CJ, Guiducci C, Hackett R, Hadley D, Hall AS, Havulinna AS, Hebebrand J, Hofman A, Isomaa B, Jacobs KB, Johnson T, Jousilahti P, Jovanovic Z, Khaw KT, Kraft P, Kuokkanen M, Kuusisto J, Laitinen J, Lakatta EG, Luan J, Luben RN, Mangino M, McArdle WL, Meitinger T, Mulas A, Munroe PB, Narisu N, Ness AR, Northstone K, O'Rahilly S, Purmann C, Rees MG, Ridderstrale M, Ring SM, Rivadeneira F, Ruokonen A, Sandhu MS, Saramies J, Scott LJ, Scuteri A, Silander K, Sims MA, Song K, Stephens J, Stevens S, Stringham HM, Tung YC, Valle TT, Van Duijn CM, Vimaleswaran KS, Vollenweider P, Waeber G, Wallace C, Watanabe RM, Waterworth DM, Watkins N, Witteman JC, Zeggini E, Zhai G, Zillikens MC, Altshuler D, Caulfield MJ, Chanock SJ, Farooqi IS, Ferrucci L, Guralnik JM, Hattersley AT, Hu FB, Jarvelin MR, Laakso M, Mooser V, Ong KK, Ouwehand WH, Salomaa V, Samani NJ, Spector TD, Tuomi T, Tuomilehto J, Uda M, Uitterlinden AG, Wareham NJ, Deloukas P, Frayling TM, Groop LC, Hayes RB, Hunter DJ, Mohlke KL, Peltonen L, Schlessinger D, Strachan DP, Wichmann HE, McCarthy MI, Boehnke M, Barroso I, Abecasis GR, Hirschhorn JN
Genetic Investigation of Anthropometric Traits Consortium
Nat Genet 2009;41:25–34

Background: Common genetic variants at only two loci, FTO and MC4R, have been reproducibly associated with body mass index (BMI) in humans.

Methods: To identify additional reproducible loci, the authors performed a meta-analysis of 15 genome-wide association studies for adult BMI (n > 32,000). The top signals were tested for replication of association with adult BMI in 14 additional cohorts (n > 59,000).

Results: The findings strongly confirmed FTO and MC4R and identified 6 additional loci (p < 5 × 10^{-8}): TMEM18, KCTD15, GNPDA2, SH2B1, MTCH2 and NEGR1 (where a 45-kb deletion polymorphism is a candidate causal variant).

Conclusions: Several of the likely causal genes in these loci are highly expressed or are known to act in the central nervous system (CNS). These findings emphasize, as in rare monogenic forms of obesity, the likely major role of the CNS in predisposition to obesity.

Genome-wide association yields new sequence variants at seven loci that associate with measures of obesity

Thorleifsson G, Walters GB, Gudbjartsson DF, Steinthorsdottir V, Sulem P, Helgadottir A, Styrkarsdottir U, Gretarsdottir S, Thorlacius S, Jonsdottir I, Jonsdottir T, Olafsdottir EJ, Olafsdottir GH, Jonsson T, Jonsson F, Borch-Johnsen K, Hansen T, Andersen G, Jorgensen T, Lauritzen T, Aben KK, Verbeek AL, Roeleveld N, Kampman E, Yanek LR, Becker LC, Tryggvadottir L, Rafnar T, Becker DM, Gulcher J, Kiemeney LA, Pedersen O, Kong A, Thorsteinsdottir U, Stefansson K
deCODE Genetics, Reykjavik, Iceland

Nat Genet 2009;41:18–24

Background: Obesity results from the interaction of genetic and environmental factors. Two common measures of obesity, weight and body mass index (BMI), are both highly heritable.

Methods: In order to identify sequence variants that influence variation in adult weight and BMI, the authors performed a genome-wide association (GWA) study with 305,846 SNPs genotyped in 25,344 Icelandic, 2,998 Dutch, 1,890 European Americans and 1,160 African American individuals. These results were combined with previously published results from the Diabetes Genetics Initiative (DGI) on 3,024 Scandinavians. 43 variants in 19 genomic regions were selected for follow-up in 5,586 Danish individuals and the results were also compared to a genome-wide study on obesity-related traits from the GIANT consortium.

Results: In total, 29 variants in 11 genomic regions reached a genome-wide statistical significance threshold of p < 1.6 × 10⁻⁷.

Conclusions: This study identified variants close to or in the FTO, MC4R, BDNF and SH2B1 genes, and also at a further 7 previously unsuspected loci, were associated with adult obesity risk.

These two papers were published back-to-back and they describe the largest GWA studies to date for adult BMI with over 25,000 individuals in the first 'genome-wide' phase of each study. Together, they identified at least 10 new loci associated with BMI. These studies confirm the principle that performing larger GWA analyses, by combining existing data from individual studies, can markedly increase the yield of true-positive signals, i.e. genetic variants that are reproducibly associated with BMI or other outcomes. By comparison, the previous GWA study of BMI based on ~17,000 individuals identified only 2 loci, FTO and MC4R. Other examples of recent highly fruitful international collaborations include studies on blood pressure [8] and type 1 diabetes [1]. As more 'meta-GWA' studies appear, undoubtedly the new loci will have smaller and smaller effects. In the above papers on BMI, the effect sizes of individual variants ranged from 0.06 to 0.33 per allele, and even together they only explained a very small proportion of the variance in adult BMI. However, major benefits are the identification of new, previously unsuspected pathways to obesity, the demonstrated relevance of many of these variants also to childhood BMI and childhood obesity, and the consistent relevance of many of these BMI variants to adult type 2 diabetes risk. Most genes in these loci are expressed or are known to act in the CNS. As in rare monogenic forms of obesity, this emphasizes the major role of the CNS in predisposition to obesity.

Ken K. Ong

Genome-wide association study for early-onset and morbid adult obesity identifies three new risk loci in European populations

Meyre D, Delplanque J, Chevre JC, Lecoeur C, Lobbens S, Gallina S, Durand E, Vatin V, Degraeve F, Proenca C, Gaget S, Korner A, Kovacs P, Kiess W, Tichet J, Marre M, Hartikainen AL, Horber F, Potoczna N, Hercberg S, Levy-Marchal C, Pattou F, Heude B, Tauber M, McCarthy MI, Blakemore AI, Montpetit A, Polychronakos C, Weill J, Coin LJ, Asher J, Elliott P, Jarvelin MR, Visvikis-Siest S, Balkau B, Sladek R, Balding D, Walley A, Dina C, Froguel P
CNRS 8090-Institute of Biology, Pasteur Institute, Lille, France
Nat Genet 2009;41:157–159

Background: Children with early-onset (before the age of 6 years) or adults with morbid obesity (body mass index (BMI) ≥40) may be enriched for genetic variants that influence the risk of obesity in the general population.

Methods: The authors analyzed genome-wide association (GWA) data from 1,380 Europeans with early-onset and morbid adult obesity compared to 1,416 age-matched normal-weight controls. Thirty-eight markers showing strong association were further evaluated in 14,186 individuals of European origin.

Results: In addition to FTO and MC4R, we detected a significant association of obesity with 3 new risk loci in NPC1 (endosomal/lysosomal Niemann-Pick C1 gene, $p = 2.9 \times 0^{-7}$), near MAF (encoding the transcription factor c-MAF, $p = 3.8 \times 10^{-13}$) and near PTER (phosphotriesterase-related gene, $p = 2.1 \times 10^{-7}$).

Conclusions: This study demonstrates the value of studying groups with early-onset, morbid adult obesity and familial recurrence to identify new susceptibility loci. The study also provides further evidence that obesity in adults and children likely share the same genetic factors.

Common nonsynonymous variants in PCSK1 confer risk of obesity

Benzinou M, Creemers JW, Choquet H, Lobbens S, Dina C, Durand E, Guerardel A, Boutin P, Jouret B, Heude B, Balkau B, Tichet J, Marre M, Potoczna N, Horber F, Le Stunff C, Czernichow S, Sandbaek A, Lauritzen T, Borch-Johnsen K, Andersen G, Kiess W, Korner A, Kovacs P, Jacobson P, Carlsson LM, Walley AJ, Jorgensen T, Hansen T, Pedersen O, Meyre D, Froguel P
Genomic Medicine, Imperial College London, Hammersmith Hospital, London, UK
Nat Genet 2008;40:943–945

Background: Mutations in PCSK1 cause monogenic obesity. To assess the contribution of PCSK1 to polygenic obesity risk.

Methods: The authors genotyped tag SNPs in a total of 13,659 individuals of European ancestry from 8 independent case-control or family-based cohorts.

Results: The nonsynonymous variants rs6232, encoding N221D, and rs6234-rs6235, encoding the Q665E-S690T pair, were consistently associated with obesity in adults and children ($p = 7.27 \times 10^{-8}$ and $p = 2.31 \times 10^{-12}$, respectively). Functional analysis showed a significant impairment of the N221D-mutant PC1/3 protein catalytic activity.

Conclusions: Although additional functional analysis and replication in other cohorts will be needed, these findings firmly place PCSK1 on the short list of genes reproducibly associated with obesity.

An alternative approach to finding genes for obesity is to specifically study children with early-onset obesity or adults with morbid obesity. Such an approach had been profitable for the identification of genes for rare monogenic obesity and has now also been shown to pay off for common variants. The sample sizes required are much smaller than in studies of whole populations, however international collaborations are still needed to achieve informative numbers of severely affected individuals. However it is still unclear whether such minority groups are indeed enriched for variants that influence weight gain and susceptibility to overweight and obesity in the general population, or whether very early onset and morbid obesity are influenced by determinants that are more specific to these traits. The second study selected as a candidate the PCSK1 gene which encodes prohormone convertase 1/3, the enzyme that converts prohormones into functional key hormones. Loss of function mutations of PCSK1 lead to a rare phenotype including early-onset obesity, ACTH deficiency and diabetes with an increased proinsulin/insulin ratio [11]. Frequent variants in genes that are causal for rare diseases have increasingly been associated with common traits (see for instance MC4R). Only 3 cases of deleterious PCSK1 mutations have yet been reported, but the findings of a robust association with common variants described here place PCSK1 on the growing short-list of genes that influence normal variations in childhood and adult obesity risk. Whether the other traits associated with the severe PCSK1 mutations will be reflected in carriers of the common variants remains to be evaluated.

New paradigms: clinical phenotypes of obesity genes

An obesity-associated FTO gene variant and increased energy intake in children

Cecil JE, Tavendale R, Watt P, Hetherington MM, Palmer CN
Bute Medical School, University of St Andrews, St Andrews, UK
N Engl J Med 2008;359:2558–2566

Background: Variation in the fat mass and obesity-associated (FTO) gene has provided the most robust associations with common obesity to date. However, the role of FTO variants in modulating specific components of energy balance is unknown.
Methods: 2,726 Scottish children, aged 4–10 years old, had weight and height measured and DNA genotyped for FTO variant rs9939609. A subsample of 97 children was examined for FTO association with adiposity, energy expenditure, and food intake.
Results: In the total group and the subsample, the A allele of rs9939609 was associated with increased weight (p = 0.003 and p = 0.049, respectively) and BMI (p = 0.003 and p = 0.03). In the subsample, although total and resting energy expenditures were increased in children with the A allele (p = 0.009 and p = 0.03, respectively), resting energy expenditure was identical to that predicted for the age and weight of the child. Independent of body weight, the A allele was associated with increased energy intake (p = 0.006) but not the weight of food ingested (p = 0.82).
Conclusions: The FTO variant does not appear to predispose to obesity by regulating lower energy expenditure. Rather it may play a role in the control of food intake and food choice, such as hyperphagia or a preference for energy-dense foods.

This is the most prominent of a number of papers over the last year describing childhood phenotypes associated with the FTO obesity susceptibility variant. On a general point, it demonstrates that while tens of thousands of individuals were required to initially identify the FTO locus [12], subsequent highly informative physiological studies of the same variants are possible in far fewer numbers if you use precise and robust methods. This study used indirect calorimetry to assess resting metabolic rate, doubly labeled water to assess total energy expenditure, and standardized test meals performed in triplicate to assess eating behavior. The findings, plus results from 2 other childhood studies, which showed associations with reduced 'satiety responsiveness' [13] and increased total energy and fat intakes [14], consistently suggest that the FTO variant influences obesity risk by central regulation of appetite. However there is a major disparity between these human associations and mouse gene knockout studies. The latter suggest that FTO leads to obesity by reducing energy expenditure and downregulation of sympathetic activation rather than increasing appetite [9]. One problem may be that the human studies have so far all been cross-sectional and it remains difficult to truly determine the causal directions between these behaviors and BMI. In addition to robust measurements, there are no shortcuts to applying robust prospective study designs to understand the genetic etiology of obesity.

Ken K. Ong

Genetic determinants of height growth assessed longitudinally from infancy to adulthood in the northern Finland birth cohort 1966

Sovio U, Bennett AJ, Millwood IY, Molitor J, O'Reilly PF, Timpson NJ, Kaakinen M, Laitinen J, Haukka J, Pillas D, Tzoulaki I, Molitor J, Hoggart C, Coin LJ, Whittaker J, Pouta A, Hartikainen AL, Freimer NB, Widen E, Peltonen L, Elliott P, McCarthy MI, Jarvelin MR
Department of Epidemiology and Public Health, Imperial College London, London, UK
PLoS Genet 2009;5:e1000409

Background: Recent genome-wide association (GWA) studies have identified several common variants associated with adult height. However, it is unknown how these variants influence childhood growth.
Methods: The study comprised 3,538 singletons with genotype data and frequent height measurements between 0 and 20 years (average 20 measurements/person). The authors calculated peak height velocity in infancy (PHV1) and in puberty (PHV2) and timing of pubertal height growth spurt from parametric growth curves fitted to longitudinal height growth data.
Results: 26 of the 48 known height genetic variants tested were associated with adult height (p < 0.05, adjusted for sex and principal components), reflecting the limited power to detect these associations in this dataset. 7 variants (in/near HHIP, DLEU7, UQCC, SF3B4/SV2A, LCORL, and HIST1H1D) were associated with PHV1. 5 variants (in/near SOCS2, SF3B4/SV2A, C17orf67, CABLES1, and DOT1L) were associated with PHV2. There was statistical evidence for age-dependent effects for the variants in SOCS2 (p = 0.003) and in HHIP (p = 0.045). None of the variants was associated with timing of the pubertal height growth spurt after correction for multiple testing.
Conclusions: This is the first genetic association analysis on longitudinal height growth in a prospective cohort from birth to adulthood. The findings support the rationale for future research on the genetic regulation of human height during different periods of growth.

This study demonstrates the very interesting potential for pediatric endocrinologists to dissect out the specific relationships of genetic variants that have recently been identified mainly for adult outcomes. Adult height is of course the sum of length at birth plus statural growth during childhood. From our understanding of the different stages of growth and modeling of these specific components [15], it should come as little surprise that genetic variants for adult height may be partitioned into subgroups that regulate specific stages. Nearly half of the genetic variants associated with adult height in this sample had a detectable effect on PHV in infancy or puberty. While they found statistical evidence for age-specific effects of two variants, the authors acknowledge that their study size lacked the power to fully explore the potential effects of many of the other variants. However, this study demonstrates the concept, and indicates that further large genetic association studies plus future characterization of the actions of these genes will undoubtedly reveal significant insights into the mechanisms that regulate the specific phases of growth and its transitions.

Genome-wide association study identifies sequence variants on 6q21 associated with age at menarche

Sulem P, Gudbjartsson DF, Rafnar T, Holm H, Olafsdottir EJ, Olafsdottir GH, Jonsson T, Alexandersen P, Feenstra B, Boyd HA, Aben KK, Verbeek AL, Roeleveld N, Jonasdottir A, Styrkarsdottir U, Steinthorsdottir V, Karason A, Stacey SN, Gudmundsson J, Jakobsdottir M, Thorleifsson G, Hardarson G, Gulcher J, Kong A, Kiemeney LA, Melbye M, Christiansen C, Tryggvadottir L, Thorsteinsdottir U, Stefansson K
deCODE Genetics, Reykjavik, Iceland
Nat Genet 2009; Epub ahead of print

Background: Earlier age at menarche (AAM) correlates with shorter adult height and higher childhood body fat. Despite a large genetic component, no common genetic variant that associates with AAM has been reported.

Methods: The authors performed a genome-wide association study of AAM in 15,297 Icelandic women. Findings were replicated in further study populations from Iceland, Denmark and the Netherlands (n = 10,040).

Results: Combined analyses of all study populations showed an association between rs314280[T] on 6q21, near the LIN28B gene, and AAM (effect = 1.2 months later per allele; p = 1.8×10^{-14}). A second SNP within the same linkage disequilibrium (LD) block, rs314277, splits rs314280[T] into two haplotypes with different effects (0.9 and 1.9 months per allele). These variants have been associated with greater adult height. Other variants, previously associated with height, did not associate with AAM. Of 11 variants recently associated with higher body mass index (BMI), 5 were associated with earlier AAM.

Conclusions: Sequence variants at 6q21 were associated with AAM in Iceland and replicated consistently in populations from Denmark and the Netherlands. In addition, many of the SNPs that have recently been associated with increased adult BMI also associate with earlier AAM.

Meta-analysis of genome-wide association data identifies two loci influencing age at menarche

Perry JR, Stolk L, Franceschini N, Lunetta KL, Zhai G, McArdle PF, Smith AV, Aspelund T, Bandinelli S, Boerwinkle E, Cherkas L, Eiriksdottir G, Estrada K, Ferrucci L, Folsom AR, Garcia M, Gudnason V, Hofman A, Karasik D, Kiel DP, Launer LJ, van Meurs J, Nalls MA, Rivadeneira F, Shuldiner AR, Singleton A, Soranzo N, Tanaka T, Visser JA, Weedon MN, Wilson SG, Zhuang V, Streeten EA, Harris TB, Murray A, Spector TD, Demerath EW, Uitterlinden AG, Murabito JM
Institute of Biomedical and Clinical Science, Peninsula Medical School, Plymouth, UK
Nat Genet 2009; Epub ahead of print

Background: Twin and family studies suggest a significant genetic component to menarcheal age, with at least 50% heritability.

Methods: The authors conducted a meta-analysis of genome-wide association data to detect genes influencing age at menarche in 17,510 women.

Results: The strongest signal was at 9q31.2 (p = 1.7×10^{-9}), where the nearest genes include TMEM38B, FKTN, FSD1L, TAL2 and ZNF462. The next best signal was near the LIN28B gene (rs7759938; p = 7.0×10^{-9}), which also influences adult height.

Conclusions: This study provides the first evidence for common genetic variants influencing the timing of female sexual maturation.

These studies were part of a handful of GWA reports published concordantly, which describe the first common polymorphisms associated with age at menarche and also their influence on the timing of the onset of puberty and pubertal growth in both boys and girls [16, 17]. Previously, linkage and candidate gene studies had not confirmed any specific loci that were reproducibly associated with normal variation in the timing of puberty [18], and therefore these studies point to new mechanisms that regulate the timing of puberty (see chapter on Reproductive Endocrinology). In addition, the two studies described above had sufficiently large GWA datasets to explore in silico the potential effects of other variants associated with BMI and height. These results show that there are causal

Ken K. Ong

inter-relationships between the timing of puberty, BMI and adult height. For example, we had long assumed that normal variation in the timing of puberty had little effect on adult height, but very large population studies also indicate that early maturers tend to be slightly shorter [19]. The study by Sulem et al. attempted to demonstrate the direction of these relationships by adjusting the genetic associations (e.g. with adult height) for other outcomes (e.g. age at menarche), however such approaches can be biased towards the outcome which is measured with better precision. Application of Mendelian randomization principles, where genetic variants are modeled as the 'instrumental variable' that randomly changes the exposure, relies on certain assumptions [20], but provides a more robust framework to make causal inferences about the association between a risk factor and disease [21].

New genetic associations: lean body mass

Genome-wide association and replication studies identified TRHR as an important gene for lean body mass

Liu XG, Tan LJ, Lei SF, Liu YJ, Shen H, Wang L, Yan H, Guo YF, Xiong DH, Chen XD, Pan F, Yang TL, Zhang YP, Guo Y, Tang NL, Zhu XZ, Deng HY, Levy S, Recker RR, Papasian CJ, Deng HW
Key Laboratory of Biomedical Information Engineering, Ministry of Education, Institute of Molecular Genetics, School of Life Science and Technology, Xi'an Jiaotong University, Xi'an Shaanxi, PR China
Am J Hum Genet 2009;84:418–423

Background: Low lean body mass (LBM) is related to a series of health problems, such as osteoporotic fracture and sarcopenia. This paper reports a genome-wide association (GWA) study on LBM variation.
Methods: The authors performed a GWA scan using the Affymetrix 500K single-nucleotide polymorphism (SNP) array. A total of 379,319 eligible SNPs were analyzed in 1,000 unrelated US whites. Associations were replicated in 3 independent samples: (1) 1,488 unrelated US whites; (2) 2,955 Chinese unrelated subjects, and (3) 593 nuclear families comprising 1,972 US whites.
Results: Two SNPs in the thyrotropin-releasing hormone receptor (TRHR) gene were associated with LBM: rs16892496 (p = 7.55 × 10^{-8}) and rs7832552 (p = 7.58 × 10^{-8}). Subjects carrying unfavorable genotypes at rs16892496 and rs7832552 had, on average, 2.70 and 2.55 kg lower LBM, respectively, compared to other individuals. Meta-analyses of the GWA scan and the replication studies yielded p values of 5.53 × 10^{-9} for rs16892496 and 3.88 × 10^{-10} for rs7832552. In addition, there were significant interactions between rs16892496 and polymorphisms in several other genes involved in the hypothalamic-pituitary-thyroid and the growth hormone-insulin-like growth factor-I axes.
Conclusions: These findings, together with the biological relevance of TRHR in muscle metabolism, support an important role for the TRHR gene in the regulation of LBM variation.

It is always reassuring when GWA studies identify genes that are clearly involved in known hormone pathways. It is certainly much easier to visualize the Mendelian randomization arguments linking the thyroid hormone axis to lean body mass and other outcomes. In addition, such findings may be the closest to providing new treatment strategies. These findings support a clear physiological role of the thyroid axis in promoting lean body mass. Previously, the evidence from clinical observations and trials was limited by clinical context and small numbers and the findings are inconsistent. For example, in clinical trials in hypothyroid adults, higher doses of thyroid hormone lead to greater reductions in BMI, but studies of hypothyroid patients or euthyroid volunteers showed no detectable effects of thyroxine on body composition. Furthermore, hyperthyroidism is associated with reduced muscle mass and strength. Possibly the bodybuilding fraternity could have told us these answers many years ago: 'Thyroid medication is frequently used by bodybuilders who are getting ready for a contest', and 'T4 has found a bit of a niche for those using GH and dieting' (author's undisclosed online sources). Higher doses of thyroid hormone have also been associated with improvements in ankle reflex time and working memory; Mendelian randomization studies could substantiate those findings and also suggest other effects of thyroid hormone. Finally, the growth hormone (GH) gene was the first to be discovered to have a thyroid response element, and the IGF1 receptor and GHRH genes were also linked to lean body mass in previous studies. The current paper indicates a thyroid-GH co-regulation of lean body mass.

New genetic associations: serum estrogen levels

Genetic variations in sex steroid-related genes as predictors of serum estrogen levels in men

Eriksson AL, Lorentzon M, Vandenput L, Labrie F, Lindersson M, Syvanen AC, Orwoll ES, Cummings SR, Zmuda JM, Ljunggren O, Karlsson MK, Mellstrom D, Ohlsson C
Center for Bone Research, Sahlgrenska Academy, Department of Internal Medicine, Gothenburg University, Gothenburg, Sweden
J Clin Endocrinol Metab 2009;94:1033–1041

Background: The risk of many conditions, including prostate cancer, breast cancer, and osteoporosis, is associated with serum levels of sex steroids. The aim of the study was to identify genetic variations in sex steroid-related genes that are associated with serum levels of estradiol (E_2), estrone (E_1) and/or testosterone in men.
Methods: The authors genotyped 604 single nucleotide polymorphisms (SNPs) in 50 sex steroid-related candidate genes in 1,041 men (age 18.9 ± 0.6 years) in the Gothenburg Osteoporosis and Obesity Determinants (GOOD) study. Significant associations were replicated in the Osteoporotic Fractures in Men (MrOS) Sweden study (n = 2,568; age 75.5 ± 3.2 years) and in the MrOS US study (n = 1,922 men; age 73.5 ± 5.8 years). Serum E_2, E_1 and testosterone levels were analyzed using gas chromatography/ mass spectrometry.
Results: In the initial phase, one SNP rs2470152 in intron 1 of the CYP19 (aromatase) gene was the most strongly associated with serum E_2 levels (p = 2 × 10^{-6}). This association was confirmed both in the MrOS Sweden study (p = 9 × 10^{-7}) and in the MrOS US study (p = 1 × 10^{-4}). In combined analyses of all populations (n = 5,531), rs2470152 was clearly associated with both E_2 (p = 2 × 10^{-14}) and E_1 (p = 8 × 10^{-19}) levels. In addition, this polymorphism was modestly associated with lumbar spine BMD (p < 0.01) and prevalent self-reported fractures (p < 0.05).
Conclusions: rs2470152 of the CYP19 gene, which encodes the aromatase enzyme responsible for the final step of the biosynthesis of E_2 and E_1, is clearly associated with serum E_2 and E_1 levels in men.

This paper reports a thorough candidate gene study to identify variants associated with serum estrogen and testosterone levels. It illustrates that in addition to the large GWA approach, smaller more focused and hypothesis-driven genetic studies can also be invaluable, particularly if the relatively smaller numbers allow investment in more precise phenotypic measurements, in this case more accurate hormone assays. It also illustrates the concept that identification of robust genetic markers of metabolic variables, or other specific traits, can then be used to infer causality between those variables and other clinically important outcomes. In this case, rs2470152 was associated with lumbar spine BMD, but not femoral neck BMD, which strongly supports the notion that the lumbar spine is a more estrogen-responsive bone site than the femoral neck. The compelling evidence that rs2470152 is a marker of serum E_2 and E_1 levels in men allows its use in future Mendelian randomization studies to evaluate the causal effects of normal variations in estrogen levels on various important phenotypic traits and disease risks in men.

Ken K. Ong

Interaction effect of genetic polymorphisms in glucokinase (GCK) and glucokinase regulatory protein (GCKR) on metabolic traits in healthy Chinese adults and adolescents

Tam CH, Ma RC, So WY, Wang Y, Lam VK, Germer S, Martin M, Chan JC, Ng MC
Department of Medicine and Therapeutics, Chinese University of Hong Kong, Prince of Wales Hospital, Shatin, Hong Kong, SAR, China
Diabetes 2009;58:765–769

Background: Glucokinase regulatory protein (GCKR) is a rate-limiting factor of glucokinase (GCK), which functions as a key glycolytic enzyme for maintaining glucose homeostasis. Recent studies in European populations have reported associations between a common intronic polymorphism (rs780094) at GCKR with higher levels of triglyceride but lower fasting plasma glucose (FPG) levels and type 2 diabetes risk.

Methods: In order to examine their associations with metabolic traits in a healthy Chinese population, the authors genotyped two single nucleotide polymorphisms (SNPs), rs780094 at GCKR and rs1799884 at GCK, in 600 adults and 986 adolescents. Associations were adjusted for age, sex, and/or BMI. Interaction between these two SNPs was also tested, and a meta-analysis among European and Asian populations was performed.

Results: The T-allele of GCKR rs780094 was associated with increased triglycerides (p = 5.4 × 10^{-7}), while the A-allele of GCK rs1799884 was associated with higher FPG (p = 3.1 × 10^{-7}). A novel interaction effect between the two SNPs on FPG was also observed (p = 0.0025). Meta-analyses strongly supported the additive effects of GCKR rs780094 and GCK rs1799884 on FPG and triglycerides, respectively.

Conclusions: In support of the intimate relationship between glucose and lipid metabolisms, GCKR and GCK genetic polymorphisms interact to increase FPG in healthy adults and adolescents. These risk alleles may contribute to increased diabetes risk in subjects who harbor other genetic or environmental/lifestyle risk factors.

So far, the main findings of GWA studies have come from individual analyses of each genetic variant considered on its own. Subsequent analyses, for example using risk-allele or risk-genotype scores [22], have shown that these individual genetic effects do indeed appear to be simply additive. The opposite scenario, that some genes can modify the effects of other genes seems more plausible from a systems biology perspective. However, the tests for gene–gene modification (which are detected by statistical interaction or epistasis) are relatively underpowered, and in general require samples sizes around four times larger than those needed for simple associations. The results of this study only add to that complexity. The rs780094 variant in GCKR is primarily associated with higher triglyceride levels, but contrary to initial expectation, is also associated with lower glucose and insulin levels [23]. In this Chinese population, GCKR rs780094 showed no direct association with FPG levels, but modified the effect of another well-established variant GCK rs1799884 on FPG. However, no such interaction was seen on triglyceride levels. The meta-analysis found no other reports of any interactions between these two variants in Europeans, possibly due to lower allele frequencies and reduced power. This paper suggests that gene–gene interactions may be specific to each trait and also to each population, which makes their detection and validation even more challenging.

Clinical risk factors, DNA variants, and the development of type 2 diabetes

Lyssenko V, Jonsson A, Almgren P, Pulizzi N, Isomaa B, Tuomi T, Berglund G, Altshuler D, Nilsson P, Groop L
Department of Clinical Sciences, Lund University, Malmö, Sweden
N Engl J Med 2008;359:2220–2232

Background: Type 2 diabetes mellitus (T2DM) results from an interaction between environmental and genetic factors. The combination of clinical and genetic factors could predict progression to diabetes. *Methods:* The authors genotyped 16 single-nucleotide polymorphisms (SNPs) and examined clinical factors in two prospective cohorts of 16,061 Swedish and 2,770 Finnish subjects. T2DM developed in 2,201 (11.7%) during a median follow-up of 23.5 years. *Results:* Strong predictors of diabetes were: family history of the disease, increased BMI, elevated liver-enzyme levels, baseline smoking status, and reduced measures of insulin secretion and action. Variants in 11 genes (TCF7L2, PPARG, FTO, KCNJ11, NOTCH2, WFS1, CDKAL1, IGF2BP2, SLC30A8, JAZF1, and HHEX) were associated with the risk of T2DM independent of the clinical risk factors. The addition of genotype information to clinical factors slightly improved the prediction of future diabetes (area under the receiver-operating-characteristic curve increased from 0.74 to 0.75; p = 1.0×10^{-4}). *Conclusions:* Common genetic variants had a small effect on the ability to predict the future development of T2DM, compared with clinical risk factors. The value of genetic factors increased with an increasing duration of follow-up.

Genotype score in addition to common risk factors for prediction of type 2 diabetes

Meigs JB, Shrader P, Sullivan LM, McAteer JB, Fox CS, Dupuis J, Manning AK, Florez JC, Wilson PW, D'Agostino RB, Sr., Cupples LA
General Medicine Division, Department of Medicine, Massachusetts General Hospital, Boston, Mass., USA
N Engl J Med 2008;359:2208–2219

Background: Multiple genetic loci have been robustly associated with the risk of type 2 diabetes mellitus (T2DM). Knowledge of these loci may allow better prediction of risk than knowledge of common phenotypic risk factors alone. *Methods:* The authors genotyped single-nucleotide polymorphisms (SNPs) at 18 loci associated with diabetes in 2,377 participants of the Framingham Offspring Study. There were 255 new cases of T2DM during 28 years of follow-up. A genotype score was calculated from the number of risk alleles. Logistic regression was used to generate C statistics indicating how well the genotype score can discriminate the risk of T2DM when used alone and in addition to clinical risk factors. *Results:* The mean (± SD) genotype score was higher 17.7 ± 2.7 among those who developed T2DM than in the others 17.1 ± 2.6 (p < 0.001). The sex-adjusted odds ratio for diabetes was 1.12 per risk allele (95% confidence interval 1.07–1.17). The C statistic was 0.534 without the genotype score and 0.581 with the score (p = 0.01). In a model adjusted for sex and self-reported family history of diabetes, the C statistic was 0.595 without the genotype score and 0.615 with the score (p = 0.11). In a model adjusted for age, sex, family history, body mass index, fasting glucose level, systolic blood pressure, high-density lipoprotein cholesterol level, and triglyceride level, the C statistic was 0.900 without the genotype score and 0.901 with the score (p = 0.49). The genotype score resulted in the appropriate risk reclassification of, at most, 4% of the subjects. *Conclusions:* A genotype score based on 18 risk alleles predicted new cases of diabetes but provided only a slightly better prediction of risk than knowledge of common risk factors alone.

The recent haul of highly reproducibly disease susceptibility genes or loci has raised the possibility of using DNA-based tests to help predict future disease risk in individuals from the general population. Already, consumer genomic companies, such as 23andMe, deCODE Genetics and Navigenics, are offering direct-to-consumer genome-wide scans for USD 399–2,500. Fear of genetic discrimination has lead to recent new legislation to protect individuals from use of their genetic information by insurers to deny, limit or cancel health insurance, and by employers to discriminate in the workplace.

However, the results of these 2 studies, and also a 3rd large study from the Netherlands [24], show that currently available genetic information provides only a negligible improvement in the prediction of T2DM compared to using routinely available clinical information. In addition to T2DM, commercial DNA tests are currently also available for myocardial infarction, atrial fibrillation, glaucoma, prostate cancer and breast cancer. The strongest scientific data available are for the relatively rare breast cancer genes BRCA1 and BRCA2, which have far stronger effects on individual risks compared to common polymorphisms. However, even in that case the prediction data are based on studies only of high risk families, and the utility of positive and negative test results in the general population remains unclear. In addition to these long-term studies of disease prediction and legislation to prevent genetic discrimination, ethical issues regarding effects of genetic testing on anxiety, false assurance, and implications for other family members need to be addressed.

New concepts: overcoming your genetic predisposition

The association of ENPP1 K121Q with diabetes incidence is abolished by lifestyle modification in the diabetes prevention program

Moore AF, Jablonski KA, Mason CC, McAteer JB, Arakaki RF, Goldstein BJ, Kahn SE, Kitabchi AE, Hanson RL, Knowler WC, Florez JC
Center for Human Genetic Research, Massachusetts General Hospital, Boston, Mass., USA
J Clin Endocrinol Metab 2009;94 449–455

Background: Ectoenzyme nucleotide pyrophosphatase phosphodiesterase 1 (ENPP1) inhibits insulin signaling. In a recent meta-analysis the Q allele in the K121Q (rs1044498) single nucleotide polymorphism in the ENPP1 gene was associated with increased risk of type 2 diabetes (T2DM).
Methods: The authors genotyped the ENPP1 K121Q variant in 3,548 adults at risk for T2DM who had participated in the Diabetes Prevention Program (DPP) study of lifestyle intervention or metformin vs. placebo. They explored genotype, intervention, and interactions as potential predictors of diabetes incidence.
Results: Fasting glucose and glycated hemoglobin were higher in QQ homozygotes at baseline (p < 0.001 for both). There was a significant interaction between genotype at rs1044498 and intervention under the dominant model (p = 0.03). In analyses stratified by treatment arm, a positive association with diabetes incidence was found in Q allele carriers compared to KK homozygotes [hazard ratio (HR) 1.38; 95% confidence interval (CI) 1.08–1.76; p = 0.009] in the placebo arm (n = 996). Lifestyle modification eliminated this increased risk. These findings persisted after adjustment for body mass index and race/ethnicity. Association of ENPP1 K121Q genotype with diabetes incidence under the additive and recessive genetic models showed consistent trends (HR 1.10, 95% CI 0.99–1.23, p = 0.08, and HR 1.16, 95% CI 0.92–1.45, p = 0.20, respectively) but did not reach statistical significance.
Conclusions: ENPP1 K121Q is associated with increased diabetes incidence; the DPP lifestyle intervention eliminates this increased risk.

Firstly, this study confirms the association between the ENPP1 K121Q variant and increased risk of T2DM. However, the association was completely confined to those adults at risk for T2DM who were in the placebo arm of this 3-year diabetes prevention study. In contrast, the effect of the variant appeared to be completely abolished in those who were randomized to lifestyle intervention or metformin therapy. With the recent high-profile discoveries of robust genetic factors for many complex disease and traits it is important that we clearly communicate the public health message that genetic predisposition does not mean that disease risks are fixed and unchangeable. Similar misconceptions may arise from studies which demonstrate developmental programming by fetal or early life growth – 'determinism', either by genes or early environmental exposures, may lead to a misguided sense of fatalism. Rather, these genetic factors could potentially help to inform risk prediction [see Lyssenko et al. and Meigs et al., above] and could even help to guide the most efficient preventative strategies. For example, as this ENPP1 variant appears to confer increased risk of insulin resistance then strategies to promote insulin sensitivity, as used in this study, may be particularly effective.

Genetic compensation in a human genomic disorder

Carelle-Calmels N, Saugier-Veber P, Girard-Lemaire F, Rudolf G, Doray B, Guerin E, Kuhn P, Arrive M, Gilch C, Schmitt E, Fehrenbach S, Schnebelen A, Frebourg T, Flori E
Department of Cytogenetics, Strasbourg University Hospital, Strasbourg, France
N Engl J Med 2009;360:1211–1216

Background: Deletions at 22q11.2 result in the DiGeorge (or velocardiofacial) syndrome. Duplications of the same 22q11.2 region result in a phenotype that has some features in common with DiGeorge. *Methods:* Cytogenetic studies were performed for the purpose of genetic counseling in the parents of a girl with the DiGeorge syndrome, who carried a deletion at 22q11.2, *Results:* The unaffected father showed an unexpected rearrangement of both 22q11.2 regions. He carried a 22q11.2 deletion on one copy of chromosome 22 and a reciprocal 22q11.2 duplication on the other copy of chromosome 22. Genetic compensation, which is consistent with the normal phenotype of the father, was shown through quantitative expression analyses of genes located within the DiGeorge genetic region. *Conclusions:* This finding has implications for genetic counseling and represents a case of genetic compensation in a human genomic disorder.

DiGeorge syndrome is the most common microdeletion syndrome in humans, with an estimated frequency of 1 in 4,000 live births. Most cases occur sporadically, indicating that the deletion occurs recurrently in the population. More than 90% of patients with a 22q11 deletion have the same 3-Mb hemizygous deletion, suggesting that sequences at the breakpoints are susceptible to rearrangements. This study describes that in an unaffected father the phenotypic effects of the 22q11.2 deletion were balanced by a 22q11.2 duplication on the other chromosome and resulted in normal gene expression levels in the father's lymphocytes. The authors discuss that copy number variations are highly common in the human genome and therefore compensatory copy number variations may explain why some loss-of-function mutations have low penetrance. The phenotype of a dominant loss-of-function mutation could be rescued by a reciprocal gain of a copy number variation. This finding also has major clinical relevance as this father's children would have a near 100% risk of unbalanced outcomes. The authors recommend that, for genetic counseling, genetic investigations should be performed in both parents even if they have normal phenotypes.

References
1. Barrett JC, Clayton DG, Concannon P, Akolkar B, Cooper JD, Erlich HA, et al: Genome-wide association study and meta-analysis find that over 40 loci affect risk of type 1 diabetes. Nat Genet 2009 [Epub ahead of print].
2. Smyth DJ, Plagnol V, Walker NM, Cooper JD, Downes K, Yang JH, et al: Shared and distinct genetic variants in type 1 diabetes and celiac disease. N Engl J Med 2008;359:2767–2777.
3. Cooper JD, Smyth DJ, Smiles AM, Plagnol V, Walker NM, Allen JE, et al: Meta-analysis of genome-wide association study data identifies additional type 1 diabetes risk loci. Nat Genet 2008;40:1399–1401.
4. Bouatia-Naji N, Bonnefond A, Cavalcanti-Proenca C, Sparso T, Holmkvist J, Marchand M, et al: A variant near MTNR1B is associated with increased fasting plasma glucose levels and type 2 diabetes risk. Nat Genet 2009;41:89–94.
5. Prokopenko I, Langenberg C, Florez JC, Saxena R, Soranzo N, Thorleifsson G, et al: Variants in MTNR1B influence fasting glucose levels. Nat Genet 2009;41:77–81.
6. Styrkarsdottir U, Halldorsson BV, Gretarsdottir S, Gudbjartsson DF, Walters GB, Ingvarsson T, et al: New sequence variants associated with bone mineral density. Nat Genet 2009;41:15–17.
7. Jehan F, Gaucher C, Nguyen TM, Walrant-Debray O, Lahlou N, Sinding C, et al: Vitamin D receptor genotype in hypophosphatemic rickets as a predictor of growth and response to treatment. J Clin Endocrinol Metab 2008;93:4672–4682.
8. Newton-Cheh C, Johnson T, Gateva V, Tobin MD, Bochud M, Coin L, et al: Genome-wide association study identifies eight loci associated with blood pressure. Nat Genet 2009 [Epub ahead of print].
9. Fischer J, Koch L, Emmerling C, Vierkotten J, Peters T, Bruning JC, et al: Inactivation of the Fto gene protects from obesity. Nature 2009;458:894–898.
10. Wheeler DA, Srinivasan M, Egholm M, Shen Y, Chen L, McGuire A, et al: The complete genome of an individual by massively parallel DNA sequencing. Nature 2008;452:872–876.
11. Jackson RS, Creemers JW, Ohagi S, Raffin-Sanson ML, Sanders L, Montague CT, et al: Obesity and impaired prohormone processing associated with mutations in the human prohormone convertase 1 gene. Nat Genet 1997;16:303–306.
12. Frayling TM, Timpson NJ, Weedon MN, Zeggini E, Freathy RM, Lindgren CM, et al: A common variant in the FTO gene is associated with body mass index and predisposes to childhood and adult obesity. Science 2007;316:889–894.

Ken K. Ong

13. Wardle J, Carnell S, Haworth CM, Farooqi IS, O'Rahilly S, Plomin R: Obesity associated genetic variation in FTO is associated with diminished satiety. J Clin Endocrinol Metab 2008;93:3640–3643.
14. Timpson NJ, Emmett PM, Frayling TM, Rogers I, Hattersley AT, McCarthy MI, et al: The fat mass- and obesity-associated locus and dietary intake in children. Am J Clin Nutr 2008;88:971–978.
15. Karlberg J: On the modelling of human growth. Stat Med 1987;6:185–192.
16. Ong KK, Elks CE, Li S, Zhao JH, Luan J, Andersen LB, et al: Genetic variation in LIN28B is associated with the timing of puberty. Nat Genet 2009;41:729–733.
17. He C, Kraft P, Chen C, Buring JE, Pare G, Hankinson SE, et al: Genome-wide association studies identify loci associated with age at menarche and age at natural menopause. Nat Genet 2009 [Epub ahead of print].
18. Gajdos ZK, Butler JL, Henderson KD, He C, Supelak PJ, Egyud M, et al: Association studies of common variants in 10 hypogonadotropic hypogonadism genes with age at menarche. J Clin Endocrinol Metab 2008;93:4290–4298.
19. Onland-Moret NC, Peeters PH, van Gils CH, Clavel-Chapelon F, Key T, Tjonneland A, et al: Age at menarche in relation to adult height: the EPIC study. Am J Epidemiol 2005;162:623–632.
20. Sandhu MS, Debenham SL, Barroso I, Loos RJ: Mendelian randomisation studies of type 2 diabetes: future prospects. Diabetologia 2008;51:211–213.
21. Sheehan NA, Didelez V, Burton PR, Tobin MD: Mendelian randomisation and causal inference in observational epidemiology. PLoS Med 2008;5:e177.
22. Willer CJ, Speliotes EK, Loos RJ, Li S, Lindgren CM, Heid IM, et al: Six new loci associated with body mass index highlight a neuronal influence on body weight regulation. Nat Genet 2009;41:25–34.
23. Saxena R, Voight BF, Lyssenko V, Burtt NP, de Bakker PI, Chen H, et al: Genome-wide association analysis identifies loci for type 2 diabetes and triglyceride levels. Science 2007;316:1331–1336.
24. van Hoek M, Dehghan A, Witteman JC, van Duijn CM, Uitterlinden AG, Oostra BA, et al: Predicting type 2 diabetes based on polymorphisms from genome-wide association studies: a population-based study. Diabetes 2008;57:3122–3128.

Evidence-Based Medicine in Pediatric Endocrinology

Stephen O'Riordan[a] and Gary Butler[a,b]

[a]Institute of Child Health University College London and [b]University College London Hospital, UK

This has been an outstanding year of publications in pediatric endocrinology and diabetes since last year's *Yearbook* chapter on evidence-based medicine [1]. The selection process has been very challenging given the space available but we have endeavored to feature the key publications, chosen on the quality of the methodology, and the significance of the outcome, especially with regard to day-to-day clinical practice. Additionally, we have tried to produce a balance of topics in pediatric endocrinology and diabetes. Many other high-quality evidence-based studies, however, can also be found in other chapters in this book. There have also been consensus statements published on the diagnosis and management of children with idiopathic short stature, and optimal management of undescended testes [2, 3]. This chapter contains a selection of important RCTs, but also randomized trials of other designs, more appropriate for the population under study. This year we are beginning to see the first reports of well-designed clinical studies of growth hormone treatment that include final adult height status, which is surely the best evidence of efficacy of any growth intervention. We also include systematic reviews and very large-scale population studies. We hope these selected publications will help with understanding and improve both knowledge and the clinical care of patients.

Mechanism of the year – new technologies in diabetes

Continuous glucose monitoring and intensive treatment of type 1 diabetes

Tamborlane WV, Beck RW, Bode BW, Buckingham B, Chase HP, Clemons R, Fiallo-Scharer R, Fox LA, Gilliam LK, Hirsch IB, Huang ES, Kollman C, Kowalski AJ, Laffel L, Lawrence JM, Lee J, Mauras N, O'Grady M, Ruedy KJ, Tansey M, Tsalikian E, Weinzimer S, Wilson DM, Wolpert H, Wysocki T, Xing D
Juvenile Diabetes Research Foundation Continuous Glucose Monitoring Study Group
N Engl J Med 2008;359:1464–1476

Background: The value of continuous glucose monitoring (CGM) in the management of type 1 diabetes has not yet been determined.
Methods: A multicenter clinical trial randomly assigned 322 adults and children already receiving intensive therapy for type 1 diabetes to CGM or a control group performing home monitoring. Patients were stratified into three groups according to age and had a glycated hemoglobin level of 7.0–10.0%. The primary outcome was the change in the HbA1c at 26 weeks.
Results: The changes in HbA1c levels in the two study groups varied markedly according to age group (p = 0.003), with a significant difference among patients 25 years of age or older that favored the continuous-monitoring group (mean difference in change –0.53%; 95% confidence interval [CI] –0.71 to –0.35; p < 0.001). The between-group difference was not significant among those who were 15–24 years of age (mean difference 0.08; 95% CI –0.17 to 0.33; p = 0.52) or among those who were 8–14 years of age (mean difference –0.13; 95% CI, –0.38 to 0.11; p = 0.29). Secondary HbA1c outcomes were better in the CGM group than in the control group among the oldest and youngest patients but not among those who were 15–24 years of age. The use of CGM averaged ≥6.0 days/week for 83% of patients 25 years of age or older, 30% of those 15–24 years of age, and 50% of those 8–14 years of age. The rate of severe hypoglycemia was low and did not differ between the two study groups.
Conclusions: CGM can be associated with improved glycemic control in adults with type 1 diabetes. Future research is warranted to identify barriers to effective continuous monitoring in children and adolescents.

Continuous glucose monitoring system in children with type 1 diabetes mellitus: a systematic review and meta-analysis

Golicki DT, Golicka D, Groele L, Pankowska E
Department of Pharmacoeconomics, Medical University of Warsaw, Warsaw, Poland
dgolicki@amwaw.edu.pl
Diabetologia 2008;51:233–240

Background: The authors investigated the potential effects of the Continuous Glucose Monitoring System (CGMS), as compared with self-monitoring of blood glucose (SMBG), on glycemic control in children with type 1 diabetes.

Methods: MEDLINE, EMBASE and The Cochrane Library electronic databases were searched in June 2007. Additional references were obtained from reviewed articles. Only randomized controlled trials were included.

Results: Five trials involving 131 type 1 diabetic patients were included in the study. Combined data from all trials showed that the CGMS did not significantly reduce HbA1c levels compared with control groups. The pooled weighted mean difference was –0.02% (95% CI –0.29 to 0.25) with a fixed model and remained insignificant in the random effect model. Sensitivity analysis-determined results were stable. There was a trend towards a longer time under the CGMS curve for glucose <3.89 mmol/l in the CGMS group compared with the control group (mean difference 49.00 min, 95% CI –18.00 to 116.00). The CGMS significantly increased the number of insulin dose changes per patient per month for those managed with CGMS compared with the control groups (mean difference 6.3 changes, 95% CI 2.88–9.72).

Conclusions: The CGMS is not better than SMBG with regard to improvement of metabolic control in children with type 1 diabetes. Because of the small number of participants and methodological limitations of the studies included, findings of this meta-analysis must be interpreted with care.

Validation of continuous glucose monitoring in children and adolescents with cystic fibrosis: a prospective cohort study

O'Riordan SM, Hindmarsh P, Hill NR, Matthews DR, George S, Greally P, Canny G, Slattery D, Murphy N, Roche E, Costigan C, Hoey H
National Children's Hospital, Tallaght, Dublin, Ireland
s.oriordan@ich.ucl.ac.uk
Diabetes Care 2009;32:1020–1022

Background: This study aimed to validate continuous glucose monitoring (CGM) in children and adolescents with cystic fibrosis.

Methods: Over a 24-month period, 102 children (aged 9.5–19.0 years) with cystic fibrosis (CF) undertook oral glucose tolerance tests (OGTTs) and CGM monitoring at the same time. These paired tests were completed at baseline (CGM1) and 12 months later (CGM2). CGM validity was assessed by reliability, reproducibility, and repeatability.

Results: Bland-Altman agreement analysis was undertaken to assess reliability. CGM was found to be reliable with a between CGM and OGTT of 0.81 mmol/l (95% CI for bias ±2.90 mmol/l) and a good correlation coefficient between the OGTT and CGM (r = 0.74–0.9; p < 0.01). CGM was reproducible with no significant differences in the coefficient of variation of the CGM assessment between visits and repeatable with a mean difference between CGM1 and CGM2 of 0.09 mmol/l (95% CI for difference ±0.46 mmol/l). Discriminant ratios were also undertaken to confirm reproducibility, the results were of 13.0 at visit 1 and 15.1 at visit 2.

Conclusions: In children and adolescents with CF, CGM performed on two occasions over a 12-month period was reliable, reproducible, and repeatable.

All three papers above highlight the utility of new technology in the form of continuous glucose monitoring (CGM) in the modern management of intensive diabetes care. When CGM technology was introduced it was supposed to revolutionize the safety and effectiveness of intensive insulin therapy in type 1 diabetes. This new tool could allow patients with diabetes to optimize basal insulin requirements and precisely define mealtime insulin boluses. However, the initial CGM system was suboptimal and sensor accuracy was in question. Today, real-time glucose sensing allows CGM integration into the everyday intensive management of children and adolescents with diabetes, allowing for improved mean glucose, reduction in glycemic variability and reduction in HbA1c.

The recent paper by Tamborlane et al. highlights the utility of CGM in young adults (>25 years) when used continuously. However, the use of CGM averaged ≥6.0 days/week for 83% of patients >25 years age, 30% of those 15–24 years old, and 50% of the children in the age group 8–14 years. These results were disappointing for the child and adolescent arm of this cohort study, however there were not separate child and adolescent age groups but a combination of both. Based on the evidence suggested from this paper, CGM does not have a role in everyday management of children (8–14 years) unless used continuously. However, the *NEJM* paper reveals significant bias in its selection criteria and in the HbA1c start point for the children and adolescent (60 and 57% HbA1c <8.0%) versus the very well-controlled adult cohort (83% HbA1c <8.0%) [4].

Based on current evidence, CGM is useful in adults when used continuously and there is not enough evidence for children and adolescents. However, new data presented at the American Diabetes Association in New Orleans in 2009 highlights that patients of all ages including children and adolescents who were willing to use CGM 6/7days over a 6-month period showed an equal reduction in HbA1c of 0.5%. All three age groups were followed for a further 6 months, i.e. 12 months in total and sustained these lower HbA1c when CGM was in high use [5]. These results are more positive and conclude that CGM does have sustained and long-term beneficial effects on glycemic control in all age groups.

A small meta-analysis by Golicki et al. reports that CGM is no better than routine home blood glucose monitoring in children with type 1 diabetes. Once again, this is a good study design; however there were very few studies, five in total, able to be included in this meta-analysis. The authors admit that due to the small number of participants and methodological limitations of the studies included, findings of this meta-analysis must be interpreted with care. We await other ongoing prospective trials on CGM utility in the care of children and adolescents with diabetes.

CGM is being used in a wide variety of scenarios in pediatric endocrinology, one of these specialized areas is cystic fibrosis and cystic fibrosis-related diabetes (CFRD). The authors report that CGM is valid for use in children with CF and CFRD. The paper by O'Riordan et al. describes the valid components of CGM for use in children with CF under the headings: reliability, reproducibility and repeatability. The study was a prospective multicenter cohort study of 102 children and adolescents with CF and CFRD. The study was undertaken over a 24-month period with two glycemic measures, OGTT and CGM, at the same time 12 months apart. When CGM was performed on two occasions over a 12-month period, it was found to be reliable, reproducible, and repeatable. Thus the novel use of CGM in assessment of glycemic dysregulation is valid in children and adolescents with CF.

These papers provide different and sometimes conflicting evidence focused on the utility and validity of CGM in childhood diabetes. All three papers provide food for thought and acknowledge that this new technology may be useful and valid in diabetes management in certain populations (type 1 diabetes and CFRD). Until large international prospective randomized control trials in children and adolescents are done, CGM cannot be regarded as fully effective by evidence-based criteria.

Control of childhood congenital adrenal hyperplasia and sleep activity and quality with morning or evening glucocorticoid therapy

German A, Suraiya S, Tenenbaum-Rakover Y, Koren I, Pillar G, Hochberg Z
Pediatric Endocrinology, Rambam Medical Center, Haifa, Israel
J Clin Endocrinol Metab 2008;93:4707–4710

Background: In most patients with congenital adrenal hyperplasia (CAH), hydrocortisone (HC) replacement therapy is given three times a day. Although a higher morning dose mimics physiological diurnal variation in cortisol secretion, giving the higher dose in the evening has been advocated to suppress the early morning surge in adrenal activity. However, giving larger doses of HC later on has been claimed to be associated with sleep disturbances and insomnia. This study aimed to evaluate giving the high HC dose in the evening versus morning with respect to disease control, sleep pattern, and daytime activity in children with CAH.

Methods: This study was an open-label, cross-over, randomized trial in 15 children with classical CAH. Patients were randomized to receive 50% of the daily HC either in the morning or in the evening for 2 weeks; the other two doses each containing 25% of the total daily dose. Disease control was assessed by 08:00 h 17-hydroxyprogesterone, testosterone, androstenedione, and dehydroepiandrosterone sulfate levels on the last day of each treatment schedule. Sleep and daytime activity were assessed by a 7-day ActiGraph.

Results: There were no significant differences in basal hormone values between the high-morning and high-evening HC treatment schedules. No significant differences in sleep or daytime activity between the schedules were recorded.

Conclusions: Neither disease control, sleep quality nor daytime activity were affected by the timing of the peak HC dose. The authors recommend the high-morning dose schedule in replacement therapy of children with CAH as being more physiological.

Managing replacement HC well in children and adolescents with CAH is one of the biggest challenges facing a pediatric endocrinologist. This elegant and well-designed randomized cross-over trial aimed at answering a simple and practical question. Does giving a reverse physiological HC dosing schedule in order to achieve better disease control cause upset to sleep parameters and changes to a child's waking activity levels? The ActiGraph was able to record time in bed, total sleep time, total wake time, sleep onset latency, sleep efficiency, arousal and activity indices. No differences were recorded between the different treatment schedules. Single morning hormone profiles could not distinguish differences in disease control between the schedules, although, as the authors admit, this does not reflect hormone status throughout the day. However, the hypothesis that a reverse HC regimen causes disturbances in wakefulness in children as has been reported in adults can therefore be rejected. Answering this simple question can bring us the evidence for reassuring our patients and families that any necessary alterations in HC schedule merited on clinical or biochemical grounds should not cause disturbance to a child's lifestyle. Very important for clinical practice.

Bone mineral density in adolescent females using injectable or oral contraceptives: a 24-month prospective study

Cromer BA, Bonny AE, Stager M, Lazebnik R, Rome E, Ziegler J, Camlin-Shingler K, Secic M
Department of Pediatrics, Division of Adolescent Medicine, MetroHealth Medical Center, Cleveland, Ohio, USA
bcromer@metrohealth.org
Fertil Steril 2008;90:2060–2067

Background: This study aimed to determine whether young female adolescents using hormonal-contraceptive methods have a lower bone mineral density (BMD) than an untreated comparison group.

Methods: This was an observational, prospective cohort study of 24-month duration in adolescent clinics in a Midwestern US city. 433 postmenarcheal girls, 12–18 years of age, who were on depot medroxyprogesterone acetate (DMPA; n = 58), or were on oral contraceptives containing 100 µg of levonorgestrel and 20 µg of ethinyl estradiol (OCs; n = 187), or were untreated (n = 188) were studied. Measurements of BMD at spine and femoral neck were obtained by using dual x-ray absorptiometry at baseline and 6-month intervals and were corrected for volumetric variations in bone content.

Results: Over the 24-month period, the mean percentage change in spine BMD in each group was: DMPA –1.5%, OC +4.2%, and untreated +6.3%. The mean percentage change in femoral neck BMD in each group was: DMPA –5.2%, OC +3.0%, and untreated +3.8%. A statistical significant fall in BMD was seen between the DMPA group and the other two groups. In the DMPA group, the mean percentage change in spine BMD over the first 12 months was –1.4%, but the rate of change slowed to –0.1% over the second 12 months. No measures of bone density loss reached the level of clinical osteopenia.

Conclusions: Adolescent girls receiving DMPA showed a significant loss in BMD, in contrast with the bone gain in both the OC and the untreated groups. However, the clinical significance of this finding is mitigated by slowed bone loss after the first year of DMPA use and general maintenance of bone density values within the normal range in the DMPA group over time.

Why has this paper been included in the *Yearbook*, as it is a report from adolescent medical services? We as pediatric endocrinologists are keen to optimize bone health in our adolescent patients. This observational, prospective cohort study was conducted principally to examine the effect of DMPA on bone health. The reduction in BMD should sound a note of caution, despite the unlikelihood of reaching clinical osteopenia. No increased fracture rate has been reported in premenopausal adult women. However, the 20 µg of ethinyl estradiol combined OC is the mainstay of most sex steroid replacement regimens in hypogonadism and ovarian dysfunction disorders, for example, in Turner syndrome. This study states that this treatment regimen is likely to be satisfactory to develop adequate bone mineralization in the 12- to 18-year group, but that further studies are required using different OC doses and estrogen types. DMPA is prescribed as it is the most effective contraceptive in adolescent girls. If we are required to consider this treatment in the presence of other risk factors for osteopenia such as immobility or dietary disorders, then the authors recommend that BMD status should be assessed. Yet, osteopenia has to be prevented rather than treated, and assessing alone is a poor preventive measure. There was no discussion of either the etiology or an approach to the prevention of progestagen-induced osteopenia. This requires further evaluation via appropriately designed clinical trials.

New hope – prolonging endogenous insulin secretion

Etanercept treatment in children with new onset type 1 diabetes: pilot randomized, placebo-controlled, double-blind study

Mastrandrea L, Yu J, Behrens T, Buchlis J, Albini C, Fourtner S, Quattrin T
Department of Pediatrics, School of Medicine and Biomedical Sciences, University of at Buffalo, Buffalo, N.Y., USA
tquattrin@upa.chob.edu

Diabetes Care 2009;32:1244–1249

Background: The authors conducted a feasibility and efficacy study of etanercept therapy to prolong endogenous insulin production in newly diagnosed pediatric patients with type 1 diabetes mellitus.
Methods: A 24-week double-blind, randomized, placebo-controlled study was undertaken in 18 children (11 M/7 F, age 7.8–18.2 years). Children were randomized to receive either placebo (P) or etanercept (E). Inclusion criteria were age 3–18 years, GAD-65 and/or ICA positivity, HbA1c >6%, 3 insulin injections per day, WBC 3,000–10,000, platelets >100,000, and normal liver and renal function. Intention-to-treat analysis was used.
Results: HbA1c at week 24 was lower in the etanercept (5.91 ± 0.5%) compared with the placebo group (6.98 ± 1.2%; p < 0.05) with a higher percent decrease from baseline compared with the placebo (E 0.41 ± 0.1 vs. P 0.18 ± 0.21%; p < 0.01). The percent change in C-peptide AUC from baseline to week 24 showed a 39% increase in the etanercept group and a 20% decrease in the placebo group (p < 0.05). Baseline to week 24 insulin dose decreased 18% in the etanercept group compared with a 23% increase in the placebo group (p < 0.05).
Conclusions: In this small pilot study, treatment of pediatric patients newly diagnosed with type 1 diabetes with etanercept reduced HbA1c, increased endogenous insulin production, suggesting preservation of β-cell function.

Etanercept is a subcutaneously administered biological response modifier that binds and inactivates tumor necrosis factor-α, a proinflammatory cytokine. In patients with early active rheumatoid arthritis, etanercept is associated with rapid improvement in disease activity. This is a double-blind, randomized, placebo-controlled study. Although only a small pilot study of the use of etanercept as a novel therapy in newly diagnosed children with type 1 diabetes, the results are promising; suggesting lower HbA1c, increased endogenous insulin production and β-cell preservation. One case in the literature highlighted that etanercept may be associated with the onset of type 1 diabetes in a 7-year-old girl, 5 months after the initiation of etanercept therapy. However, larger randomized controlled trials are warranted to confirm these preliminary results and to explore the safety and efficacy profiles in childhood.

Management and 1-year outcome for UK children with type 2 diabetes

Shield JP, Lynn R, Wan KC, Haines L, Barrett TG
Education Centre, University of Bristol, and Bristol Royal Hospital for Children, Bristol, UK
j.p.h.shield@bristol.ac.uk
Arch Dis Child 2009;94:206–209

Background: This paper is a report of the 1-year outcome in the UK for children newly diagnosed with type 2 diabetes.

Methods: All children under the age of 17 years diagnosed as having type 2 diabetes from 1 October 2004 to 31 October 2005 were reported as part of a follow-up study of a UK national cohort.

Results: Follow-up data were available on 73 of 76 children. The mean age at follow-up was 14.5 years, with mean duration of diabetes 1 year. The revised incidence of type 2 diabetes in the UK in children under 17 years is 0.6/100,000/year. The mean body mass index (BMI) SDS at diagnosis was 2.89, and mean change at 1 year was –0.11 (range –1.53 to +1.37). At 1 year, only 58% achieved within target HbA1c <=7.0% (ADA and EASD). No relationship between improvement in BMI and improvement in HbA1c was identified. There was wide variation in choice of treatments and regimens. Hypertension was a common comorbidity (34%) and nephropathy less common (4%). Evidence of polycystic ovarian disease was identified in 26% of girls. In the first year after diagnosis, 22% of children had not been screened for nephropathy or retinopathy.

Conclusions: Pediatricians use a wide variety of treatment regimens to reduce HbA1c, however systematic screening for complications of diabetes is incomplete. Evidence-based treatment and management protocols are urgently needed to reduce the risks of long-term micro- and macrovascular complications of diabetes.

Shield et al. describe the difficulties young children have in the first year after diagnosis with type 2 diabetes, indicating that many children find it hard to make the necessary lifestyle changes needed to positively affect metabolic health. This follow-up national cohort study redefines the UK incidence of childhood type 2 diabetes in children under 17 years is 0.6/100,000/year. Pediatricians are noted to use a wide variety of treatment regimens to reduce HbA1c, however systematic screening for complications of diabetes is lacking. In the USA among African-American youths aged 10–19 years, prevalence (per 1,000) of type 2 diabetes was 1.06 (0.93–1.22) with an annual incidence of 19.0/100,000. Although the age ranges (<17 vs. 10–19 years) do not allow exact comparison, it seems that the USA is farther ahead with more new cases of type 2 diabetes in childhood. This paper is important as the epidemic of type 2 diabetes continues to emerge across Europe. It highlights the urgent need for evidence-based treatment and management protocols to reduce the risks of long-term complications of type 2 diabetes in these children. Large national-based audits and follow-up audits are essential to develop evidence-based treatment and management protocols in this challenging group of children.

Perinatal outcome of children born to mothers with thyroid dysfunction or antibodies: a prospective population-based cohort study

Mannisto T, Vaarasmaki M, Pouta A, Hartikainen AL, Ruokonen A, Surcel HM, Bloigu A, Jarvelin MR, Suvanto-Luukkonen E
Department of Obstetrics and Gynecology, University of Oulu, Oulu, Finland
J Clin Endocrinol Metab 2009;94:772–779

Background: The authors prospectively investigated the effects of thyroid dysfunction or antibody positivity on perinatal outcome.

Methods: Population was the Northern Finland Birth Cohort 1986 (9,247 singleton pregnancies). First-trimester maternal serum samples were analyzed for thyroid hormones [TSH, free T_4 (fT_4)] and antibodies [thyroid-peroxidase antibody (TPO-Ab) and thyroglobulin antibody (TG-Ab)]. Mothers were classified by their hormone and antibody status into percentile categories based on laboratory data and compared. Outcome variables were perinatal mortality, preterm delivery, absolute and gestational age-adjusted birth weight, and absolute and relative placental weight.

Results: Children from TPO-Ab- and TG-Ab-positive mothers had higher perinatal mortality which was not affected by thyroid hormone status. Unadjusted and adjusted (for maternal age and parity) risk for increased perinatal mortality was an odds ratio of 3.1 and 3.2 (1.4–7.1) in TPO-Ab- and 2.6 and 2.5 (1.1–5.9) in TG-Ab-positive mothers. TPO-Ab-positive mothers had more large infants, p = 0.017, as did mothers with low TSH and high fT_4 concentrations vs. reference group (6.6 vs. 2.5%, p = 0.045). Significantly higher placental weights were observed in mothers with low TSH and high fT_4 or high TSH and low fT_4 levels as well as among TPO-Ab-positive mothers.

Conclusions: First-trimester antibody positivity is a risk factor for perinatal death but not altered thyroid hormone status. Thyroid dysfunction early in pregnancy affects fetal and placental growth.

Thyroid autoimmunity in schoolchildren in an area with long-standing iodine sufficiency: correlation with gender, pubertal stage, and maternal thyroid autoimmunity

Kaloumenou I, Mastorakos G, Alevizaki M, Duntas LH, Mantzou E, Ladopoulos C, Antoniou A, Chiotis D, Papassotiriou I, Chrousos GP, Dacou-Voutetakis C
Endocrine Unit, First Department of Pediatrics, Athens University School of Medicine, Athens, Greece
Thyroid 2008;18:747–754

Background: The aim of this study was to determine the prevalence of thyroid autoimmunity (TA) in children and adolescents, and to determine if there are relationships between the period of onset of TA and gender and between TA and maternal autoimmunity.

Methods: Antithyroperoxidase antibodies (anti-TPO Ab), antithyroglobulin antibodies (anti-Tg Ab), thyrotropin, thyroxine, triiodothyronine, and urinary iodine were determined in 440 healthy schoolchildren (200 boys and 240 girls), aged 5–18 years, and in 123 mothers.

Results: The prevalence of positive anti-TPO and anti-Tg Ab was 4.6 and 4.3%, respectively. In girls, the prevalence of positive anti-TPO Ab was higher in Tanner stage 2–5 compared with Tanner stage 1 (8.2 vs. 2.2%; p < 0.05). No difference was detected with regard to anti-Tg Ab. In girls, positive anti-TPO and anti-Tg Ab levels were associated with significantly greater thyroid volume. Hypoechogenicity was detected in 52.6 and 36.8% of the children with positive anti-TPO or anti-Tg Ab, respectively (p = 0.0005). The prevalence of autoimmune thyroiditis, as defined by positive serum anti-TPO and/or anti-Tg and an echographic pattern of the thyroid gland having diffuse or irregular hypoechogenicity, was 2.5%. Mothers of anti-TPO Ab-positive children had positive anti-TPO Ab more frequently compared with mothers of anti-TPO Ab-negative children (82 vs. 18%; p = 0.0005). Mothers of anti-Tg Ab-positive children had positive anti-Tg Ab more frequently compared to mothers of anti-Tg Ab-negative children (75 vs. 25%; p = 0.0005).

Conclusions: These findings demonstrate that TA positivity in children was significantly associated with maternal autoimmunity and their development in girls emerges at puberty. Because genetic background, female gender and puberty are strongly associated with TA, girls with a family history of TA should be reassessed at the onset of puberty.

Two different papers were reviewed together as these disorders of the thyroid are common in childhood. There are few large population-based studies assessing the effects of thyroid antibody positivity on perinatal outcome. This work by Mannisto et al. is a prospective population-based Northern Finland Birth Cohort 1986, including 9,247 singleton pregnancies. The increased risk of perinatal mortality quoted in this paper is high with odds ratios of 3.1 and 2.5 for TPO and TG antibody-positive mothers. The authors conclude that first-trimester antibody positivity is a risk factor for perinatal death but not altered thyroid hormone status. Thus, thyroid dysfunction early in pregnancy affects fetal and placental growth. The next report from Athens, Greece, demonstrates that thyroid autoimmunity (TA) positivity in children was significantly associated with maternal autoimmunity and their development in girls emerges at puberty. These data are derived from thyroid autoantibodies, thyroxine, triiodothyronine, and urinary iodine measurements which were determined in a large cohort of 440 healthy schoolchildren (200 boys and 240 girls), aged 5–18 years, and in 123 mothers. Hypoechogenicity was detected in more than one-half and one-third of the children found to be positive anti-TPO or anti-Tg Ab, respectively (p = 0.0005). The prevalence of TA, defined by positive serum anti-TPO and/or anti-Tg and an echographic pattern of the thyroid gland being diffuse or irregular hypoechogenicity was 2.5%. The authors conclude that because genetic background, female gender, and puberty are strongly associated with TA; girls with a family history of TA should be reassessed at the onset of puberty. These papers were chosen based on good study design, large population-based datasets or large cohort studies. All describe known anecdotal associations in various aspects in thyroid disease in childhood and adolescence. However, these reports provide good evidence to support and confirm these associations.

Concepts revised – GH treatment to final adult height

Dose-dependent effect of growth hormone on final height in children with short stature without growth hormone deficiency

Albertsson-Wikland K, Aronson AS, Gustafsson J, Hagenas L, Ivarsson SA, Jonsson B, Kristrom B, Marcus C, Nilsson KO, Ritzen EM, Tuvemo T, Westphal O, Aman J
Goteborg Pediatric Growth Research Center/Vaxthuset, Department of Pediatrics, The Sahlgrenska Academy at University of Gothenburg, and The Queen Silvia Children's Hospital, Goteborg, Sweden
kerstin.albertsson-wikland@pediat.gu.se
J Clin Endocrinol Metab 2008;93:4342–4350

Background: This study aimed at defining the response to GH treatment in children without GH deficiency, focusing especially in those described as having idiopathic short stature (ISS) who were treated in a controlled trial until final height. The study also aimed at examining the effect of two different doses of GH.

Methods: This was a randomized controlled, long-term, multicenter trial from Sweden. Children were all short (–2 SD) and GH deficiency and organic disease were excluded. Although 177 subjects were initially enrolled, after exclusion of those born small for gestational age (SGA) the final group included 126 children in the intention-to-treat population and 68 subjects who observed the study protocol exactly. The principal outcomes were final height SD score (SDS), difference in SDS to midparenteral height, and gain in height SDS. Two doses of GH (Genotropin) were administered, 33 or 67 µg/kg/day; control subjects were untreated.

Results: GH therapy was given for a mean of 5.9 ± 1.1 years. The final height SDS in the protocol observing population treated with GH was –1.5 ± 0.81 (33 µg/kg/day –1.7 ± 0.70, and 67 µg/kg/day –1.4 ± 0.86; p < 0.032) vs. –2.4 ± 0.85 in the controls (p < 0.001). The difference in SDS to midparenteral height was –0.2 ± 1.0 vs. –1.0 ± 0.74 (p < 0.001), and the gain in height SDS was 1.3 ± 0.78 vs. 0.2 ± 0.69 (p < 0.001). The time to the onset of puberty was unchanged. A dose-response relationship identified after 1 year continued to final height for all growth outcome variables in all populations studied.

Conclusions: GH treatment significantly increased final height in ISS children with a clear dose responsiveness. Although the mean treatment gain was 1.3 SDS (8 cm), there was a broad range of response from no gain to +3 SDS compared with a mean increase of +0.2 SDS in the untreated controls. The distance from initial target height predicted greater gains in height. GH therapy was monitored and found to be safe.

A randomised study of the effect of two doses of biosynthetic human growth hormone on final height of children with familial short stature

Elder CJ, Barton JS, Brook CG, Preece MA, Dattani MT, Hindmarsh PC
Great Ormond Street Hospital for Children NHS Trust, University College Hospital, London, UK
Horm Res 2008;70:89–92

Background: This randomized trial aimed to ascertain the dose-dependent effect of two different doses of recombinant human GH in children with familial short stature (FSS) who were not GH-deficient.
Methods: The age range of the 29 (24 male, 5 female) FSS children at presentation was 5.1–10.5 years, height <1.5 standard deviation scores (SDS) below the mean, height velocity SDS >–1.5 and peak growth hormone response to provocative testing >13.5 mU/l. GH was randomized in two doses, 20 or 40 IU/m^2 body surface area/week (33 or 67 µg/kg/day) by daily subcutaneous injection of GH and continued until the endpoint which was assessment of adult height.
Results: Adult height data (SDS) were similar at 16.5 ± 2.1 years for the low-dose group –1.06 (SD 0.75) and at 16.1 ± 1.1 years for the high-dose group –1.02 (SD 0.83) (no significant difference, p = 0.88 for adult height). The incremental effect of both doses on stature was minimal (low-dose actual minus predicted difference in height 0.79 (SD 0.94), high dose 1.27 (SD 0.88); p = 0.12).
Conclusions: Neither GH dosing schedule produced beneficial effects either in short-term gains in height or in long-term increases in adult stature in this group of children with FSS.

These two papers reporting randomized trials of GH treatment in non-GH-deficient short statured children followed up to adult height seem at first glance to show opposite results. However, on closer inspection that is not the case. They represent carefully designed and executed clinical trials begun over 20 years ago which have run to completion with the ultimate endpoint of measured adult height thus providing the highest level of evidence in this situation. Albertsson-Wikland's paper is a remarkable achievement, as it has a randomized untreated group. In what ways are they similar? Both studies randomized patients to the same standard and high doses of GH, and one of the studies showed a dose-dependent increase in stature with a similar non-significant trend in the other study. In the study of Coelho et al. the recruited patients were more homogeneous, being less short and not as far below target height as those in Albertsson-Wikland et al. In this latter study there was a greater range of responses to GH with short children of non-familial short stature families showing the best height gains on GH treatment in a dose-dependent manner. Thus the conclusions of both trials is that slightly short children of short parents do not show good responsiveness to GH treatment, whereas Albertsson-Wikland et al. demonstrate that ISS patients furthest below target height at diagnosis gain the most in height. However, despite the demonstration of gains in height, additional evidence is needed on cost effectiveness and quality-of-life gains before GH can be advocated.

A randomised study of two doses of biosynthetic human growth hormone on final height of pubertal children with growth hormone deficiency

Coelho R, Brook CG, Preece MA, Stanhope RG, Dattani MT, Hindmarsh PC
Great Ormond Street Hospital for Children NHS Trust, and University College Hospital, London, UK
Horm Res 2008;70:85–88

Background: This study was a randomized clinical trial to determine the effectiveness of two different doses of GH therapy (standard and high dose) during puberty in children undergoing treatment for growth hormone deficiency (GHD).
Methods: 49 children with GHD who showed a spontaneous onset of puberty were allocated randomly using a random number table to one of two groups: 15 IU/m^2/week (25 µg/kg/day) or 30 IU/m^2/week (50 µg/kg/day). Patients were also included if they had received hGH daily at a dose of 15 IU/m^2/week for at least 1 year before randomization.
Results: Both groups showed similar height standard deviation score (SDS) increases (standard dose: 1.1; high dose: 1.2; p = 0.81). Time to mid-puberty was similar, but the high-dose group attained adult height 1.1 year earlier at 16.1 years (p = 0.026).
Conclusions: Doubling the dose GH from the start of puberty until adult height does not appear to have a significant effect on adult height of children with GH deficiency.

Studies of the nocturnal physiological pattern of GH secretion during puberty have demonstrated a 2- to 4-fold increase in total GH secretion. The corollary of this is that this physiological pattern of normal growth should be reproduced by doubling the pubertal GH replacement dose in patients with GHD. Interestingly, this common sense idea is rejected by this study, and has not been upheld in earlier short-term studies. The GH dose has not previously been found to be a significant factor in modeling total pubertal growth gains. Although there was a reduction in the duration of the pubertal growth spurt with high-dose treatment, this was not during the acceleration phase, time to mid-puberty being similar between the groups. This lack of ability to significantly manipulate the magnitude of adolescent growth remains one of the unmet challenges of pediatric endocrinology. The authors suggest that altering pubertal tempo with GnRH analogues or aromatase inhibitors, or intensifying prepubertal hGH therapy may be more promising approaches to improving final height in children with GH deficiency, but this remains speculative until evidence is provided.

Important for clinical practice – highs, lows and carbs!

Cognitive function is disrupted by both hypo- and hyperglycemia in school-aged children with type 1 diabetes: a field study

Gonder-Frederick LA, Zrebiec JF, Bauchowitz AU, Ritterband LM, Magee JC, Cox DJ, Clarke WL
Behavioral Medicine Center, Department of Psychiatric Medicine and Neurobehavioral Science, Department of Pediatrics, University of Virginia Health Sciences Center, Charlottesville, Va., USA
lag3g@virginia.edu
Diabetes Care 2009;32:1001–1006

Background: The authors developed a field procedure using personal digital assistant (PDA) technology to test the hypothesis that naturally occurring episodes of hypo- and hyperglycemia are associated with deterioration in cognitive function in children with type 1 diabetes.

Methods: A total of 61 children aged 6–11 years with type 1 diabetes received a PDA programmed with two brief cognitive tests (mental maths and choice reaction time), which they completed just before home glucose readings. The computer recorded speed of each test and number of correct answers. Children undertook multiple tests daily over 4–6 weeks for a total of 70 tests. Performance variables were compared across glucose ranges. Individual impairment scores were calculated from the SD between performance during euglycemia and that during glucose extremes.

Results: Hypoglycemia increased time to complete both mental maths and reaction time. During hyperglycemic episodes, time to complete maths was significantly longer and there was a trend towards increased reaction time (p = 0.053). No differences on task accuracy were found. Decline in mental maths performance was equal at glucose levels <3.0 and >22.2 mmol/l. Individual impairment scores varied greatly across children, with no age or sex differences.

Conclusions: Mental efficiency declines with naturally occurring hypoglycemic and hyperglycemic fluctuations in children with type 1 diabetes. There are equal declines in performance for low and high blood glucose concentrations >22.2 mmol/l. These effects can be detected using PDA technology.

Impact of carbohydrate counting on glycemic control in children with type 1 diabetes

Mehta SN, Quinn N, Volkening LK, Laffel LM
Pediatric, Adolescent, and Young Adult Section, Joslin Diabetes Center, Boston, Mass., USA
sanjeev.mehta@joslin.harvard.edu
Diabetes Care 2009;32:1014–1016

Background: To study the association between parent carbohydrate counting knowledge and glycemic control in children with type 1 diabetes (T1D).

Methods: The authors assessed 67 youth ages 4–12 years with T1D (duration ≥1 year). Parents estimated carbohydrate content of children's meals. The ratio of parent estimates to computer analysis defined carbohydrate counting knowledge; the mean and SD of these ratios defined accuracy and precision, respectively. HbA1c defined glycemic control.

Results: Better accuracy and precision were associated with lower HbA1c in bivariate analyses (p < 0.05). In a multivariate analysis (R^2 = 0.25, p = 0.007) adjusting for child age, sex, and type 1 diabetes duration, precision (p = 0.02) and more frequent blood glucose monitoring (p = 0.04), but not accuracy (p = 0.9), were associated with lower HbA1c. HbA1c was 0.8% lower among youth whose parents demonstrated precise knowledge of carbohydrate counting.

Conclusions: Parental precision with carbohydrate counting and increased blood glucose monitoring were associated with lower HbA1c in children with type 1 diabetes.

The first report by Gonder-Frederick et al. provides good evidence on practical everyday management of patients in the pediatric diabetes clinic. The authors report declining mental performance and efficiency with naturally occurring hypo- and hyperglycemic glucose fluctuations in children with type 1 diabetes. However, what is most interesting about this paper is that the authors highlight the equal decline in performance for low (<3.0 mmol/l) and high blood glucose concentrations >22.2 mmol/l. These effects can be detected using PDA technology. The impact of severe hypoglycemic episodes on cognitive development in children with diabetes is well known; however, practical demonstration of similar effects from hyperglycemia >22.2 mmol/l has not been previously described. Prevention of extremes of hypo- and hyperglycemia are important as both impact equally on the mental performance and efficiency of the developing brain in childhood diabetes. Mehta et al. demonstrate that precision with carbohydrate counting by parents and increased blood glucose monitoring were associated with lower HbA1c in children with type 1 diabetes. This paper reminds us that in this age group <12 years old, the parent is the primary caregiver and the huge responsibilities that are included in intensive diabetes care for children, including precise carbohydrate counting. The reported reduction in HbA1c by 0.8% was significantly associated with precise carbohydrate counting and more frequent blood glucose measurements. This reduction in HbA1c (almost 1%) is important, according to the Diabetes Complications and Controls Trial (DCCT), which demonstrated that intensive diabetes care effectively delays the onset and slows the progression of diabetic retinopathy (76%), nephropathy (39%), and neuropathy (60%) in patients with type 1 diabetes [6]. These two papers report practical data for the everyday management of children and highlight the importance of carbohydrate counting and prevention of extremes of glucose fluctuations. These papers reflect some of the NICE guidelines [7]. These papers are neither randomized nor population-based but both provide sound important practical evidence on more than 60 children in each cohort <12 years old with type 1 diabetes.

Clinical trials, new treatments

Nasal insulin to prevent type 1 diabetes in children with HLA genotypes and autoantibodies conferring increased risk of disease: a double-blind, randomised controlled trial

Nanto-Salonen K, Kupila A, Simell S, Siljander H, Salonsaari T, Hekkala A, Korhonen S, Erkkola R, Sipila JI, Haavisto L, Siltala M, Tuominen J, Hakalax J, Hyoty H, Ilonen J, Veijola R, Simell T, Knip M, Simell O
Department of Paediatrics, University of Turku, Turku, Finland
Lancet 2008;372:1746–1755

Background: In mouse models of diabetes, prophylactic insulin reduced incidence of the disease. The authors investigated whether administration of nasal insulin decreased the incidence of type 1 diabetes, in children with HLA genotypes and susceptibility autoantibodies.

Methods: At three university hospitals in Turku, Oulu, and Tampere (Finland), cord blood samples were analyzed of 116,720 consecutively born infants, and 3,430 of their siblings, for the HLA-DQB1 susceptibility alleles for type 1 diabetes. 17,397 infants and 1,613 siblings had increased genetic risk, of whom 11,225 and 1,574, respectively, consented to screening of diabetes-associated autoantibodies at every 3–12 months. During this double-blind trial, patients were randomly assigned 224 infants and 40 siblings positive for two or more autoantibodies, in consecutive samples, to receive short-acting human insulin (1 unit/kg; n = 115 and n = 22) or placebo (n = 109 and n = 18) once a day intranasally. Restricted randomization was used, stratified by site, with permuted blocks of size two. Primary end-point was diagnosis of diabetes. Analysis was by intention to treat. The study was terminated early because insulin had no beneficial effect.

Results: Median duration of the intervention was 1.8 years (range 0–9.7). Diabetes was diagnosed in 49 index children randomized to receive insulin, and in 47 randomized to placebo (hazard ratio [HR] 1.14; 95% CI 0.73–1.77). 42 and 38 of these children, respectively, continued treatment until diagnosis, with yearly rates of diabetes onset of 16.8% (95% CI 11.7–21.9) and 15.3% (10.5–20.2). Seven siblings were diagnosed with diabetes in the insulin group, versus 6 in the placebo group (HR 1.93; 0.56–6.77). In all randomized children, diabetes was diagnosed in 56 in the insulin group, and 53 in the placebo group (HR 0.98; 0.67–1.43, p = 0.91).

Conclusions: In children with HLA-conferred susceptibility to diabetes, administration of nasal insulin, started soon after detection of autoantibodies, does not prevent or delay type 1 diabetes.

In this large double-blinded randomized controlled trial from Finland, 11 225 and 1574 infants and their siblings were finally included to assess their HLA susceptibility to diabetes. Administration of nasal insulin, started soon after detection of autoantibodies does not prevent or delay type 1 diabetes. This paper has a good study design but the problem lies in the very indirect assessment (diabetes or not) of the immune tolerance that is meant to be induced by intra-nasal administration. At time of writing, nasal insulin that was meant to deliver hormonally active (rather than immunologically active) insulin has been withdrawn from the retail market. Perhaps if rapid acting analogues were used instead of nasal insulin the results might be more relevant to clinical practice and diabetes care. This study highlights that even with national screening in Finland and early autoantibody susceptibility screening the prophylactic use of nasal insulin does not prevent the onset of diabetes and that new schemes should be evaluated to induce immune tolerance in type 1 diabetes.

Growth response to an individualised versus fixed dose GH treatment in short children born small for gestational age: the OPTIMA study

Jung H, Land C, Nicolay C, De Schepper J, Blum WF, Schonau E
Lilly Research Laboratories, Bad Homburg, Germany
jung_heike@lilly.com
Eur J Endocrinol 2009;160:149–156

Background: This randomized, open-label, multicenter study compared the effect of an individually adjusted GH dose versus a fixed high GH dose over 1 year in 194 prepubertal children born small for gestational age (SGA) who failed to show catch-up growth and were severely short. Initial GH-induced catch-up growth is highly variable in short SGA children and is mainly influenced by age at start of therapy and GH dose.

Methods: The fixed high GH dose group received 67 µg/kg/day GH continuously throughout the 12-month study. The individually adjusted GH dose group initially received 35 µg/kg/day GH. After 3 months of treatment, if predicted annual change was <0.75 SDS using the Cologne Growth-Prediction Model, then the dose of GH was increased to 67 µg/kg/day for the remaining 9 months, otherwise the initial dose was continued.

Results: In the individually adjusted GH dose group, 38 out of the 80 patients required a GH dose increase from month 3 following the prediction model application. From an ANCOVA for non-inferiority, mean difference in change in height SDS between individually adjusted GH dose and fixed high GH dose groups was –0.24 (95% confidence interval (CI) –0.35: –0.12), the CI for height SDS being above the predefined non-inferiority margin of –0.5 SDS based on reasonable expectations. Safety data were similar between groups but a reduction of GH dose due to IGF-I SDS >0.5 and IGFBP-3 SDS <–0.5 was made in 4/99 fixed high GH dose patients, but not in any of the individually adjusted GH dose group patients.

Conclusions: There was a statistically significant mean difference of 1 cm lower total growth over the full year in the individually adjusted GH dose compared with the fixed high GH dose group, although this was considered non-inferior as per the predetermined endpoint. The authors suggest that early growth prediction may be used to tailor the dose to the individual patient's needs, thus resulting in a lower overall GH dose.

European multicentre study in children born small for gestational age with persistent short stature: comparison of continuous and discontinuous growth hormone treatment regimens

Phillip M, Lebenthal Y, Lebl J, Zuckerman-Levin N, Korpal-Szczyrska M, Marques JS, Steensberg A, Jons K, Kappelgaard AM, Ibanez L, European Norditropin SGASG
Institute for Endocrinology and Diabetes, Schneider Children's Medical Center of Israel and Sackler Faculty of Medicine, Tel-Aviv University, Tel-Aviv, Israel
mosheph@post.tau.ac.il
Horm Res 2009;71:52–59

Background: This was a multinational randomized, prospective, 2-year parallel group study designed to investigate the most effective GH treatment regimen for increasing height in short children born SGA.
Methods: A total of 151 SGA children aged 3–8 years, height below –2.5 standard deviation scores) were randomized into three groups: low-dose GH continuously for 2 years (33 µg/kg/day, n = 51); high-dose GH for 1 year (100 µg/kg/day, n = 51) and then no treatment for 1 year; or were left untreated for 1 year then received mid-dose GH for 1 year (67 µg/kg/day, n = 47). Height, bone age and adverse events were determined during 3 monthly assessments.
Results: The additional height increase with GH after 1 year, compared with untreated controls, was greater with high-dose than with low-dose GH (mean (SD) gain 6.5 ± 0.2 vs. 3.3 ± 0.2 cm). After 2 years, the additional height gain was similar between high- and low-dose GH groups (between-group treatment difference = 0.2 cm, 95% CI = –0.8 to 1.2 cm, p = 0.702). Patients treated exclusively in the last year with mid-dose GH had a similar height gain to those in the other treatment groups (p = 0.604). The total height gain in all three groups was 1.1–1.2 SDS. Maximum IGF-1 levels rose to 0.9 SD in the low-dose group, 3.3 SD in the high-dose group, and 2.9 SD in the mid-dose group.
Conclusions: In short SGA children, continuous low-dose and discontinuous high-dose GH regimens were associated with similar height gain. Treatment with mid-dose GH for 1 year also led to a similar improvement in growth. GH treatment allowed approximately half the children in each group to achieve a stature above –2 SDS after 2 years from pretreatment values below –3.1 SDS.

Maximizing height gain with the minimum of GH dosing in short SGA children who demonstrate a degree of GH resistance is a tricky challenge, and these two studies show imaginative, yet different approaches. Each is a large-scale multinational randomized trial with novel treatment strategies. Both sought to augment the all-important period of catch-up growth over the first 2 years. Phillip et al. confirmed that double and triple the conventional dose of GH for 1 year achieved similar height gains to 2 years' treatment at standard low dose (33 µg/kg/day), but at what cost? The high-dose regimen produced impressively quick catch-up growth, showing that supraphysiological GH doses can overdrive the GH-IGF axis into a maximal response mode, but despite no significant metabolic disturbance being demonstrated, concern must remain with the rise of IGF-1 levels to +3.3 SD, and unknown long-term consequences.

Jung et al. employed a prediction algorithm, the Cologne Growth-Prediction Model, for first year GH responsiveness. The predicted height velocity after 3 months' GH treatment can be calculated from HV response, pretreatment IGF-1 levels, bone age retardation and urinary deoxypyridinoline levels 1 month into treatment. If this value was below the predetermined level of 0.75 SDS, then the GH dosage regimen was doubled from the standard 35 µg/kg/day. Only half of the study limb needed dose adjustments upwards, and although this approach produced a smaller growth increment, the authors argue this was not of major clinical relevance. Additionally, although the higher dosing regimen in both limbs increased IGF-1 levels, maximum levels of +1.1 SDS, only 4% required a GH dose reduction. This type of approach may herald a more economical and safe approach to improved therapeutic efficacy. However, we now have half a dozen prediction models, yet too many of them include parameters that are not readily available – urinary deoxypyridinoline levels in this report. We look forward for a model based on simple auxology and minimal laboratory workup.

Long-term follow-up and comparison between genotype and phenotype in 29 cases of complete androgen insensitivity syndrome

Cheikhelard A, Morel Y, Thibaud E, Lortat-Jacob S, Jaubert F, Polak M, Nihoul-Fekete C
Department of Pediatric Surgery, APHP Hôpital Necker-Enfants Malades and Université Paris Descartes, Paris, France
J Urol 2008;180:1496–1501

Background: The aim of this study was to assess the safety of keeping gonads in place for spontaneous puberty in a consecutive cohort of patients with complete androgen insensitivity syndrome confirmed by genetic analysis as the diagnosis and management has dramatically changed over the last few decades, with earlier diagnosis and the development of molecular biology. Some patients maintaining wolffian and müllerian remnants may have subtle residual androgen activity. Variations of these features clearly exist among patients and may influence treatment. The need for vaginal surgery and gonadectomy was investigated on account of the potential risks of virilization at puberty and gonadal tumor development.

Methods: The authors reported the clinical outcome of 29 cases of complete androgen insensitivity syndrome managed by the same team from diagnosis (frequently in early childhood) to adulthood. They studied the genotype, phenotype, anatomy of the internal and external genitalia.

Results: All of the patients had a complete female phenotype. 19 different mutations (including 7 unreported) were found. Each family presented with a different mutation. No somatic mosaicism was detected. Vas deferens and epididymis were found in all types of mutations (missense, nonsense and frameshift). 23 patients were postpubertal at the time of reporting. Of those 19 with spontaneous pubertal development, no virilization was seen. Only 1 patient developed carcinoma in situ when the gonad was removed prophylactically once puberty was complete. Vaginal surgery was rarely necessary.

Conclusions: The authors recommend that removal of the gonads in the complete androgen insensitivity syndrome need only take place once spontaneous puberty is complete. The risk of virilization at puberty should be ruled out for each individual androgen receptor mutation before management decisions and genetic counseling are undertaken. Vaginal surgery is not necessary as first-line treatment.

Detailed long-term studies of relatively unselected cohorts combining genetic and clinical outcomes are rare, and that is why this report provides a valuable and unique insight into the management of females with CAIS. The general feeling of anxiety to remove the gonads at the earliest opportunity may have arisen from confusion with the clear association of dysgenetic gonads with the risk of gonadoblastoma. This has not been reported in CAIS. Carcinoma in situ and seminoma may occur, but mainly after 18 years of age, and carcinoma in situ was found in only 1 postpubertal patient in this cohort, hence the recommendation they make is to leave gonads in situ until after puberty has completed spontaneously, although the authors admitted this study did not look in detail at the psychological consequences of doing this. Benign testicular changes such as Sertoli adenomas and polar hamartomas were found more frequently in the postpubertal gonads. In the testes which were left, spermatic tubules tended to deteriorate in shape and germ cells disappeared progressively after 1 year of age. Inguinal hernia was the commonest form of presentation of childhood CAIS, none progressing beyond the inguinal ring. This was followed by prenatal diagnosis as the second most frequent where a mismatch between karyotype and ultrasonic phenotype was seen. This contrasts with the typical mode of presentation in late adolescence and adulthood of primary amenorrhea. Although the degree of wolffian duct remnants in 69% was very variable, there was no association with virilization (as in CAH) or genotype. Pubic or axillary hair development (if any) was not regarded as a sign of virilization, and was not associated with any particular genotype. Müllerian duct remnants were seen associated with the gonad in 38%, but complete uteri or fallopian tubes have never been reported in cases of CAIS. All of the patients had a completely normal female phenotype with a vagina of variable length. Androgen receptor mutations were identified in all patients, 17 cases occurring in 8 families, and there was only one de novo mutation. There was no association between anatomy and genotype.

Long-term GH treatment improves adult height in children with Noonan syndrome with and without mutations in protein tyrosine phosphatase, non-receptor type 11

Noordam C, Peer PG, Francois I, De Schepper J, van den Burgt I, Otten BJ
Department of Metabolic and Endocrine Diseases 833, Radboud University Medical Centre, Nijmegen, the Netherlands
c.noordam@cukz.umcn.nl
Eur J Endocrinol 2008;159:203–208

Background: Noonan syndrome (NS) is characterized by short stature, typical facial dysmorphology and mostly right-sided congenital heart defects. GH therapy in NS may produce short-term gains in height, but reports on the effect on adult height are scarce. This study aimed to determine the effect of long-term GH therapy in children with NS.

Methods: 29 children with the clinical diagnosis of NS from endocrinology departments in the Netherlands and Belgium were treated with GH until final height was reached. At the mean age of 11.0 years at the start of therapy, GH was administered subcutaneously at 50 µg/kg/day until growth velocity was 1 cm/6 months. Height was measured at 3-month intervals in the first year and at 6-month intervals thereafter until final height. 22 out of 27 tested children had a mutation in the protein tyrosine phosphatase, non-receptor type 11 gene (PTPN11 gene).

Results: At the start of treatment, median height SDS was –2.8 (–4.1 to –1.8) and 0.0 (–1.4 to +1.2), based on National Dutch/Belgian and Noonan standards respectively. GH therapy continued for 3.0–10.3 years (median 6.4 years), producing mean height gains of +1.3 SDS (+0.2 to +2.7) and +1.3 SDS (–0.6 to +2.4), compared with the National and Noonan standards respectively. In 22 children with a mutation in PTPN11 the mean gain for national standards was +1.3 SDS and not different from the mean height gain in the 5 children who did not show this mutation in PTPN11 of also +1.3 SDS (p = 0.98).

Conclusions: Long-term GH treatment in NS leads to attainment of adult height within the normal range in most patients (22/29). Safety monitoring revealed no concerns on carbohydrate metabolism or cardiovascular status.

This is the final report of a cohort study of pre- and peripubertal patients with NS, who did not have hypertrophic cardiomyopathy and whose height at referral was –2 SDS. Although this was not a randomized or controlled trial, the patients followed a carefully conducted protocol of a relatively high-dose GH, and this report of adult height must surely provide the best evidence of outcome. This in fact does represent the type of patient who would potentially be considered for GH therapy. The gain of +1.3 SDS represents about a 9.5 cm increase in boys and 9 cm in girls. Height gain after 4 years on treatment was maintained until adult height. The authors recommend that the use of Noonan-specific standards is a better predictor of height gain than bone age. This study provides the first report of adult height in long-term GH treatment where genetic analysis was performed. This study had a preponderance of children with PTPN11 mutations, thus it is not possible to state the magnitude of the effect of GH in children with ras and SOS1 and BRAF mutations. However, PTPN11 and thus SHP-2 mutations may be associated with mild GH resistance on account of a postreceptor signaling defect, and that this may have a transient influence on GH treatment. More data on the outcome of GH treatment in children with other NS mutations are needed to explore this further.

High versus low dose of initial thyroid hormone replacement for congenital hypothyroidism

Ng SM, Anand D, Weindling AM
School of Reproductive and Developmental Medicine, University of Liverpool, Liverpool Women's Hospital, Liverpool, UK
ngszemay@yahoo.com
Cochrane Database Syst Rev 2009(1):CD006972

Background: Congenital hypothyroidism (CHT) is one of the most common preventable causes of learning difficulties, affecting 1 in 4,000 infants. This systematic review aimed to determine the effects of high versus low dose of initial thyroid hormone replacement for CHT.
Methods: Randomized controlled trials were identified by searching The Cochrane Library, Medline and Embase. Randomized controlled clinical trials assessing the effects of high versus low dose of initial thyroid hormone replacement for CHT were chosen. Authors independently selected trials, assessed risk of bias and extracted data.
Results: The initial search identified 1,014 records which identified 13 publications for further examination. After screening the full text of the 13 selected papers, only one study evaluating 47 babies finally met the inclusion criteria. Using the same cohort at two different time periods, the study investigated the effects of high- versus low-dose thyroid hormone replacement in relation to (1) time taken to achieve euthyroid state and (2) neurodevelopmental outcome. The authors reported that a high dose is more effective at establishing free thyroxine concentrations in the normal range and also allows earlier normalization of thyroid-stimulating hormone compared with a lower dose. Intelligence quotient was significantly higher in children who received the high dose compared with the lower dose. No growth and adverse effects were reported.
Conclusions: Currently there is only one randomized controlled trial evaluating the effects of high versus low dose of initial thyroid hormone replacement for CHT. Current evidence is inadequate to confirm that a high dose is more beneficial than low dose as initial thyroid hormone replacement in the management of CHT.

Effect of high versus low initial doses of l-thyroxine for congenital hypothyroidism on thyroid function and somatic growth

Jones JH, Gellen B, Paterson WF, Beaton S, Donaldson MD
Royal Hospital for Sick Children, Glasgow, UK
Arch Dis Child 2008;93:940–944

Background: The optimal dose of thyroxine (T_4) in congenital hypothyroidism (CH) during infancy is controversial. Higher doses lead to improvement in cognitive scores, but have been linked to later behavioral difficulties. The authors examined the effects of initial T_4 dose on somatic growth – a marker of overtreatment.
Methods: 314 CH children (214 girls, 100 boys) were analyzed according to initial daily dose of T_4: group 1 (25 µg, n = 152), group 2 (30-40 µg, n = 63) and group 3 (50 µg, n = 99). Thyroid function and weight, length and occipito-frontal head circumference (OFC) standard deviation score (SDS) were compared at 3, 6, 12, 18, 24 and 36 months of age. Linear growth SDS was compared between the three groups using a regression adjustment model. Thyroid function was compared at diagnosis (T0), 7–21 days and after the start of treatment (T1).
Results: At T1, median thyroid-stimulating hormone (TSH) for groups 1, 2 and 3 was 58, 29 and 4.1 mU/l, respectively (p < 0.001), group 3 values remaining significantly lower at 3 and 6 months. Median free T_4 (fT_4) was within or just above the reference range in all groups at T1, but 7.4% of group 1 had values <9 pmol/l compared with 5.1 and 0% for groups 2 and 3. At 3 months, weight, length and OFC SDS values were −0.39, −0.35, 0.09; −0.30, −0.47, 0.32; and −0.03, −0.13, 0.18 for groups 1, 2 and 3, respectively, reporting a relatively large OFC in these infants. Regression analysis revealed no significant difference in growth rate from baseline and 12 or 18 months of age, between the three groups.
Conclusions: A T_4 dose of 50 µg daily at onset of disease normalizes thyroid function several months earlier than lower doses, with no evidence of somatic overgrowth between 3 months and 3 years.

These two papers were reviewed under the common endocrine disorder of congenital hypothyroidism (CHT). A Cochrane systematic review highlighted that only one randomized controlled trial was available to evaluate the effects of high- versus low-dose thyroxine for CHT. The authors concluded from this one trial that there was inadequate evidence to confirm that a high dose is more beneficial than low dose as initial thyroid hormone replacement in the management of CHT. The paper by Jones et al., on the other hand, used a different approach to explore the evidence for an initial higher dose regimen. They retrospectively analyzed 26 years' detailed data from a national database. Although no information on neurodevelopmental outcome was available, Jones et al. conclude that an initial thyroxine dose of 50 µg/day normalizes thyroid function several months earlier than lower doses with no evidence of somatic overgrowth between 3 months and 3 years.

The conflicting conclusions from these papers highlight that optimal initial management of CHT with high dose (50 µg/day) thyroid hormone remains controversial. This controversy remains largely on account of the paucity of well-conducted RCTs to definitively prove the point that high-dose treatment can achieve optimal intellectual development with no adverse sequelae. This contrasts with our current clinical understanding and practice, and underlines why it is important to gather evidence for therapeutic approaches in a systematic manner.

References

1. O'Riordan SM, Butler G: Evidence-based medicine in pediatric endocrinology; in Carel JC, Hochberg Z (eds): Yearbook of Pediatric Endocrinology. Basel, Karger, 2008, pp 177–193.
2. Cohen P, Rogol AD, Deal CL, Saenger P, Reiter EO, Ross JL, et al: Consensus statement on the diagnosis and treatment of children with idiopathic short stature: a summary of the Growth Hormone Research Society, the Lawson Wilkins Pediatric Endocrine Society, and the European Society for Paediatric Endocrinology Workshop. J Clin Endocrinol Metab 2008;93:4210–4217.
3. Ritzen EM: Undescended testes: a consensus on management. Eur J Endocrinol 2008;159(suppl 1):S87–S90.
4. Tamborlane WV, Beck RW: Continuous glucose monitoring in type 1 diabetes mellitus. Lancet 2009;373:1744–1746.
5. Bode BW: Sustained benefits of continuous glucose monitoring through 12 months of sensor use in the JDRF CGM Randomized Clinical Trial. American Diabetes Assoication, New Orleans, June 204-OR2009.
6. DCCT: The effect of intensive treatment of diabetes on the development and progression of long-term complications in insulin-dependent diabetes mellitus – Diabetes Control and Complications (DCCT) Research Group. N Engl J Med 1993;329:977–986.
7. Pickup JC, Hammond P: NICE guidance on continuous subcutaneous insulin infusion 2008: review of the technology appraisal guidance. Diabet Med 2009;26:1–4.

Editors' Choice

Jean-Claude Carel and Ze'ev Hochberg

Clinical trials: turn off the sugar high but do no harm

Intensive insulin therapy for patients in paediatric intensive care: a prospective, randomised controlled study

Vlasselaers D, Milants I, Desmet L, Wouters PJ, Vanhorebeek I, van den Heuvel I, Mesotten D, Casaer MP, Meyfroidt G, Ingels C, Muller J, Van Cromphaut S, Schetz M, Van den Berghe G
Department of Intensive Care Medicine (Paediatric Intensive Care Unit), Catholic University Leuven, Leuven, Belgium
Lancet 2009;373:547–556

Background: Critically ill infants and children often develop hyperglycemia, which is associated with adverse outcome; however, whether lowering blood glucose concentrations to age-adjusted normal fasting values improves outcome is unknown. We investigated the effect of targeting age-adjusted normoglycemia with insulin infusion in critically ill infants and children on outcome.

Methods: In a prospective, randomized controlled study, this project enrolled 700 critically ill patients, 317 infants (aged <1 year) and 383 children (aged ≥1 year), who were admitted to the pediatric intensive care unit (PICU) of the University Hospital of Leuven, Belgium. Patients were randomly assigned by blinded envelopes to target blood glucose concentrations of 2.8–4.4 mmol/l in infants and 3.9–5.6 mmol/l in children with insulin infusion throughout PICU stay (intensive group [n = 349]), or to insulin infusion only to prevent blood glucose from exceeding 11.9 mmol/l (conventional group [n = 351]). Patients and laboratory staff were blinded to treatment allocation. Primary endpoints were duration of PICU stay and inflammation. Analysis was by intention-to-treat. This study is registered with ClinicalTrials.gov, number NCT00214916.

Findings: Mean blood glucose concentrations were lower in the intensive group than in the conventional group (infants: 4.8 [SD 1.2] vs. 6.4 [1.2] mmol/l, p < 0.0001; children: 5.3 [1.1] vs. 8.2 [3.3] mmol/l, p < 0.0001). Hypoglycemia (defined as blood glucose ≤2.2 mmol/l) occurred in 87 (25%) patients in the intensive group (p < 0.0001) versus 5 (1%) patients in the conventional group; hypoglycemia defined as blood glucose <1.7 mmol/l arose in 17 (5%) patients versus 3 (1%; p = 0.001). Duration of PICU stay was shortest in the intensively treated group (5.51 [95% CI 4.65–6.37] vs. 6.15 days [5.25–7.05], p = 0.017). The inflammatory response was attenuated at day 5, as indicated by lower C-reactive protein in the intensive group compared with baseline (–9.75 [95% CI –19.93 to 0.43] vs. 8.97 mg/l [–0.9 to 18.84], p = 0.007). The number of patients with extended (>median) stay in PICU was 132 (38%) in the intensive group versus 165 (47%) in the conventional group (p = 0.013). Nine (3%) patients died in the intensively treated group versus 20 (6%) in the conventional group (p = 0.038).

Conclusion: Targeting of blood glucose concentrations to age-adjusted normal fasting concentrations improved short-term outcome of patients in PICU. The effect on long-term survival, morbidity, and neurocognitive development needs to be investigated.

Early insulin therapy in very-low-birth-weight infants

Beardsall K, Vanhaesebrouck S, Ogilvy-Stuart AL, Vanhole C, Palmer CR, van Weissenbruch M, Midgley P, Thompson M, Thio M, Cornette L, Ossuetta I, Iglesias I, Theyskens C, de Jong M, Ahluwalia JS, de Zegher F, Dunger DB
University of Cambridge, Cambridge, UK
N Engl J Med 2008;359:1873–1884

Background: Studies involving adults and children being treated in intensive care units indicate that insulin therapy and glucose control may influence survival. Hyperglycemia is also associated with morbidity and mortality. An international randomized, controlled trial aimed to determine whether early insulin replacement reduced hyperglycemia and affected outcomes in such very-low-birth-weight neonates.

Methods: In this multicenter trial, 195 infants were assigned to continuous infusion of insulin at a dose of 0.05 U/kg/h with 20% dextrose support and 194 to standard neonatal care on days 1–7. The efficacy of glucose control was assessed by continuous glucose monitoring. The primary outcome was mortality at the expected date of delivery. The study was discontinued early because of concerns about futility with regard to the primary outcome and potential harm.

Results: As compared with infants in the control group, infants in the early-insulin group had lower mean (±SD) glucose levels (6.2 ± 1.4 vs. 6.7 ± 2.2 mmol/l, p = 0.007). Fewer infants in the early-insulin group had hyperglycemia for more than 10% of the first week of life (21 vs. 33%, p = 0.008). The early-insulin group had significantly more carbohydrate infused (51 ± 13 vs. 43 ± 10 kcal/kg/day, p < 0.001) and less weight loss in the first week (standard-deviation score for change in weight, –0.55 ± 0.52 vs. –0.70 ± 0.47; p = 0.006). More infants in the early-insulin group had episodes of hypoglycemia (defined as a blood glucose level of <2.6 mmol/l for >1 h; 29% in the early-insulin group vs. 17% in the control group, p = 0.005), and the increase in hypoglycemia was significant in infants with birth weights of more than 1 kg. There were no differences in the intention-to-treat analyses for the primary outcome (mortality at the expected date of delivery) and the secondary outcome (morbidity). In the intention-to-treat analysis, mortality at 28 days was higher in the early-insulin group than in the control group (p = 0.04).

Conclusions: Early insulin therapy offers little clinical benefit in very-low-birth-weight infants. It reduces hyperglycemia but may increase hypoglycemia.

Hyperglycemia is prevalent in patients in pediatric ICUs and in premature very low birth weight infants. The extent of hyperglycemia correlates with adverse outcome of a critical illness. Whether these associations are an indicator of the severity of the underlying illness, or rather that hyperglycemia or hypoglycemia in themselves are risk factors, is unclear. Two large studies this year postulated that targeting age-adjusted normoglycemia with insulin infusion in critically ill infants and children in the ICU would improve outcome, and designed randomized controlled studies to test this hypothesis. Quite interestingly, the 2 studies yielded quite radically different results. In the pediatric ICU, intensive insulin therapy protected the cardiovascular system, prevented secondary infections, and attenuated the inflammatory response, reducing the need for extended stay in the ICU. Mortality was lowered by 3.1% due to prevention of lethal neurological and pulmonary damage, and possibly prevention of infection. In contrast, in very low birth weight premature babies, although glucose targets were nicely reached, the overall outcome was unfavorable and the study had to be discontinued due to concerns about potential harm, although a preliminary study had given positive results [1]. The risk of hypoglycemia with insulin therapy in these young patient populations necessitates a long-term follow-up study to quantify late survival and morbidity, especially the effect of hyperglycemia and hypoglycemia on the developing brain. Overall these 2 studies illustrate the difficulties of addressing important questions regarding management through ambitious randomized controlled trials. Unavoidable biases (for instance the study by Vlasselaers et al. had 75% of the patients in the ICU after heart surgery) might affect the outcomes and practical problems with managing insulin and glucose infusion might also affect the outcomes. In any case, the authors of the positive study admit that the findings cannot be generalized at this time and that tight blood glucose control requires exceptional expertise of the nursing team.

Mechanism of the year: on the benefits of eating oneself

Autophagy regulates lipid metabolism

Singh R, Kaushik S, Wang Y, Xiang Y, Novak I, Komatsu M, Tanaka K, Cuervo AM, Czaja MJ
Department of Medicine, Albert Einstein College of Medicine, Bronx, New York, N.Y., USA
Nature 2009;458:1131–1135

Context: The intracellular storage and utilization of lipids are critical to maintain cellular energy homeostasis. During nutrient deprivation, cellular lipids stored as triglycerides in lipid droplets are hydrolyzed into fatty acids for energy. A second cellular response to starvation is the induction of autophagy, which

                                                Jean-Claude Carel/Ze'ev Hochberg

delivers intracellular proteins and organelles sequestered in double-membrane vesicles (autophago-somes) to lysosomes for degradation and use as an energy source. Lipolysis and autophagy share simi-larities in regulation and function but are not known to be interrelated.

Aim: The authors show a previously unknown function for autophagy in regulating intracellular lipid stores (macrolipophagy).

Results: Lipid droplets and autophagic components associated during nutrient deprivation, and inhibi-tion of autophagy in cultured hepatocytes and mouse liver increased triglyceride storage in lipid drop-lets.

Conclusions: This study identifies a critical function for autophagy in lipid metabolism that could have important implications for human diseases with lipid over-accumulation such as those that comprise the metabolic syndrome.

When starved, cells degrade proteins, lipids and even whole organelles. Autophagy targets all three cellular components. Fatty acids are stored as triglycerides in dynamic lipid droplets, and, when nec-essary, are released by lipolysis. Established models of lipid storage and breakdown have undergone substantial revision in recent years. For many years it was believed that hormone-sensitive lipase acted alone lipolysis. The discovery of the regulatory proteins of the fat drop perilipin and CGI-58 encouraged a new look at lipolysis.

We now learn that autophagy, the pathway by which excess or damaged organelles and proteins are degraded, also mediates fat mobilization and breakdown in hepatocytes. In autophagy, destined cel-lular organelles are trapped in double-membrane-bound autophagosomes, and are then broken down in lysosomes. Singh et al. show that, under fasting conditions, specific cytoplasmic proteins are recruited to lipid droplets, where they form a double membrane that encloses droplet parts that fuse with lysosomes, and their contents are degraded. They also show that feeding the animals a high-fat diet impairs autophagy-mediated breakdown, so that increased fat consumption may be associated with decreased fat removal and excessive lipid deposition. A similar response in obese people would explain how they might develop fatty-liver disease.

A new hormone: a lipid posing

N-acylphosphatidylethanolamine, a gut-derived circulating factor induced by fat ingestion, inhibits food intake

Gillum MP, Zhang D, Zhang XM, Erion DM, Jamison RA, Choi C, Dong J, Shanabrough M, Duenas HR, Frederick DW, Hsiao JJ, Horvath TL, Lo CM, Tso P, Cline GW, Shulman GI
Howard Hughes Medical Institute, Yale University School of Medicine, New Haven, Conn., USA
Cell 2008;135:813–824

Context: N-acylphosphatidylethanolamines (NAPEs) are a relatively abundant group of plasma lipids of unknown physiological significance.

Results: NAPEs were secreted into circulation from the small intestine in response to ingested fat. Systemic administration of the most abundant circulating NAPE, at physiologic doses, decreased food intake in rats without causing conditioned taste aversion. Radiolabeled NAPE entered the brain and was concen-trated in the hypothalamus. Intracerebroventicular infusions of nanomolar amounts of NAPE reduce food intake. Chronic NAPE infusion results in a reduction of both food intake and body weight,

Conclusions: NAPE effects may be mediated through direct interactions with the central nervous system. NAPE and long-acting NAPE analogs may be novel therapeutic targets for the treatment of obesity.

Neuronal sensing of fatty acids (FAs) has been implicated in the regulation of feeding behavior by studies demonstrating that food intake can be reduced through inhibition of FA synthase or intrath-ecal oleic acid infusion. In contrast to plasma glucose and amino acids, which increase after meals, plasma FAs typically decrease with feeding and rise with fasting, contrary to what is expected of a negative regulator of appetite. Furthermore, intravenous infusions of lipid do not affect food intake, and thus it was unclear how either circulating triglyceride or FA signal lipid surfeit to the CNS under physiological conditions. This group hypothesized that food intake could be modified by circulating nutrient signals reflective of meal fat content. Screening lipid derivatives that increased in plasma after high-fat feeding, they discovered a class of phospholipids, the N-acylphosphatidylethanolamines (NAPEs), of previously unknown physiologic function in plasma, whose hydrolysis products, the N-acylethanolamines, have been implicated in the peripheral control of food intake. They found that, at physiologic doses, intraperitoneal and intravenous injection of the most abundant plasma NAPE reduced food intake. NAPE levels increased consistently in rats and mice that had eaten a fatty meal. When synthesized and injected into the laboratory rodents, NAPEs concentrated in the hypothalamus and shut down the rodent's food intake, with one dose lasting 12 h or longer. A curious property of C16:0 NAPE was its ability to reduce locomotor activity in rodents when given systemically or centrally. This may play a physiologic role in mediating the lethargy typically observed in rodents (and humans) during the postabsorptive state. There is precedent for interactions between circulating regulators of appetite and the motor circuits in the brain; acute knockdown of the leptin receptor has been shown to increase locomotor activity in rodents, and the association of lassitude and voracious appetite is the whole mark of hypothalamic obesity. NAPEs is a new circulating FA, synthesized in the small intestine from ingested fat, and may be part of an important physiologic negative feedback loop that serves to reduce food intake and arousal after a fat-containing meal.

New therapy mode: Marfan's syndrome

Angiotensin II blockade and aortic-root dilation in Marfan's syndrome

Brooke BS, Habashi JP, Judge DP, Patel N, Loeys B, Dietz HC, 3rd
McKusick-Nathans Institute of Genetic Medicine, Johns Hopkins University School of Medicine, Baltimore, Md., USA
N Engl J Med 2008;358:2787–2795

Context: Progressive enlargement of the aortic root, leading to dissection, is the main cause of premature death in patients with Marfan's syndrome. Recent data from mouse models of Marfan's syndrome suggest that aortic-root enlargement is caused by excessive signaling by TGF-β that can be mitigated by treatment with TGF-β antagonists, including angiotensin II-receptor blockers (ARBs).
Aim: The authors evaluated the clinical response to ARBs in pediatric patients with Marfan's syndrome who had severe aortic-root enlargement.
Methods: They identified 18 pediatric patients with Marfan's syndrome who had been followed during 12–47 months of therapy with ARBs after other medical therapy had failed to prevent progressive aortic-root enlargement. The ARB was losartan in 17 patients and irbesartan in 1 patient. They evaluated the efficacy of ARB therapy by comparing the rates of change in aortic-root diameter before and after the initiation of treatment with ARBs.
Results: The rate of change in aortic-root diameter decreased significantly from 3.54 ± 2.87 mm/year during previous medical therapy to 0.46 ± 0.62 mm/year during ARB therapy (p < 0.001). The deviation of aortic-root enlargement from normal, as expressed by the rate of change in z scores, was reduced by a mean difference of 1.47 z scores/year (95% CI 0.70–2.24; p < 0.001) after the initiation of ARB therapy. The sinotubular junction, which is prone to dilation in Marfan's syndrome as well, also showed a reduced rate of change in diameter during ARB therapy (p < 0.05), whereas the distal ascending aorta, which does not normally become dilated in Marfan's syndrome, was not affected by ARB therapy.
Conclusions: In a small cohort study, the use of ARB therapy in patients with Marfan's syndrome significantly slowed the rate of progressive aortic-root dilation.

Studies in a mouse model of Marfan's syndrome have shown that a deficiency of fibrillin-1 in the extracellular matrix leads to excessive signaling by TGF-β, an event that probably contributes to the pathogenesis of multiple phenotypic features of Marfan's syndrome, including progressive enlargement of the aortic root. These genetically engineered mice, in which the pathologic changes in the aortic root closely mimic those seen in humans, were subsequently used to demonstrate the therapeutic benefit of treatment with TGF-β antagonists in vivo. The development of pathologic changes in the aortic wall and the progressive dilation of the aortic root were attenuated or prevented by systemic treatment with a TGF-β-neutralizing antibody or the angiotensin-II-receptor blocker losartan, an antihypertensive medication known to inhibit TGF-β signaling. In comparison, mutant mice treated with the β-blocker propranolol continued to show substantial aortic-wall pathologic changes and had only a moderate reduction in the rate of aortic-root dilation. These findings led to this clinical trial of loasartan in patients with Marfan's syndrome. The current study provides early evidence suggesting that the addition of losartan to the traditional regimen used to treat aortic aneurysm in patients with Marfan's syndrome may be beneficial. Therapy resulted in a significant reduction in the rate of change in aortic-root diameter as compared with β-blocker therapy alone. The therapeutic effect extended to the sinotubular junction, a site also affected by Marfan's syndrome. In comparison, aortic segments not typically affected in Marfan's syndrome (e.g., the ascending aorta above the sinotubular junction) continued to show an annual rate of change in diameter that was appropriate for age and body size. Thus, losartan does not arrest aortic growth but specifically reduces the pathologic rate of increase in the diameter of aortic segments that are already of sufficient size to accommodate the physiologic demands of the tissues for blood flow. The authors suggest that despite the encouraging results of this observational study, equipoise is maintained regarding a role for this therapy in the treatment of patients with Marfan's syndrome; these findings must be confirmed by a prospective, randomized trial. Indeed, a trial coordinated by the Pediatric Heart Network of the National Heart, Lung, and Blood Institute, comparing losartan with atenolol in patients with Marfan's syndrome, began enrolling patients.

Concept recentered: adapt to starvation by stunting

Inhibition of growth hormone signaling by the fasting-induced hormone FGF21

Inagaki T, Lin VY, Goetz R, Mohammadi M, Mangelsdorf DJ, Kliewer SA
Department of Molecular Biology, University of Texas Southwestern Medical Center, Dallas, Tex., USA
Cell Metab 2008;8:77–83

Aim: The authors investigated fibroblast growth factor 21 (FGF21) effect on possible GH resistance.
Results: In liver, FGF21 reduced concentrations of the active form of STAT5, and caused corresponding decreases in the expression of its target genes, including IGF-1. FGF21 also induces hepatic expression of IGF-1-binding protein 1 and suppressor of cytokine signaling 2, which blunt GH signaling. Chronic exposure to FGF21 markedly inhibited growth in mice.
Conclusion: These data suggest a central role for FGF21 in inhibiting growth as part of its broader role in inducing the adaptive response to starvation.

Fibroblast growth factor 21 (FGF21) has recently taken center stage as a key metabolic hormone that helps the body to adapt to starvation [Yearbook 2008]. One way to adapt is to stunt growth. When mice are fasted, FGF21 expression levels in the liver rise, and in turn, FGF21 stimulates the release of fatty acids from adipose tissue and promotes their conversion in the liver to ketone bodies, which can be used as an energy source when carbohydrates are scarce. This study reports that FGF21 inhibits STAT5 signaling and the expression of IGF-1 through its PPAR effect, and thereby blunts GH action as part of its broader role in promoting energy conservation during starvation. Cross-talk between PPARα and STAT5B has been previously described in cell-based assays, with GH-activated STAT5B inhibiting PPARα-regulated gene transcription, and conversely, ligand-activated PPARα inhibiting STAT5B-regulated transcription. Thus, cross-talk between PPARα and STAT5 may occur at multiple levels. Notably, in clinical studies the PPARα agonist bezafibrate significantly lowers IGF-1 levels in patients. This finding together with data showing that FGF21 expression is induced by PPARα agonists in primary human hepatocytes suggest that the PPARα/FGF21 pathway may be operative and affect IGF-1 signaling in humans.

Aquaporin 1 is important for maintaining secretory granule biogenesis in endocrine cells

Arnaoutova I, Cawley NX, Patel N, Kim T, Rathod T, Loh YP
National Institutes of Health, Bethesda, Md., USA

Mol Endocrinol 2008;22:1924–1934

Context: Aquaporins (AQPs), a family of water channels expressed in epithelial cells, function to transport water in a bidirectional manner to facilitate transepithelial fluid absorption and secretion. Additionally, AQP1 and AQP5 are found in pancreatic zymogen granules and synaptic vesicles and are involved in vesicle swelling and exocytosis in exocrine cells and neurons.

Aim: The authors show AQP1 in dense-core secretory granule (DCSG) membranes of endocrine tissue: pituitary and adrenal medulla.

Methods and Results: The need for AQP1 in endocrine cell function was examined by stable transfection of AQP1 antisense RNA into AtT20 cells, a pituitary cell line, to downregulate AQP1 expression. These AQP1-deficient cells showed more than 60% depletion of DCSGs and significantly decreased DCSG protein levels, including proopiomelanocortin/pro-ATCH and prohormone convertase 1/3, but not non-DCSG proteins. Pulse-chase studies revealed that whereas DCSG protein synthesis was unaffected, approximately 50% of the newly synthesized proopiomelanocortin was degraded within 1 h. Low levels of ACTH were released upon stimulation, indicating that the small number of DCSGs that were made in the presence of the residual AQP1 were functionally competent for exocytosis. Analysis of anterior pituitaries from AQP1 knockout mice showed reduced prohormone convertase 1/3, carboxypeptidase E, and ACTH levels compared to wild-type mice demonstrating that our results observed in AtT20 cells can be extended to the animal model.

Conclusion: AQP1 is important for maintaining DCSG biogenesis and normal levels of hormone secretion in pituitary endocrine cells.

Secretory granules are key organelles for secretion of hormones in endocrine cells in response to stimulation. They are stored within the cell, and as water enters the granules, causing them to swell during exocytosis, they release their contents upon stimulation. AQP1 present on the granule membrane has been shown to participate in the rapid vesicular water gating and swelling during exocytosis. This study investigated the role of AQP1 in pituitary endocrine cell function. We found that induction of DCSG granule biogenesis by chromogranin A (CgA) in a mutant pituitary cell line lacking granules, which led to a significant increase in expression of AQP1 mRNA and protein. They show that AQP1 is present in the membrane fraction of pituitary secretory granules and adrenal chromaffin granules. Furthermore, downregulation of APQ1 expression led to attenuated regulated secretion of ACTH. These results corroborate with decreased ACTH levels in the pituitary and serum in the AQP1 KO mice. The findings demonstrate that AQP1 is important for maintaining secretory function and granule biogenesis, and hence normal hormone sequestration in endocrine cells.

Physiological significance of a peripheral tissue circadian clock

Lamia KA, Storch KF, Weitz CJ
Department of Neurobiology, Harvard Medical School, Boston, Mass., USA

Proc Natl Acad Sci USA 2008;105:15172–15177

Context: Mammals have circadian clocks in peripheral tissues, but there is no direct evidence of their physiological importance. Unlike the suprachiasmatic nucleus clock that is set by light and drives rest-activity and fasting-feeding cycles, peripheral clocks are set by daily feeding, suggesting that at least some contribute metabolic regulation.

Results: The liver plays a well-known role in glucose homeostasis, and the authors report here that mice with a liver-specific deletion of *Bmal*1, an essential clock component, exhibited hypoglycemia restricted to the fasting phase of the daily feeding cycle, exaggerated glucose clearance, and loss of rhythmic expression of hepatic glucose regulatory genes.

Conclusions: The liver clock is important for buffering circulating glucose in a time-of-day-dependent manner. The findings suggest that the liver clock contributes to homeostasis by driving a daily rhythm of hepatic glucose export that counterbalances the daily cycle of glucose ingestion resulting from the fasting-feeding cycle.

That hypothalamic neurons have a biological clock is well established. The current study provides persuasive evidence for a liver clock that counterbalances the fluctuating sugar supply provoked by hypothalamus-driven feeding–fasting cycles. The dependence of oscillating Glut2 transcription on hepatocyte-derived *Bmal*1 suggests that circadian glucose export is indeed driven by local liver clocks. The liver circadian clock, entrained by the feeding cycle, has daily cycles of metabolic activity that ensure a steady supply of energy for the organism.

New concepts: always look back at old things

Brain-derived neurotrophic factor and obesity in the WAGR syndrome

Han JC, Liu QR, Jones M, Levinn RL, Menzie CM, Jefferson-George KS, Adler-Wailes DC, Sanford EL, Lacbawan FL, Uhl GR, Rennert OM, Yanovski JA
Unit on Growth and Obesity, Program in Developmental Endocrinology and Genetics, Eunice Kennedy Shriver National Institute of Child Health and Human Development, National Institutes of Health, Bethesda, Md., USA
N Engl J Med 2008;359:918–927

Background: Brain-derived neurotrophic factor (BDNF) has been found to be important in energy homeostasis in animal models, but little is known about its role in energy balance in humans. Heterozygous, variably sized, contiguous gene deletions causing haploinsufficiency of the WT1 and PAX6 genes on chromosome 11p13, approximately 4 Mb centromeric to BDNF (11p14.1), result in the Wilms' tumor, aniridia, genitourinary anomalies, and mental retardation (WAGR) syndrome. Hyperphagia and obesity are observed in a subgroup of patients with the WAGR syndrome. The authors hypothesized that the subphenotype of obesity in the WAGR syndrome is attributable to deletions that induce haploinsufficiency of BDNF.

Methods: The relationship between genotype and body mass index (BMI) in 33 patients with the WAGR syndrome who were recruited through the International WAGR Syndrome Association was studied. The extent of each deletion was determined with the use of oligonucleotide comparative genomic hybridization.

Results: Deletions of chromosome 11p in the patients studied ranged from 1.0 to 26.5 Mb; 58% of the patients had heterozygous BDNF deletions. These patients had significantly higher BMI z scores throughout childhood than did patients with intact BDNF (mean [± SD] z score at 8–10 years of age, 2.08 ± 0.45 in patients with heterozygous BDNF deletions vs. 0.88 ± 1.28 in patients without BDNF deletions; p = 0.03). By 10 years of age, 100% of the patients with heterozygous BDNF deletions (95% confidence interval [CI] 77–100) were obese (BMI ≥95th percentile for age and sex) as compared with 20% of persons without BDNF deletions (95% CI 3–56; p < 0.001). The critical region for childhood-onset obesity in the WAGR syndrome was located within 80 kb of exon 1 of BDNF. Serum BDNF concentrations were approximately 50% lower among the patients with heterozygous BDNF deletions (p = 0.001).

Conclusions: Among persons with the WAGR syndrome, BDNF haploinsufficiency is associated with lower levels of serum BDNF and with childhood-onset obesity; thus, BDNF may be important for energy homeostasis in humans.

This paper started with a clinical observation that some of the patients with WAGR syndrome (Wilms' tumor, aniridia, genitourinary anomalies, and mental retardation) have hyperphagia and obesity.

Rather than dismissing the observation, the authors collected a series of patients with this rare disease, mapped the chromosome 11p13 deletion, and found that obese patients have a contiguous gene syndrome and a deletion of the BDNF (brain-derived neurotrophic factor). Functionally those with a heterozygous deletion of the BDNF gene had lower levels of circulating BDNF. The BDNF locus has been identified as being involved in the susceptibility to obesity by GWAS studies and is involved in the hypothalamus melanocortin pathway [2]. In addition, BDNF can be experimentally manipulated and modulate food intake in experimental obesity [3]. Leptin and the like have disappointed us; BDNF holds new promise in the development of pharmaceutical approaches to obesity. Beyond its result, this paper shows that careful clinical observations can lead to important findings with impacts that go well beyond the context of the initial observation.

Concepts revised: insulin resistance look at the fat

Postreceptor insulin resistance contributes to human dyslipidemia and hepatic steatosis

Semple RK, Sleigh A, Murgatroyd PR, Adams CA, Bluck L, Jackson S, Vottero A, Kanabar D, Charlton-Menys V, Durrington P, Soos MA, Carpenter TA, Lomas DJ, Cochran EK, Gorden P, O'Rahilly S, Savage DB
Metabolic Research Laboratories, Institute of Metabolic Science, University of Cambridge, Addenbrooke's Hospital, Cambridge, UK
rks16@cam.ac.uk
J Clin Invest 2009;119:315–322

Background: Metabolic dyslipidemia is characterized by high circulating triglyceride (TG) and low HDL cholesterol levels and is frequently accompanied by hepatic steatosis. Increased hepatic lipogenesis contributes to both these problems. Because insulin fails to suppress gluconeogenesis but continues to stimulate lipogenesis in both obese and lipodystrophic insulin-resistant mice, it has been proposed that a selective postreceptor defect in hepatic insulin action is central to the pathogenesis of fatty liver and hypertriglyceridemia in these mice.

Methods and Results: Humans with generalized insulin resistance caused by either mutations in the insulin receptor gene or inhibitory antibodies specific for the insulin receptor uniformly exhibited low serum TG and normal HDL cholesterol levels. This was due at least in part to surprisingly low rates of de novo lipogenesis and was associated with low liver fat content and the production of TG-depleted VLDL cholesterol particles. In contrast, humans with a selective postreceptor defect in AKT2 manifest increased lipogenesis, elevated liver fat content, TG-enriched VLDL, hypertriglyceridemia, and low HDL cholesterol levels. People with lipodystrophy, a disorder characterized by particularly severe insulin resistance and dyslipidemia, demonstrated similar abnormalities.

Conclusions: These data from humans with molecularly characterized forms of insulin resistance suggest that partial postreceptor hepatic insulin resistance is a key element in the development of metabolic dyslipidemia and hepatic steatosis.

We are used to thinking of insulin resistance as a complex picture linking deranged insulin-mediated glucose metabolism, abnormal lipid partitioning and elevated lipid levels. However the interrelationship between glucose and lipid abnormalities remains incompletely understood. Rather than using fancy knockout mouse models, these authors elected to study patients with molecularly characterized defects leading to insulin resistance. They confirm previous findings that patients with insulin receptor mutations or antibodies have high glucose but normal lipid levels whereas those affected with postreceptor defects have both. This indicates that alterations in the liver insulin signal itself are not sufficient to generate dyslipidemia, and that insulin action on liver lipid metabolism results from postreceptor modification. The interplay of glucose and lipids in type 2 diabetes is not new and was first proposed in a famous editorial by McGarry, 'What if Minkowski had been ageusic? An alternative angle on diabetes' [4]. This important aspect of pathophysiology is further discussed in a nice recent review by Brown and Goldstein [5] and will need to be sorted in order to better hierarchies the therapeutic approaches to insulin resistance.

Incidence trends for childhood type 1 diabetes in Europe during 1989–2003 and predicted new cases 2005–20: a multicentre prospective registration study

Patterson CC, Dahlquist GG, Gyurus E, Green A, Soltesz G
Epidemiology Research Group, Centre for Public Health, Queen's University Belfast, Belfast, UK
c.patterson@qub.ac.uk
Lancet 2009;373:2027–2033

Background: The incidence of type 1 diabetes in children younger than 15 years is increasing. Prediction of future incidence of this disease will enable adequate fund allocation for delivery of care to be planned. The authors aimed to establish 15-year incidence trends for childhood type 1 diabetes in European centers, and thereby predict the future burden of childhood diabetes in Europe.

Methods: 20 population-based EURODIAB registers in 17 countries registered 29,311 new cases of type 1 diabetes, diagnosed in children before their 15th birthday during a 15-year period, 1989–2003. Age-specific log linear rates of increase were estimated in 5 geographical regions, and used in conjunction with published incidence rates and population projections to predict numbers of new cases throughout Europe in 2005, 2010, 2015, and 2020.

Results: Ascertainment was better than 90% in most registers. All but 2 registers showed significant yearly increases in incidence, ranging from 0.6 to 9.3%. The overall annual increase was 3.9% (95% CI 3.6–4.2), and the increases in the age groups 0–4, 5–9, and 10–14 years were 5.4 (4.8–6.1), 4.3 (3.8–4.8), and 2.9% (2.5–3.3), respectively. The number of new cases in Europe in 2005 is estimated as 15,000, divided between the 0–4, 5–9, and 10–14 year age groups in the ratio 24, 35, and 41%, respectively. In 2020, the predicted number of new cases is 24,400, with a doubling in numbers in children younger than 5 years and a more even distribution across age-groups than at present (29, 37, and 34%, respectively). Prevalence under age 15 years is predicted to rise from 94,000 in 2005, to 160,000 in 2020.

Conclusion: If present trends continue, doubling of new cases of type 1 diabetes in European children younger than 5 years is predicted between 2005 and 2020, and prevalent cases younger than 15 years will rise by 70%. Adequate healthcare resources to meet these children's needs should be made available.

Epidemiology is often considered a 'soft' science as opposed to 'hard' laboratory work. However, it is essential not only to provide precise estimates of the number of patients affected with a disease but also to allow an evaluation of the basic concepts in light of real life data. In this study, the Eurodiab group evaluated the incidence of type 1 diabetes and its evolution over time in 17 countries of Western Europe (Spain, Luxembourg, Belgium, 2 German centers), Central Europe (Czech Republic, Austria, and Slovenia) and East Europe (Lithuania, Poland, Slovakia, Hungary, Romania). The findings confirm the marked increase in diabetes incidence, striking particularly the younger kids. Cumulatively, the data extrapolated predict about twice as many new cases annually in 2020. Together with the decreased age at onset, the number of prevalent cases is predicted to rise by more than 50% in 2020. These findings confirm previous publications [6] and importantly show that earlier predictions are true, and even exceeded. The paper has a public health perspective and its main message is towards the organization of healthcare for children with type 1 diabetes. One other aspect is the importance of basic research towards finding the genes for type 1 diabetes. Indeed, type 1 diabetes research has been a paradigm for all types of gene association studies and the last GWAS analysis by the Type 1 Diabetes Genetics Consortium, using approximately 20,000 patients and 20,000 controls revealed more than 40 loci spread throughout the genome, most of them with minuscule effect sizes [7]. It may be time to concentrate our efforts on the environmental and epigenetic modifications that have induced such a rapid change in the disease incidence?

Innate immunity and intestinal microbiota in the development of type 1 diabetes

Wen L, Ley RE, Volchkov PY, Stranges PB, Avanesyan L, Stonebraker AC, Hu C, Wong FS, Szot GL, Bluestone JA, Gordon JI, Chervonsky AV
Section of Endocrinology, Yale University School of Medicine, New Haven, Conn., USA
Nature 2008;455:1109–1113

Background: Type 1 diabetes (T1D) is a debilitating autoimmune disease that results from T-cell-mediated destruction of insulin-producing β-cells. Its incidence has increased during the past several decades in developed countries, suggesting that changes in the environment (including the human microbial environment) may influence disease pathogenesis. The incidence of spontaneous T1D in non-obese diabetic (NOD) mice can be affected by the microbial environment in the animal housing facility or by exposure to microbial stimuli, such as injection with mycobacteria or various microbial products.
Methods: Manipulation of NOD mice that are deficient in the MyD88 protein, a key element of innate immunity with various microbiota.
Results: Specific pathogen-free NOD mice lacking MyD88 protein (an adaptor for multiple innate immune receptors that recognize microbial stimuli) do not develop T1D. The effect is dependent on commensal microbes because germ-free MyD88-negative NOD mice develop robust diabetes, whereas colonization of these germ-free MyD88-negative NOD mice with a defined microbial consortium (representing bacterial phyla normally present in human gut) attenuates T1D. We also find that MyD88 deficiency changes the composition of the distal gut microbiota, and that exposure to the microbiota of specific pathogen-free MyD88-negative NOD donors attenuates T1D in germ-free NOD recipients.
Conclusions: Interaction of the intestinal microbes with the innate immune system is a critical epigenetic factor modifying T1D predisposition.

Last year, we learnt that the gut microbiome could play an important role in the pathogenesis of obesity both in mice and humans [8, 9]. The major focus of type 1 diabetes immunology research has been to identify the partners of cognate immunity, i.e. an antigen-specific immune cell with a tissue-specific antigen of antigen-derived peptide. Although some have identified a role of α-interferons, non-specifically induced by viruses or by inflammation, it must be remembered that the first step of immune activation is a non-cognate interaction of a class of 'foreign' determinants with the immune compartment called 'innate immunity'. In addition, it has been known for a long time that NOD mice raised in a clean environment had a much higher incidence of diabetes than mice raised in the presence of weak pathogens, such as gut parasites. Wen et al. manipulated the mouse microbiome to evaluate the impact of the intestinal microbes on the pathogenesis of diabetes in the NOD mouse. Their main findings are that mice that are incapable of sensing the microbiota through Myd88 are protected from diabetes and are colonized by an altered microbiota that can transfer protection against the disease. Although the exact mechanisms involved have not yet been worked out completely, this approach opens new avenues in diabetes research, and we could end up inoculating children at risk of diabetes with anti-diabetic bacteria earlier than we think.

Dysregulation of lipid and amino acid metabolism precedes islet autoimmunity in children who later progress to type 1 diabetes

Oresic M, Simell S, Sysi-Aho M, Nanto-Salonen K, Seppanen-Laakso T, Parikka V, Katajamaa M, Hekkala A, Mattila I, Keskinen P, Yetukuri L, Reinikainen A, Lahde J, Suortti T, Hakalax J, Simell T, Hyoty H, Veijola R, Ilonen J, Lahesmaa R, Knip M, Simell O
VTT Technical Research Centre of Finland, Espoo, Finland
matej.oresic@vtt.fi
J Exp Med 2008;205:2975–2984

Background: The risk determinants of type 1 diabetes, initiators of autoimmune response, mechanisms regulating progress toward β-cell failure, and factors determining time of presentation of clinical diabetes are poorly understood.

Methods: The authors investigated changes in the serum metabolome prospectively in children who later progressed to type 1 diabetes. Serum metabolite profiles were compared between sample series drawn from 56 children who progressed to type 1 diabetes and 73 controls who remained nondiabetic and permanently autoantibody negative.

Results: Individuals who developed diabetes had reduced serum levels of succinic acid and phosphatidylcholine (PC) at birth, reduced levels of triglycerides and antioxidant ether phospholipids throughout the follow-up, and increased levels of proinflammatory lysoPCs several months before seroconversion to autoantibody positivity. The lipid changes were not attributable to HLA-associated genetic risk. The appearance of insulin and glutamic acid decarboxylase autoantibodies was preceded by diminished ketoleucine and elevated glutamic acid. The metabolic profile was partially normalized after the seroconversion.

Conclusion: Autoimmunity may be a relatively late response to the early metabolic disturbances. Recognition of these pre-autoimmune alterations may aid in studies of disease pathogenesis and may open a time window for novel type 1 diabetes prevention strategies.

When we fail to understand the course of events, we postulate working hypotheses. The current dogma is that immune abnormalities precede metabolic abnormalities in type 1 diabetes, and that environmental or other triggers initiate the autoimmune process. Here, the Finnish group used a large collection of serum samples of children followed from birth to study their metabolome and try to detect early metabolic alterations prior to the appearance of diabetes-associated antibodies. Differences were found between progressors and non-progressors in terms of lipid levels (triglycerides, phosphatidylcholine, ceramides) and amino acid levels. The intriguing results suggest that the appearance of GAD- and insulin-specific autoantibodies may be a relatively late response to earlier metabolic disturbances. Glutamate, the amino acid ligand of specific brain and β-cell receptors and transporters, was much elevated in children who went on to develop diabetes. The Chinese restaurant syndrome-related monosodium leads, among others, to higher insulin concentrations. Theoretically, it is possible that a glutamate load in β cells increases the activity of GAD65, one of the major β-cell antigens. Of note, previous epidemiological data had linked the intake of ω–3 polyunsaturated fatty acid to the risk of type 1 diabetes [10]. Although no clear picture emerges from the study and no working hypothesis seems to be formulated at this time, it is clear that similar approaches will help explore new avenues in one of the major medical mysteries that has resisted the sophisticated and expensive GWAS approaches: susceptibility to autoimmune diseases and type 1 diabetes [11].

References
1. Beardsall K, Ogilvy-Stuart AL, Frystyk J, Chen JW, Thompson M, Ahluwalia J, et al: Early elective insulin therapy can reduce hyperglycemia and increase insulin-like growth factor-I levels in very low birth weight infants. J Pediatr 2007;151:611–617, 617e1.
2. Froguel P, Blakemore AI: The power of the extreme in elucidating obesity. N Engl J Med 2008;359:891–893.
3. Cao L, Lin EJ, Cahill MC, Wang C, Liu X, During MJ: Molecular therapy of obesity and diabetes by a physiological autoregulatory approach. Nat Med 2009;15:447–454.
4. McGarry JD: What if Minkowski had been ageusic? An alternative angle on diabetes. Science 1992;258:766–770.
5. Brown MS, Goldstein JL: Selective versus total insulin resistance: a pathogenic paradox. Cell Metab 2008;7:95–96.

6. Dabelea D: The accelerating epidemic of childhood diabetes. Lancet 2009;373:1999–2000.
7. Barrett JC, Clayton DG, Concannon P, Akolkar B, Cooper JD, Erlich HA, et al: Genome-wide association study and meta-analysis find that over 40 loci affect risk of type 1 diabetes. Nat Genet 2009 [Epub ahead of print].
8. Ley RE, Turnbaugh PJ, Klein S, Gordon JI: Microbial ecology: human gut microbes associated with obesity. Nature 2006;444:1022–1023.
9. Turnbaugh PJ, Ley RE, Mahowald MA, Magrini V, Mardis ER, Gordon JI: An obesity-associated gut microbiome with increased capacity for energy harvest. Nature 2006;444:1027–1031.
10. Norris JM, Yin X, Lamb MM, Barriga K, Seifert J, Hoffman M, et al: Omega-3 polyunsaturated fatty acid intake and islet autoimmunity in children at increased risk for type 1 diabetes. JAMA 2007;298:1420–1428.
11. Bougneres P, Valleron AJ: Causes of early-onset type 1 diabetes: toward data-driven environmental approaches. J Exp Med 2008;205:2953–2957.

Science and Medicine

Ze'ev Hochberg and Jean-Claude Carel

Small and variable

Origins and genetic diversity of pygmy hunter-gatherers from Western Central Africa

Verdu P, Austerlitz F, Estoup A, Vitalis R, Georges M, Thery S, Froment A, Le Bomin S, Gessain A, Hombert JM, Van der Veen L, Quintana-Murci L, Bahuchet S, Heyer E
Ecoanthropology and Ethnobiology, UMR, CNRS-MNHN-Université Paris, Paris, France
verdu@mnhn.fr
Curr Biol 2009;19:312–318

Context: Central Africa is currently peopled by numerous sedentary agriculturalist populations neighboring the largest group of mobile hunter-gatherers, the Pygmies. Although archeological remains attest to *Homo sapiens'* presence in the Congo Basin for at least 30,000 years, the demographic history of these groups, including divergence and admixture, remains widely unknown. It is still debated whether common history or convergent adaptation to a forest environment resulted in the short stature characterizing the pygmies.
Methods: The authors genotyped 604 individuals at 28 autosomal tetranucleotide microsatellite loci in 12 non-pygmy and 9 neighboring pygmy populations.
Results: They found a high level of genetic heterogeneity among Western Central African pygmies, as well as evidence of heterogeneous levels of asymmetrical gene flow from non-pygmy to pygmy, consistent with the variable sociocultural barriers against intermarriages. Using approximate bayesian, they compared several historical scenarios. The most likely points toward a unique ancestral pygmy population that diversified 2,800 years ago, contemporarily with the Neolithic expansion of non-pygmy agriculturalists.
Conclusions: The results show that recent isolation, genetic drift, and heterogeneous admixture enabled a rapid and substantial genetic differentiation among Western Central African pygmies. Such an admixture pattern is consistent with the various sociocultural behaviors related to intermarriages between pygmy and non-pygmy.

Last year this *Yearbook* cited that pygmies have not evolved through positive selection for small stature. This was a by-product of selection for early onset of reproduction in the face of short survival in a hostile environment. The authors of the current article suggest that the spread of non-pygmy farmers through Western Central Africa may have driven pygmies into isolated groups, prompting their speedy evolution into distinct populations with a huge genetic diversity. Their average height can vary by up to 20 cm.

Verdu et al. collected DNA samples from 9 pygmy and 12 nearby non-pygmy groups in Cameroon and Gabon. The genetic variation between different pygmy populations was of a similar scale to that between Europeans and Asians. The pygmy groups seem to have emerged around 2,800 years ago from a common ancestral group that likely split from other humans 54,000–90,000 years ago. The authors suggest that this coincides with the expansion of non-pygmy agriculture in the region, a process that might have driven pygmies into small, isolated hunter-gatherer groups that evolved rapidly.

Function of mitochondrial Stat3 in cellular respiration

Wegrzyn J, Potla R, Chwae YJ, Sepuri NB, Zhang Q, Koeck T, Derecka M, Szczepanek K, Szelag M, Gornicka A, Moh A, Moghaddas S, Chen Q, Bobbili S, Cichy J, Dulak J, Baker DP, Wolfman A, Stuehr D, Hassan MO, Fu XY, Avadhani N, Drake JI, Fawcett P, Lesnefsky EJ, Larner AC
Department of Biochemistry and Molecular Biology and Massey Cancer Center, Virginia Commonwealth University, Richmond, Va., USA
Science 2009;323:793–797

Context: Cytokines such as interleukin-6 induce tyrosine and serine phosphorylation of Stat3 that results in activation of Stat3-responsive genes.
Aim: To provide evidence that Stat3 is present in the mitochondria of cultured cells and primary tissues, including the liver and heart.
Results: In Stat3–/– cells, the activities of complexes I and II of the electron transport chain (ETC) were significantly decreased. We identified Stat3 mutants that selectively restored the protein's function as a transcription factor or its functions within the ETC. In mice that do not express Stat3 in the heart, there were also selective defects in the activities of complexes I and II of the ETC.
Conclusions: These data indicate that Stat3 is required for optimal function of the ETC, which may allow it to orchestrate responses to cellular homeostasis.

We recognize the Stat 3 (signal transducers and activators of transcription) as a transcription factor that is activated in response to GH and other cytokines. We now learn that Stat3 has a distinct function in the mitochondria. It interacts with a component of complex I of the electron transport chain and interferons to inhibit mitochondrial function – the authors explored a role for Stat3 in mitochondria. In a subset of mouse B lymphocytes devoid of Stat3, oxidative phosphorylation was reduced, a defect attributable to the diminished activity of complexes I and II. It is tempting to speculate that GH and other cytokines use Stat3 to regulate transcription and respiration. Yet, cytokines may not be the only, or even the major, controllers of Stat3-modulated oxidation.

> **Quixotic alright**
> **Review**

Tilting at quixotic trait loci: an evolutionary perspective on genetic causation

Weiss KM
Department of Anthropology and Integrated Biosciences Genetics Program, Pennsylvania State University, University Park, Pa., USA
kenweiss@psu.edu
Genetics 2008;179:1741–1756

Recent years have seen great advances in generating and analyzing data to identify the genetic architecture of biological traits. Human disease has understandably received intense research focus, and the genes responsible for most mendelian diseases have successfully been identified. However, the same advances have shown a consistent if less satisfying pattern in which complex traits are affected by variation in large numbers of genes, most of which have individually minor or statistically elusive effects, leaving the bulk of genetic etiology unaccounted for. This pattern applies to diverse and unrelated traits, not just disease, in basically all species, and is consistent with evolutionary expectations, raising challenging questions about the best way to approach and understand biological complexity.

Complex phenotypic or disease traits are affected by variation in large numbers of genes, most of which have individually minor or statistically intangible effects. This pattern is consistent with evolutionary expectations. Yet, if diabetes or height shows a genetic component of ~50% by twin studies, and the GWAS explain 3% of the variation, that leaves the bulk of genetic etiology unaccounted for.

The huge longitudinal biobanks being launched can be expected to do any better than they have already done. This important review suggests that the demand for increased sequence and sample size may itself be evidence that we are approaching diminishing returns. By chasing the effects most difficult to replicate, or hardest to discriminate between true and false positives, accurate risk estimation may be as small. While these efforts go on, it is time to realize time and again that we are not our gene sequence. Our DNA sequence is just part of the story, while gene expression may get us closer to understanding.

Transgenerational rescue of a genetic defect in long-term potentiation and memory formation by juvenile enrichment

Arai JA, Li S, Hartley DM, Feig LA
Sackler School of Biomedical Sciences and Department of Biochemistry, Tufts University School of Medicine, Boston, Mass., USA
J Neurosci 2009;29:1496–1502

Context: The idea that qualities acquired from experience can be transmitted to future offspring has long been considered incompatible with current understanding of genetics. However, the recent documentation of non-mendelian transgenerational inheritance makes such a 'lamarckian'-like phenomenon more plausible.

Results: This paper demonstrates that exposure of 15-day-old mice to 2 weeks of an enriched environment (EE), that includes exposure to novel objects, elevated social interactions and voluntary exercise, which enhances long-term potentiation (LTP) not only in these enriched mice but also in their future offspring through early adolescence, even if the offspring never experience EE. In both generations, LTP induction is augmented by a newly appearing cAMP/p38 MAP kinase-dependent signaling cascade. Strikingly, defective LTP and contextual fear conditioning memory normally associated with ras-grf knock-out mice are both masked in the offspring of enriched mutant parents. The transgenerational transmission of this effect occurs from the enriched mother to her offspring during embryogenesis.

Perspective: If a similar phenomenon occurs in humans, the effectiveness of one's memory during adolescence, particularly in those with defective cell signaling mechanisms that control memory, can be influenced by environmental stimulation experienced by one's mother during her youth.

An enriched environment during young age causes striking changes in brain function including enhanced learning and memory. This group showed previously that 2 weeks of enriched environment induces the expression of a signaling cascade that contributes to the induction of synaptic plasticity that is known to be important for learning and memory – the appearance of an otherwise latent NMDA receptor/cAMP/p38 MAP kinase signaling pathway. They now demonstrate the incredible power of an animal's environment to modulate this signaling network and to improve contextual fear memory formation across generations. Exposing young animals to an enriched environment enhanced long-term potentiation induction in their future offspring through adolescence, even if the offspring are not exposed to enriched environment. In both generations, this phenomenon involves the addition of cAMP and p38 MAP kinase dependence to LTP induction. If this reminds you of transgenerational transmission of epigenetic changes, such changes have not been investigated here. It was previously shown that pups, who are exposed to strong nurturing mothers, display life-long alterations in the patterns of promoter DNA methylation and changes in expression of specific genes in the hypothalamus that regulate the stress response. These offspring then become strong nurturing mothers and pass the phenotype on to the next generation by their behavior.

DNA methylation profiles in monozygotic and dizygotic twins

Kaminsky ZA, Tang T, Wang SC, Ptak C, Oh GH, Wong AH, Feldcamp LA, Virtanen C, Halfvarson J, Tysk C, McRae AF, Visscher PM, Montgomery GW, Gottesman, II, Martin NG, Petronis A
Centre for Addiction and Mental Health, Toronto, Ont., Canada
Nat Genet 2009;41:240–245

Context: Twin studies have provided the basis for genetic and epidemiological studies in human complex traits.

Methods: As epigenetic factors can contribute to phenotypic outcomes, the authors conducted a DNA methylation analysis in white blood cells (WBC), buccal epithelial cells and gut biopsies of 114 monozygotic (MZ) twins as well as WBC and buccal epithelial cells of 80 dizygotic (DZ) twins using 12K CpG island microarrays.

Results: They provide the first annotation of epigenetic metastability of 6,000 unique genomic regions in MZ twins. An intraclass correlation (ICC)-based comparison of matched MZ and DZ twins showed significantly higher epigenetic difference in buccal cells of DZ co-twins (p = 1.2 10-294).

Conclusions: Although such higher epigenetic discordance in DZ twins can result from DNA sequence differences, these in silico SNP analyses and animal studies favor the hypothesis that it is due to epigenomic differences in the zygotes, suggesting that molecular mechanisms of heritability may not be limited to DNA sequence differences.

MZ twins reared apart are generally quite similar to MZ twins reared together according to IQ, personality, social attitudes and more. Yet variations are not rare. These investigators mapped MZ twin DNA methylation differences in relatively easily accessible tissues: white blood cells, buccal epithelial cells and rectal biopsies. They detected a large degree of co-twin DNA methylation variation in all tissues investigated. The varying degrees of epigenetic dissimilarity detected between MZ twins may reflect differences in epigenetic divergence among embryonic cells at the time the twin blastomeres separated. They found greater epigenetic similarity between MZ co-twins at functionally important regions in comparison to the loci without clearly defined regulatory function, suggesting functional stratification of the epigenome. They speculate that stochastic events in epigenetically determined phenotypic differences in MZ co-twins are much more important than environment.

Human predators outpace other agents of trait change in the wild

Darimont CT, Carlson SM, Kinnison MT, Paquet PC, Reimchen TE, Wilmers CC
Department of Biology, University of Victoria, Victoria, B.C., Canada
darimont@ucsc.edu
Proc Natl Acad Sci USA 2009;106:952–954

Context: The observable traits of wild populations are continually shaped and reshaped by the environment and numerous agents of natural selection, including predators. In stark contrast with most predators, humans now typically exploit high proportions of prey populations and target large, reproductive-aged adults. Consequently, organisms subject to consistent and strong 'harvest selection' by fishers, hunters, and plant harvesters may be expected to show particularly rapid and dramatic changes in phenotype. However, a comparison of the rate at which phenotypic changes in exploited taxa occurs relative to other systems has never been undertaken.

Results: Average phenotypic changes in 40 human-harvested systems are much more rapid than changes reported in studies examining not only natural (n = 20 systems) but also other human-driven (n = 25 systems) perturbations in the wild, outpacing them by >300 and 50%, respectively. Accordingly, harvested organisms show some of the most abrupt trait changes ever observed in wild populations, providing a new appreciation for how fast phenotypes are capable of changing. These changes, which include average declines of almost 20% in size-related traits and shifts in life history traits of nearly 25%, are most rapid in commercially exploited systems and, thus, have profound conservation and economic implications.

Conclusions: The widespread potential for transitively rapid and large effects on size- or life history-mediated ecological dynamics might imperil populations, industries, and ecosystems.

Previous research has shown that in response to commercial fishing and hunting, traits such as average size at reproductive age adjust. Human prey mammals and fish turned smaller by 20% and reproduced earlier, which made them even more vulnerable. From a meta-analysis of reports on the morphology and life histories of 29 species, including fish, mammals and plants, these authors report that phenotypic changes in human-harvested organisms occurred more than 300% faster than in natural systems, and 50% faster than in systems affected by other human influences, such as pollution. Predation by humans drives phenotypic changes in exploited prey much faster than other evolutionary pressures do. Prey animals adjust their life history to a new, shorter lifespan. Why does human predation work so quickly? Apparently, because it is often felt by a large proportion of the adults in a population. Why is human prey different from wild animals prey? Whereas the latter hunt the small and weak, humans' hunting and fishing techniques and targets are the big and strong. This is paradoxically aggravated by regulations that forbid the hunting or fishing of small animals.

Artificial organism

One-step assembly in yeast of 25 overlapping DNA fragments to form a complete synthetic Mycoplasma genitalium genome

Gibson DG, Benders GA, Axelrod KC, Zaveri J, Algire MA, Moodie M, Montague MG, Venter JC, Smith HO, Hutchison CA, 3rd
The J. Craig Venter Institute, Synthetic Biology Group, Rockville, Md., USA
dgibson@jcvi.org

Proc Natl Acad Sci USA 2008;105:20404–20409

Context: This group previously reported assembly and cloning of the synthetic *Mycoplasma genitalium* JCVI-1.0 genome in the yeast *Saccharomyces cerevisiae* by recombination of six overlapping DNA fragments to produce a 592-kb circle.

Results: Here they extend this approach by demonstrating assembly of the synthetic genome from 25 overlapping fragments in a single step.

Conclusions: The use of yeast recombination greatly simplifies the assembly of large DNA molecules from both synthetic and natural fragments.

The *Yearbook 2008* missed this breakthrough, published in February 2008 [Gibson DG, et al: Science 2008;319(5867):1215–1220], but this latest in the series cannot go unmentioned. By stitching together more than 500,000 bp of DNA, they created the first synthetic genome as a step towards the construction of the world's first artificial organism.

Speciation through sensory drive in cichlid fish

Seehausen O, Terai Y, Magalhaes IS, Carleton KL, Mrosso HD, Miyagi R, van der Sluijs I, Schneider MV, Maan ME, Tachida H, Imai H, Okada N
Institute of Zoology, University of Bern, Bern, Switzerland
ole.seehausen@aqua.unibe.ch
Nature 2008;455:620–626

Context: Theoretically, divergent selection on sensory systems can cause speciation through sensory drive. However, empirical evidence is rare and incomplete.

Results: This study demonstrates sensory drive speciation within island populations of cichlid fish. They identify the ecological and molecular basis of divergent evolution in the cichlid visual system, demonstrate associated divergence in male coloration and female preferences, and show subsequent differentiation at neutral loci, indicating reproductive isolation. Evidence is replicated in several pairs of sympatric populations and species. Variation in the slope of the environmental gradients explains variation in the progress towards speciation: speciation occurs on all but the steepest gradients.

Conclusions: This is the most complete demonstration so far of speciation through sensory drive without geographical isolation. The results also provide a mechanistic explanation for the collapse of cichlid fish species diversity during the anthropogenic eutrophication of Lake Victoria.

Classically, geographical isolation was considered to be the main drive for speciation. We now learn of a sensory drive that leads to the evolution of color polymorphisms and speciation, even in the absence of geographical isolation, when the light environment is heterogeneous. The cichlids of the African lakes are the most rapidly speciating species known. Males are either red or blue, and females have genetic variation for visual sensitivity to those colors. Females with blue-biased vision seem to mate only with blue males, whereas red-biased females mate only with red males. The implication is that natural selection acting on the visual system contributes to the formation of new species.

Genetic variation in the vasopressin receptor 1a gene (AVPR1A) associates with pair-bonding behavior in humans

Walum H, Westberg L, Henningsson S, Neiderhiser JM, Reiss D, Igl W, Ganiban JM, Spotts EL, Pedersen NL, Eriksson E, Lichtenstein P
Department of Medical Epidemiology and Biostatistics, Karolinska Institutet, Stockholm, Sweden
hasse.walum@ki.se
Proc Natl Acad Sci USA 2008;105:14153–14156

Context: Pair-bonding has been suggested to be a critical factor in the evolutionary development of the social brain. The brain neuropeptide arginine vasopressin (AVP) exerts an important influence on pair-bonding behavior in voles. There is a strong association between a polymorphic repeat sequence in the 5′-flanking region of the gene (AVPR1A) encoding one of the AVP receptor subtypes (V1aR), and proneness for monogamous behavior in males of this species. It is not yet known whether similar mechanisms are important also for human pair-bonding.

Results: This report shows an association between one of the human AVPR1A repeat polymorphisms (RS3) and traits reflecting pair-bonding behavior in men, including partner bonding, perceived marital problems, and marital status. It shows that the RS3 genotype of the males also affects marital quality as perceived by their spouses.

Conclusions: These results suggest an association between a single gene and pair-bonding behavior in humans, and indicate that the well-characterized influence of AVP on pair-bonding in voles may be of relevance also for humans.

The topic here is pair-bonded relationships, or what we call love. It may have been the demands for pair-bonding behavior that triggered the evolutionary development of the primate social brain. It has known for some time that oxytocin is involved in mother-infant bonding, but also between man and woman. We now learn that AVP, acting through the pressor receptor V1aR, plays a role in the regulation of love behaviors. Polymorphisms of the receptor gene are associated with variation in relation quality; men with a certain repeat polymorphism were twice as likely to remain unmarried, or when married, twice as likely to report marriage crises. You can already purchase on the internet a love-boosting oxytocin and pheromones preparation. AVP may make this love mixture more effective. You may wish to study the bonding of your patients with diabetes insipidus.

A second hit

Persistent hypomethylation in the promoter of nucleosomal binding protein 1 (Nsbp1) correlates with overexpression of Nsbp1 in mouse uteri neonatally exposed to diethylstilbestrol or genistein

Tang WY, Newbold R, Mardilovich K, Jefferson W, Cheng RY, Medvedovic M, Ho SM
Department of Environmental Health, Kettering Complex, University of Cincinnati Medical Center, Cincinnati, Ohio, USA
Endocrinology 2008;149:5922–5931

Context: Neonatal exposure of CD-1 mice to diethylstilbestrol (DES) or genistein (GEN) induces uterine adenocarcinoma in aging animals. Uterine carcinogenesis in this model is ovarian dependent because its evolution is blocked by prepubertal ovariectomy.

Aim: This study seeks to discover novel uterine genes whose expression is altered by such early endocrine disruption via an epigenetic mechanism.

Methods: Neonatal mice were treated with 1 or 1,000 µg/kg DES, 50 mg/kg GEN, or oil (control) on days 1–5. One group of treated mice was killed before puberty on day 19. Others were ovariectomized or left intact, and killed at 6 and 18 months of age. Methylation-sensitive restriction fingerprinting was performed to identify differentially methylated sequences associated with neonatal exposure to DES/GEN.

Results: Among 14 candidates, *nucleosomal binding protein* 1 (*Nsbp*1), the gene for a nucleosome-core-particle binding protein, was selected for further study because of its central role in chromatin remodeling. In uteri of immature control mice, *Nsbp*1 promoter CpG island (CGI) was minimally methylated. Once control mice reached puberty, the *Nsbp*1 CGI became hypermethylated, and gene expression declined further. In contrast, in neonatal DES/GEN-treated mice, the *Nsbp*1 CGI stayed anomalously hypomethylated, and the gene exhibited persistent overexpression throughout life. However, if neonatal DES/GEN-treated mice were ovariectomized before puberty, the CGI remained minimally to moderately methylated, and gene expression was subdued except in the group treated with 1,000 µg/kg DES.

Conclusions: The life reprogramming of uterine *Nsbp*1 expression by neonatal DES/GEN exposure appears to be mediated by an epigenetic mechanism that interacts with ovarian hormones in adulthood.

Exposure to estrogenic chemicals during critical stages of development exerts long-lasting effects on male and female reproductive organs. The best-studied example is exposure to diethylstilbestrol (DES) and the risk for clear cell adenocarcinoma of the vagina and cervix in female offspring (DES daughters). In contrast to in utero exposure to xenoestrogens, peripubertal human exposures to dietary phytoestrogens such as genistein (GEN) appear to reduce later-life breast cancer risk. Yet, questions related to the safety of early-life exposure to phytoestrogens remain unanswered. Infants exposed to high levels of dietary phytoestrogens have an increased risk of developing type 1 diabetes. This study aimed to determine whether neonatal exposure to DES/GEN can alter gene expression in the mouse uterus in later life via an epigenetic mechanism such as DNA methylation, and looked for interaction between adult ovarian hormones and neonatal DES/GEN reprogramming. The study identified 14 candidate genes that encode proteins involved in signal transduction, receptor activation, tumor angiogenesis/metastasis, cell proliferation, apoptosis, intracellular trafficking, DNA repair, and chromatin remodeling, whose methylation status in the mature mouse uterus was altered by neonatal exposure of the pups to DES and/or GEN. The discovery of these genes has strengthened the claim of an epigenetic basis for the developmental effects of DES, and has provided much needed initial evidence that a phytoestrogen such as GEN may possess a similar potential. The complex interplay among the type of estrogen, timing of exposure, reproductive status, and aging time line all significantly contribute to the phenotypical outcome of the epigenetic reprogramming in this model system.

The main novelty of this article is in the demonstration that epigenetic reprogramming requires a 'second hit'. The onset of uterine adenocarcinoma in neonatal DES-exposed mice required a secondary hormonal 'push' by pubertal steroids because prepubertally ovariectomized mice did not develop cancers. This is a direct function of specific DNA methylation changes induced by the secondary pubertal hormones that occur only in mice that were first exposed neonatally to DES or GEN.

Reduced by fat

7-Oxysterols modulate glucocorticoid activity in adipocytes through competition for 11β-hydroxysteroid dehydrogenase type 1

Wamil M, Andrew R, Chapman KE, Street J, Morton NM, Seckl JR
Endocrinology Unit, Centre for Cardiovascular Science, The Queen's Medical Research Institute, University of Edinburgh, Edinburgh, UK
Endocrinology 2008;149:5909–5918

Context: Obesity is associated with an increased risk of diabetes type 2, dyslipidemia, and atherosclerosis. These cardiovascular and metabolic abnormalities are exacerbated by excessive dietary fat, particularly cholesterol and its metabolites. High adipose tissue glucocorticoid levels, generated by the intracellular enzyme 11β-hydroxysteroid dehydrogenase type 1 (11β-HSD1), are also implicated in the pathogenesis of obesity, metabolic syndrome, and atherosclerosis. 11β-HSD1 also interconverts the atherogenic oxysterols 7-ketocholesterol (7KC) and 7β-hydroxycholesterol (7β-HC).

Aim: Here, they report that 11β-HSD1 catalyzes the reduction of 7KC to 7β-HC in mature 3T3-L1 and 3T3-F442A adipocytes, leading to cellular accumulation of 7β-HC.

Results: Approximately 73% of added 7KC was reduced to 7β-HC within 24 h; this conversion was prevented by selective inhibition of 11β-HSD1. Oxysterol and glucocorticoid conversion by 11β-HSD1 was competitive and occurred with a physiologically relevant IC_{50} range of 450 nm for 7KC inhibition of glucocorticoid metabolism. Working as an inhibitor of 11β-reductase activity, 7KC decreased the regeneration of active glucocorticoid and limited the process of differentiation of 3T3-L1 preadipocytes. 7KC and 7β-HC did not activate liver X receptor in a transactivation assay, nor did they display intrinsic activation of the glucocorticoid receptor. However, when coincubated with glucocorticoid (10 nm), 7KC repressed, and 7β-HC enhanced glucocorticoid receptor transcriptional activity. The effect of 7-oxysterols resulted from the modulation of 11β-HSD1 reaction direction, and could be ameliorated by overexpression of hexose 6-phosphate dehydrogenase, which supplies reduced nicotinamide adenine dinucleotide phosphate to 11β-HSD1.

Conclusions: The activity and reaction direction of adipose 11β-HSD1 is altered under conditions of oxysterol excess, and could impact upon the pathophysiology of obesity and its complications.

The reduction of inert cortisone to active cortisol by 11β-HSD1, which is elevated specifically in adipose tissue of obese humans and rodents, was suggested to cause 'Cushing's syndrome of adipose tissue' in idiopathic obesity. Transgenic mice overexpressing 11β-HSD1 selectively in adipose tissue develop many features of the metabolic syndrome, including glucose intolerance, insulin resistance, dyslipidemia, and hypertension, whereas 11β-HSD1 null mice are protected from these deleterious effects upon high-fat feeding and have an atheroprotective phenotype, with increased plasma HDL cholesterol and lower free fatty acid levels. It was reported recently that 11β-HSD1 interconverts in the liver 7-ketocholesterol (7KC) and 7β-hydroxycholesterol (7β-HC), which are the most abundant oxysterols in oxLDL, and their concentrations correlate with atherosclerosis risk. Given the key role of adipose tissue in modulating whole-body cholesterol homeostasis, the study hypothesized that metabolism of these oxysterols by 11β-HSD1 might provide a novel link between obesity, adipose glucocorticoid action, and atherogenesis. The findings show that 7-oxysterols are produced enzymatically in adipocytes, regulate 11β-HSD1-dependent conversion of glucocorticoids, and, therefore, signaling by glucocorticoid receptor, and when in excess may inhibit the differentiation of preadipocytes. The effects appear to occur predominantly through substrate competition at the enzyme activity level, and may also include reversal of 11β-HSD1 reaction direction (reductase) if 7KC levels are high and reduced nicotinamide adenine dinucleotide phosphate cofactor levels are limiting within the cell. These data could lead to a revision of our understanding of the association between glucocorticoids and atherogenesis.

Whereas essential for preadipocyte differentiation, in the mature adipocytes glucocorticoids promote lipolysis, increasing glycerol release that can lead to insulin resistance under states of pathogenic excess. The data presented here further define the mechanisms and components underlying this biology in which increased levels of oxysterols, such as that found in dyslipidemia and obesity, can modulate the enzymatic activity controlling glucocorticoid production.

A pluripotent future: three papers on stem cells

Induction of pluripotent stem cells from primary human fibroblasts with only Oct4 and Sox2

Huangfu D, Osafune K, Maehr R, Guo W, Eijkelenboom A, Chen S, Muhlestein W, Melton DA
Department of Stem Cell and Regenerative Biology, Howard Hughes Medical Institute, Harvard Stem Cell Institute, Harvard University, Cambridge, Mass., USA
Nat Biotechnol 2008;26:1269–1275

Context: Ectopic expression of defined sets of genetic factors can reprogram somatic cells to induced pluripotent stem (iPS) cells that closely resemble embryonic stem (ES) cells. The low efficiency with which iPS cells are derived hinders studies on the molecular mechanism of reprogramming, and integration of viral transgenes, in particular the oncogenes c-Myc and Klf4, may handicap this method for human therapeutic applications.

Results: Valproic acid (VPA), a histone deacetylase inhibitor, enables reprogramming of primary human fibroblasts with only two factors, Oct4 and Sox2, without the need for the oncogenes c-Myc or Klf4. The two factor-induced human iPS cells resemble human ES cells in pluripotency, global gene expression profiles and epigenetic states.

Conclusions: These results support the possibility of reprogramming through purely chemical means, which would make therapeutic use of reprogrammed cells safer and more practical.

Induced pluripotent stem cells generated without viral integration

Stadtfeld M, Nagaya M, Utikal J, Weir G, Hochedlinger K
Massachusetts General Hospital Cancer Center and Center for Regenerative Medicine, Boston, Mass., USA
Science 2008;322:945–949

Pluripotent stem cells have been generated from mouse and human somatic cells by viral expression of the transcription factors Oct4, Sox2, Klf4, and c-Myc. A major limitation of this technology is the use of potentially harmful genome-integrating viruses. We generated mouse-induced pluripotent stem (iPS) cells from fibroblasts and liver cells by using nonintegrating adenoviruses transiently expressing Oct4, Sox2, Klf4, and c-Myc. These adenoviral iPS (adeno-iPS) cells show DNA demethylation characteristic of reprogrammed cells, express endogenous pluripotency genes, form teratomas, and contribute to multiple tissues, including the germ line, in chimeric mice. Our results provide strong evidence that insertional mutagenesis is not required for in vitro reprogramming. Adenoviral reprogramming may provide an improved method for generating and studying patient-specific stem cells and for comparing embryonic stem cells and iPS cells.

Disease-specific induced pluripotent stem cells

Park IH, Arora N, Huo H, Maherali N, Ahfeldt T, Shimamura A, Lensch MW, Cowan C, Hochedlinger K, Daley GQ
Department of Medicine, Division of Pediatric Hematology Oncology, Children's Hospital Boston, and Dana-Farber Cancer Institute, Boston, Mass., USA
Cell 2008;134:877–886

Context: Tissue culture of immortal cell strains from diseased patients is an invaluable resource for medical research but is largely limited to tumor cell lines or transformed derivatives of native tissues. *Aim:* The authors describe the generation of induced pluripotent stem (iPS) cells from patients with a variety of genetic diseases with either mendelian or complex inheritance; these diseases include adenosine deaminase deficiency-related severe combined immunodeficiency (ADA-SCID), Shwachman-Bodian-Diamond syndrome (SBDS), Gaucher disease (GD) type III, Duchenne (DMD) and Becker muscular dystrophy (BMD), Parkinson disease (PD), Huntington disease (HD), juvenile-onset, type 1 diabetes mellitus (JDM), Down syndrome (DS)/trisomy 21, and the carrier state of Lesch-Nyhan syndrome. *Conclusions:* Such disease-specific stem cells offer an unprecedented opportunity to recapitulate both normal and pathologic human tissue formation in vitro, thereby enabling disease investigation and drug development.

Following the reprogramming of human skin cells to imitate embryonic stem cells, researches have now used adult skin cells and by adding valproic acid they reverted the cells back into a stem cell-like state. Scientists were also able to reprogram adult cells into pluripotent stem cells without utilization of retroviruses. Stem cell researchers believe that patient-derived stem cells will be needed to develop into different tissue types, hoping to identify the biological errors that contribute to these diseases. This is now achieved for disorders such as Parkinson's disease and Down's syndrome.

Correcting for purifying selection: an improved human mitochondrial molecular clock

Soares P, Ermini L, Thomson N, Mormina M, Rito T, Rohl A, Salas A, Oppenheimer S, Macaulay V, Richards MB
Institute of Integrative and Comparative Biology, Faculty of Biological Sciences, University of Leeds, Leeds, UK
Am J Hum Genet 2009;84:740–759

Context: There is currently no calibration available for the whole human mtDNA genome, incorporating both coding and control regions. Furthermore, as several authors have pointed out recently, linear molecular clocks that incorporate selectable characters are in any case problematic. *Objective:* This paper confirms a modest effect of purifying selection on the mtDNA coding region and proposes an improved molecular clock for dating human mtDNA, based on a worldwide phylogeny of >2,000 complete mtDNA genomes and calibrating against recent evidence for the divergence time of humans and chimpanzees. *Results:* They focus on a time-dependent mutation rate based on the entire mtDNA genome and supported by a neutral clock based on synonymous mutations alone. They show that the corrected rate is further corroborated by archaeological dating for the settlement of the Canary Islands and Remote Oceania and also, given certain phylogeographic assumptions, by the timing of the first modern human settlement of Europe and resettlement after the Last Glacial Maximum. The corrected rate yields an age of modern human expansion in the Americas at approximately 15 thousand years that – unlike the uncorrected clock – matches the archaeological evidence, but continues to indicate an out-of-Africa dispersal at around 55–70 thousand years, 5–20 thousand years before any clear archaeological record, suggesting the need for archaeological research efforts focusing on this time window. They also present improved rates for the mtDNA control region, and the first comprehensive estimates of positional mutation rates for human mtDNA, which are essential for defining mutation models in phylogenetic analyses.

These researchers have devised a method of dating ancient human migration based on mitochondrial DNA (mtDNA) calculation by taking into account the process of natural selection, which very gradually but nonlinearly removes harmful gene mutations in the mtDNA. This produces a time-dependent effect on how many mutations you see in the family tree, to provide reliable time-depth estimates for the entire window of anatomically modern human evolution. They can now put a timescale on any part of a given family tree, right back to 'Mitochondrial Eve', who lived some 200,000 years ago. Working with published databases of more than 2,000 fully sequenced mtDNAs, the new method yielded some surprising findings. They confirm the date mankind's expansion through the Americas to be some 15,000 years ago, around the time of the first unequivocal archaeological remains, and estimate the time of the third 'out of Africa' migration around 60–70,000 years ago – some 10–20,000 years earlier than previously thought. The paper offers a calculator into which researchers can feed their data.

Concepts revised: screening for disease is not a panacea

Screening and prostate-cancer mortality in a randomized European study

Schroder FH, Hugosson J, Roobol MJ, Tammela TL, Ciatto S, Nelen V, Kwiatkowski M, Lujan M, Lilja H, Zappa M, Denis LJ, Recker F, Berenguer A, Maattanen L, Bangma CH, Aus G, Villers A, Rebillard X, van der Kwast T, Blijenberg BG, Moss SM, de Koning HJ, Auvinen A
Department of Urology, Erasmus Medical Center, Rotterdam, The Netherlands
N Engl J Med 2009;360:1320–1328

Background: The European Randomized Study of Screening for Prostate Cancer was initiated in the early 1990s to evaluate the effect of screening with prostate-specific-antigen (PSA) testing on death rates from prostate cancer.

Methods: 182,000 men between the ages of 50 and 74 years through registries in seven European countries were identified for inclusion. The men were randomly assigned to a group that was offered PSA screening at an average of once every 4 years or to a control group that did not receive such screening. The predefined core age group for this study included 162,243 men between the ages of 55 and 69 years. The primary outcome was the rate of death from prostate cancer. Mortality follow-up was identical for the two study groups and ended on December 31, 2006.

Results: In the screening group, 82% of men accepted at least one offer of screening. During a median follow-up of 9 years, the cumulative incidence of prostate cancer was 8.2% in the screening group and 4.8% in the control group. The rate ratio for death from prostate cancer in the screening group, as compared with the control group, was 0.80 (95% confidence interval [CI], 0.65–0.98; adjusted p = 0.04). The absolute risk difference was 0.71 deaths per 1,000 men. This means that 1,410 men would need to be screened and 48 additional cases of prostate cancer would need to be treated to prevent 1 death from prostate cancer. The analysis of men who were actually screened during the first round (excluding subjects with noncompliance) provided a rate ratio for death from prostate cancer of 0.73 (95% CI, 0.56–0.90).

Conclusions: PSA-based screening reduced the rate of death from prostate cancer by 20% but was associated with a high risk of overdiagnosis.

Mortality results from a randomized prostate-cancer screening trial

Andriole GL, Crawford ED, Grubb RL, 3rd, Buys SS, Chia D, Church TR, Fouad MN, Gelmann EP, Kvale PA, Reding DJ, Weissfeld JL, Yokochi LA, O'Brien B, Clapp JD, Rathmell JM, Riley TL, Hayes RB, Kramer BS, Izmirlian G, Miller AB, Pinsky PF, Prorok PC, Gohagan JK, Berg CD
Washington University School of Medicine, St. Louis, Mo.,USA
N Engl J Med 2009;360:1310–1319

Background: The effect of screening with prostate-specific-antigen (PSA) testing and digital rectal examination (DRE) on the rate of death from prostate cancer is unknown. This is the first report from the Prostate, Lung, Colorectal, and Ovarian (PLCO) Cancer Screening Trial on prostate-cancer mortality.

Methods: From 1993 through 2001, 76,693 men at 10 US study centers were randomly assigned to receive either annual screening (38,343 subjects) or usual care as the control (38,350 subjects). Men in the screening group were offered annual PSA testing for 6 years and DRE for 4 years. The subjects and healthcare providers received the results and decided on the type of follow-up evaluation. Usual care sometimes included screening, as some organizations have recommended. The numbers of all cancers and deaths and causes of death were ascertained.

Results: In the screening group, rates of compliance were 85% for PSA testing and 86% for DRE. Rates of screening in the control group increased from 40% in the first year to 52% in the sixth year for PSA testing and ranged from 41 to 46% for DRE. After 7 years of follow-up, the incidence of prostate cancer per 10,000 person-years was 116 (2,820 cancers) in the screening group and 95 (2,322 cancers) in the control group (rate ratio, 1.22; 95% confidence interval [CI], 1.16–1.29). The incidence of death per 10,000 person-years was 2.0 (50 deaths) in the screening group and 1.7 (44 deaths) in the control group (rate ratio, 1.13; 95% CI, 0.75–1.70). The data at 10 years were 67% complete and consistent with these overall findings.

Conclusions: After 7–10 years of follow-up, the rate of death from prostate cancer was very low and did not differ significantly between the two study groups.

Long-term health and quality-of-life consequences of mass screening for childhood celiac disease: a 10-year follow-up study

Van Koppen EJ, Schweizer JJ, Csizmadia CG, Krom Y, Hylkema HB, van Geel AM, Koopman HM, Verloove-Vanhorick SP, Mearin ML

Department of Paediatrics, Leiden University Medical Centre, Leiden, The Netherlands
Pediatrics 2009;123:e582–588

Objective: Mass screening for celiac disease is controversial. The objective of the study was to determine whether detection of childhood celiac disease by mass screening improves long-term health status and health-related quality of life.

Methods: A prospective 10-year follow-up study of 32 children who were aged 2–4 years, had celiac disease identified by mass screening, and had a gluten-free diet (19) or a normal gluten-containing diet (13) was conducted. The follow-up included assessments of general health status, celiac disease-associated symptoms, celiac disease-associated serum antibodies, and health-related quality of life.

Results: Ten years after mass screening, 81% of the children were adhering to a gluten-free diet. The health status improved in 66% of the treated children: in 41% by early treatment and in 25% by prevention of the gluten-dependent symptoms that they developed after diagnosis. For 19% of the children, treatment after screening would not have improved their health status, because they had no symptoms at screening and have remained symptom-free while consuming gluten. The health-related quality of life of the children with symptoms improved significantly after 1 year of gluten-free diet. Ten years after screening, the health-related quality of life of the children with celiac disease was similar to that of the reference population.

Conclusion: Identification by mass screening led 10 years later to health improvement in 66% of children without deterioration of generic health-related quality of life. There is a good compliance after mass screening. In a research setting, delaying treatment for children without symptoms seems to be an option after a positive screening test. Long-term follow-up studies are needed to assess possible long-term complications in untreated, nonsymptomatic celiac disease.

Including papers on prostate cancer screening in the Science and Medicine section of the *Yearbook* does not reflect a personal concern but rather the quality of these two papers that exemplify how an obviously good idea might in the end prove not to be so good. These two papers used screening strategies for prostate cancer in more than 200,000 subjects, based on PSA measurements, with or without rectal examination. There was a 20% reduction by screening of death related to prostate cancer in the European study and no difference in the US study. In all cases, the number of cancer cases detected was higher with screening (twice as many in the European study). In the positive European study, the estimated absolute reduction in cancer-related mortality of about 0.7 deaths per 1,000 men should be weighed against the interventions. The 73,000 men in the screening group had more than 17,000 biopsies. Diagnosis led to more treatment: 277 vs. 100 per 10,000 radical prostatectomy and 220 vs. 123 per 10,000 radiation therapy with or without hormones. Altogether, these huge studies should be praised, although specialists do not consider them as definitive [1].

The study by the Dutch group is obviously more modest (32 celiac children identified by mass screening) but asks the important question of whether the screening process has improved long-term quality of life, rather than focusing on the ability of the screening to identify the disease. The authors conclude that in 66% of the children with a diagnosis made after screening, the health status improved. However, they fail to take into account the roughly equal number of children who had a small bowel biopsy with possible impact on discomfort of an unnecessary procedure. Altogether, these studies emphasize the need for evidence: nothing should be taken for granted in the screening world. Hard and meaningful endpoints should be used to evaluate all our medical actions in that domain.

Tumours with PI3K activation are resistant to dietary restriction

Kalaany NY, Sabatini DM
Whitehead Institute for Biomedical Research, Nine Cambridge Center, Cambridge, Mass., USA
Nature 2009;458:725–731

Background: Dietary restriction delays the incidence and decreases the growth of various types of tumors, but the mechanisms underlying the sensitivity of tumors to food restriction remain unknown.
Results: Certain human cancer cell lines, when grown as tumor xenografts in mice, are highly sensitive to the anti-growth effects of dietary restriction, whereas others are resistant. Cancer cells that form dietary-restriction-resistant tumors carry mutations that cause constitutive activation of the phosphatidylinositol-3-kinase (PI3K) pathway and in culture proliferate in the absence of insulin or insulin-like growth factor 1. Substitution of an activated mutant allele of PI3K with wild-type PI3K in otherwise isogenic cancer cells, or the restoration of PTEN expression in a PTEN-null cancer cell line, is sufficient to convert a dietary-restriction-resistant tumour into one that is dietary-restriction-sensitive. Dietary restriction does not affect a PTEN-null mouse model of prostate cancer, but it significantly decreases tumour burden in a mouse model of lung cancer lacking constitutive PI3K signalling.
Conclusions: The PI3K pathway is an important determinant of the sensitivity of tumors to dietary restriction, and activating mutations in the pathway may influence the response of cancers to dietary restriction-mimetic therapies.

Dietary restriction limiting nutrient intake without reaching malnutrition extends lifespan in most if not all, species including humans [2]. This extension of lifespan is partly due to a decreased rate of cancer, and the growth of certain cancers can be limited by dietary restriction. This surprising benefit is likely to be due to the evolutionary advantage of prolonging lifespan under suboptimal nutrient availability, and postponing reproduction until food is abundant. The authors identified human cancer lines that when implanted in mice were sensitive or insensitive to the effect of dietary restriction and looked for the mechanism underlying this differential effect. They found that PI3 kinase, enzyme acting downstream of the insulin and the IGF-1 receptor is involved in this differential effect through a mechanism of apoptosis, and that constitutive activation of the PI3K pathway abolishes the effect of dietary restriction. Another component of the pathway, PTEN, is also similarly involved. These observations link once again the insulin and IGF-1 pathway to longevity and cancer [3]. Indeed, mutation of the GH receptor, which affects the production of IGF1, abrogates the dietary restriction-induced longevity in mice. These mechanisms may be related to the recent worrisome news of the potentially increased risk of cancer with the use of glargine insulin, together with the decreased risk associated with the use of metformin [4].

Pulmonary autoimmunity as a feature of autoimmune polyendocrine syndrome type 1 and identification of KCNRG as a bronchial autoantigen

Alimohammadi M, Dubois N, Skoldberg F, Hallgren A, Tardivel I, Hedstrand H, Haavik J, Husebye ES, Gustafsson J, Rorsman F, Meloni A, Janson C, Vialettes B, Kajosaari M, Egner W, Sargur R, Ponten F, Amoura Z, Grimfeld A, De Luca F, Betterle C, Perheentupa J, Kampe O, Carel JC
Department of Medical Sciences, University Hospital, Uppsala University, Uppsala, Sweden
mohammad.alimohammadi@medsci.uu.se
Proc Natl Acad Sci USA 2009;106:4396–4401

Background: Patients with autoimmune polyendocrine syndrome type 1 (APS-1) suffer from multiple organ-specific autoimmunity with autoantibodies against target tissue-specific autoantigens. Endocrine and nonendocrine organs such as skin, hair follicles, and liver are targeted by the immune system. Despite sporadic observations of pulmonary symptoms among APS-1 patients, an autoimmune mechanism for pulmonary involvement has not been elucidated.

Methods: A subset of APS-1 patients with respiratory symptoms is reported. Eight patients with pulmonary involvement were identified. Severe airway obstruction was found in 4 patients, leading to death in 2. Immunoscreening of a cDNA library using serum samples from a patient with APS-1 and obstructive respiratory symptoms identified a putative potassium channel regulator (KCNRG) as a pulmonary autoantigen. Reactivity to recombinant KCNRG was assessed in 110 APS-1 patients by using immunoprecipitation.

Results: Autoantibodies to KCNRG were present in 7 of the 8 patients with respiratory symptoms, but in only 1 of 102 APS-1 patients without respiratory symptoms. Expression of KCNRG messenger RNA and protein was found to be predominantly restricted to the epithelial cells of terminal bronchioles.

Conclusions: Autoantibodies to KCNRG, a protein mainly expressed in bronchial epithelium, are strongly associated with pulmonary involvement in APS-1. These findings may facilitate the recognition, diagnosis, characterization, and understanding of the pulmonary manifestations of APS-1.

Sorry for the lack of modesty in citing an own contribution. Starting from a single observation of an unusual component of a very rare disease, a new concept of autoimmune bronchiolitis could be proposed, and that a molecular autoimmune target could be identified. Indeed, APS-1 constitutes a constellation of autoimmune diseases with public components (i.e. hypoparathyroidism, candidaiasis, and adrenal insufficiency) and a very extensive list of private components that can be severe or life-threatening. These components are a challenge for the clinician but can be an opportunity to find new autoimmune components for the investigator. Finally, it remains to be evaluated whether more common form of bronchial manifestations have an autoimmune component and correspond to KCNRG autoimmunity.

References
1. Barry MJ: Screening for prostate cancer – the controversy that refuses to die. N Engl J Med 2009;360:1351–1354.
2. Brunet A: Cancer: when restriction is good. Nature 2009;458:713–714.
3. Holzenberger M: The role of insulin-like signalling in the regulation of ageing. Horm Res 2004;62(suppl 1):89-92.
4. Currie CJ, Poole CD, Gale EA: The influence of glucose-lowering therapies on cancer risk in type 2 diabetes. Diabetologia. 2009; [Epub ahead of print].

Author Index

Hammer, G.D. 97
Hammer, R.E. 136
Hammond, N. 41
Han, D.Y. 89
Han, J.C. 205
Han, S.J. 20
Han, Z. 21
Hancock, J.F. 47
Hanley, N.A. 93
Hannula-Jouppi, K. 52
Hansen, T. 147, 148, 168, 169
Hanson, R.L. 177
Hao, X. 21
Hardarson, G. 172
Hardy, R. 90
Harfe, B.D. 90
Hariharan, K. 53
Harmon, C.M. 157
Harnaha, J. 122
Harries, L.W. 44
Harris, T.B. 172
Hart, D.J. 41
Hartikainen, A.L. 147, 169, 171, 186
Hartley, D.M. 213
Hartmann, M.F. 103, 106
Hartoft-Nielsen, M.L. 129
Hassan, M. 135
Hassan, M.O. 212
Hattersley, A.T. 44, 167
Haukka, J. 171
Havulinna, A.S. 167
Haworth, C.M. 134
Hay, A. 58
Hay, A.C. 109
Hay, A.W. 58
Hayes, R.B. 167, 221
He, C. 85
He, H. 27
He, Y.Z. 73
Healy, B.C. 123
Heap, G.A. 128
Heaton, J.H. 97
Hebebrand, J. 139, 167
Hedstrand, H. 223
Hegedus, B. 49
Heger, S. 88
Heglind, M. 137
Heid, I.M. 167
Heino, T. 61
Heinrich, U. 103
Hekkala, A. 191, 209
Helgadottir, A. 168
Helgadottir, H. 27
Helmrath, M. 157
Henderson, B.E. 85
Henderson, J. 142
Henderson, K.D. 85

Henningsson, S. 216
Hercberg, S. 169
Hession, C. 53
Hetherington, M.M. 170
Hettinger, A. 143
Heude, B. 147, 169
Hew-Butler, T. 19
Hewitt, S.C. 82
Heyer, E. 211
Hill, E. 58
Hill, N.R. 182
Hillier, T.A. 150
Hindmarsh, P. 182
Hindmarsh, P.C. 13, 189
Hinney, A. 139
Hirsch, I.B. 181
Hirsch, J. 140
Hirschhorn, J.N. 85, 167
Hjartarsson, H. 27
Hjorth, M. 119
Ho, S.M. 217
Ho, S.N. 53
Hochberg, Z. IX, 76, 183, 199, 211
Hochedlinger, K. 219, 220
Hodder, P. 98
Hoeger, K. 156
Hoey, H. 182
Hoffman, L. 111
Hoffstedt, J. 135
Hofman, A. 41, 167, 172
Hofman, P. 155
Hogeland, K. 122
Hoggart, C. 171
Holland, J. 88
Hollowell, J.G. 38
Holly, J. 44
Holm, H. 27, 172
Holmdahl, G. 101
Holmkvist, J. 147, 148
Holzenberger, M. 25, 56
Hombert, J.M. 211
Horber, F. 169
Horenburg, S. 133
Horn, P.S. 151
Horvath, T.L. 201
Hoshino, M. 17
Hou, R. 79
Houten, S.M. 138
Hovey, K.M. 116
Howson, J.M. 128
Hrafnkelsson, J. 27
Hsiao, J.J. 201
Hu, C. 208
Hu, F.B. 133, 167
Hu, K. 16
Huang, E.S. 181
Huang, F. 53
Huang, G.C. 113

Huang, N. 96
Huangfu, D. 219
Hugosson, J. 221
Huijbregts, L. 1
Hunt, K.A. 128
Hunter, D.J. 85, 133, 167
Huo, H. 220
Husebye, E.S. 223
Hutchison 3rd, C.A. 215
Hutton, J. 149
Huynh, T. 32
Hwang, J.I. 6
Hylkema, H.B. 222
Hyoty, H. 191, 209

Ibanez, L. 193
Igl, W. 216
Iglesias, I. 199
Ihnat, M.A. 127
Ikeda, H. 48
Ilonen, J. 191, 209
Imai, H. 216
Imamoglu, S. 9
Imielinski, M. 123
Imperatore, G. 150
Inagaki, T. 203
Inge, T.H. 157
Ingels, C. 199
Inouye, M. 41
Iqbal, J. 63
Ishizu, K. 17
Isolato, G. 29
Isomaa, B. 167, 176
Ito, M. 32
Ito, Y. 48
Ivarsson, S. 119
Ivarsson, S.A. 188
Izmirlian, G. 221

Jaaskelainen, J. 105
Jablonski, K.A. 177
Jackson, A.U. 167
Jackson, S. 206
Jacobs, K.B. 167
Jacobs, L.C. 167
Jacobson, P. 169
Jahnukainen, K. 88
Jakobsdottir, M. 27, 172
Jamison, R.A. 201
Jansen, H. 144
Janson, C. 223
Janson, P.O. 101
Jarvelin, M.R. 147, 148, 167, 169, 171, 186

Sandbaek, A. 169
Sandhu, M.S. 41, 167
Sanford, E.L. 205
Sanna, S. 167
Santa, E. 123
Santos, M.G. 97
Saramies, J. 167
Sargur, R. 223
Sasaki, A. 105
Sasaki, N. 17
Sato, N. 16
Saugier-Veber, P. 178
Savage, D.B. 206
Sävendahl, L. 61, 69
Savisto, N.J. 137
Schally, A.V. 54
Scheet, P. 167
Scheideler, M. 62
Scherer, M.A. 72
Schetz, M. 199
Schlereth, F. 93
Schlessinger, D. 167
Schmidt, J.A. 85
Schmitt, E. 178
Schnebelen, A. 178
Schneck, M.E. 154
Schneider, M.V. 216
Schoenau, E. 106
Schoenherr, E. 159
Schoenle, E.J. 86
Scholl-Burgi, S. 159
Scholtens, S. 141
Schonau, E. 192
Schrauwen, P. 137
Schreiber, G.B. 151
Schroder, F.H. 221
Schuit, F. 147
Schulz, K.M. 83, 84
Schweizer, J.J. 222
Scott, L.J. 167
Scuteri, A. 167
Secco, A. 13
Secic, M. 184
Seckl, J.R. 218
Seehausen, O. 216
Sellers, E.A. 153
Semple, R.K. 9, 206
Seong, J.Y. 6
Seppanen-Laakso, T. 209
Sepuri, N.B. 212
Sereno, A. 53
Serin, A. 9
Seriwatanachai, D. 64
Serrat, M.A. 59
Sewell, A.K. 113
Shalhoub, V. 71
Shanabrough, M. 201
Shandala, T. 72
Shaner, J.L. 123

Shapiro, A.M. 126
Sharma, S. 11
Shaw, C. 4
Shen, H. 173
Sherins, R.J. 87
Shestowsky, W.S. 53
Shi, H. 111
Shi, L. 79
Shi, S. 74
Shi, Y. 87
Shield, J.P. 186
Shields, M. 53
Shimamura, A. 220
Shinawi, M. 42
Shiojima, I. 48
Shires, S. 58
Shoback, D. 65
Shrader, P. 176
Shrewsbury, V.A. 144
Shuldiner, A.R. 172
Shulman, D. 88
Shulman, G.I. 201
Shum, C.K. 28
Siegel, A.J. 19
Sigurdsson, A. 27
Silander, K. 167
Siljander, H. 191
Siltala, M. 191
Silverstein, J.H. 143
Simell, O. 191, 209
Simell, S. 191, 209
Simell, T. 191, 209
Simonet, W.S. 71
Simpson, N. 58
Sims, M.A. 90, 167
Sinaii, N. 66, 98
Sinclair, L. 67
Sinding, C. 72
Singh, R. 200
Singhal, V. 143
Singleton, A. 172
Sinkevicius, K.W. 82
Sipila, J.I. 191
Sisk, C.L. 83
Sisk C.L 84
Skakkebaek, N.E. 91
Skarphedinsson, O.B. 27
Skoldberg, F. 223
Skowera, A. 113
Skraban, R. 123
Sladek, R. 147, 169
Slattery, D. 182
Sleigh, A. 206
Smeets, R. 93
Smeitink, J.A. 93
Smiles, A. 124
Smiles, A.M. 123
Smit, H.A. 141
Smith, A.V. 172

Smith, E.P. 68
Smith, G.D. 90, 167
Smith, H.O. 215
Smith, J.T. 7
Smith, R.M. 123
Smith, R.W. 161
Smulders, N.M. 137
Smyth, D.J. 123, 128
Snider, W.D. 32
Snipas, T. 53
Snyder, P. 16
Snyder, W. 53
So, M.T. 28
So, W.Y. 175
Soares, P. 220
Söder, O. 79
Soldin, S.J. 19
Solis, A.S. 45
Soltesz, G. 207
Son, G.H. 99
Song, K. 90, 167
Song, S. 21
Sonoyama, W. 74
Sonzogni, A. 95
Soos, M.A. 206
Soranzo, N. 41, 167, 172
Sørensen, K. 91
Soty, M. 140
Soule, S.G. 108
Sovio, U. 171
Spalding, A.C. 97
Spalding, K.L. 135
Sparsø T 147, 148
Specker, B. 68
Spector, T.D. 41, 167, 172
Speedy, D.B. 19
Speiser, P.W. 143
Speliotes, E.K. 167
Spirin, P. 107
Spotts, E.L. 216
Stacey, S.N. 27, 172
Stadtfeld, M. 219
Stager, M. 184
Stamp, G.W. 8
Stanhope, R.G. 189
Stanley, C.A. 123
Starost, M.F. 20
Steck, A.K. 149
Steensberg, A. 193
Stefansson, K. 27, 168, 172
Steiner, R.A. 7
Steinthorsdottir, V. 168, 172
Stephens, J. 41, 167
Stevens, H. 128
Stevens, S. 167
Stolk, L. 41, 172
Stolk, R.P. 144
Stonebraker, A.C. 208
Storch, K.F. 204